Audiology

Audiology

Third Edition

HAYES A. NEWBY
University of Maryland

Prentice-Hall, Inc.
Englewood Cliffs, New Jersey

Printed in the United States of America

ISBN: 0-13-050799-7

Library of Congress Catalog Card Number: 74-180172

10 9 8 7 6 5 4 3 2

PRENTICE-HALL INTERNATIONAL, INC., *London*
PRENTICE-HALL OF AUSTRALIA, PTY. LTD., *Sydney*
PRENTICE-HALL OF CANADA, LTD., *Toronto*
PRENTICE-HALL OF INDIA PRIVATE LIMITED, *New Delhi*
PRENTICE-HALL OF JAPAN, INC., *Tokyo*

Preface

Except for the table of Contents, this edition of *Audiology* bears little resemblance to the first one, published in 1958, and there have been substantial revisions from the 1964 edition. For the most part the changes consist of additions to the text and updating and adding illustrations. Not only does the subject matter of the field of audiology constantly expand, but terminology changes, calibration standards are altered, and equipment is improved, so that periodic revision of a book such as this is mandatory to keep it from becoming hopelessly outdated.

This book was written as a textbook primarily for the beginning student in audiology. Usually the first course is designed to give students an overview of the entire field of audiology without going into detail on any one aspect. In some universities, however, the emphasis in the beginning course is on audiometry, particularly when only one or two courses in the field are offered.

This book can be used as a textbook for the beginning course regardless of the way it is taught. For a survey course, the instructor probably should not assign chapters 5 through 9. Chapters 5, 6, and 8 can form the core for an entire second course in basic hearing measurement. If the beginning course emphasizes audiometry, however, and the student is expected to understand and obtain practice in the administration of hearing tests, then the instructor should assign these chapters also. Chapters 7 and 9 will be useful as the bases for courses in advanced clinical audiology and industrial audiology, respectively.

It was my thought that this book would be supplemented as a text by the assignment of pertinent chapters from other books and articles from current issues of professional journals. These collateral reading assignments should be revised annually to keep up to date with the current literature.

I hope that this book will serve not only as a textbook for students of audiology but also as a reference for other professional people, such as physicians, psychologists, educators, and speech pathologists, and as a source of information on problems of hearing for interested laymen. The book has grown out of my more than twenty-five years of experience as a teacher and clinician. The subject matter of the field of audiology is so vast that no single individual can hope to be an expert in all its aspects. If I have appeared presumptuous in undertaking to write of the whole field, I apologize.

I am grateful to all those individuals who assisted me in the preparation of the first two editions, and especially to my wife, Jean, for her constant encouragement and patience.

H.A.N.

Contents

Audiology

1

THE LINEAGE OF AUDIOLOGY

"Audiology" refers to the study of hearing and hearing disorders. The field of audiology is a broad one which can be approached from many aspects and to which varied specialists contribute their knowledge and skills. So far as these specialists make contributions to this field, they are properly designated as audiologists, even though audiology may be a secondary interest with them. Generally, however, the term *audiologist* is reserved for the individual whose primary interest is in the identification and measurement of hearing loss and the rehabilitation of those with hearing impairments.[1] Usually his training has been academic rather than medical, although there are a few notable exceptions. Most audiologists are products of university graduate training programs in speech and hearing, and many have Ph.D. degrees in this field.

Speaking figuratively, audiology is the offspring of two parents: speech pathology and otology. Speech pathology deals with the diagnosis and treatment of individuals who suffer from disorders in oral language. Otology is concerned with the diagnosis and treatment of individuals who have an ear disease or disorders of the peripheral mechanism of hearing. Speech pathology is primarily a nonmedical specialty, whereas otology is purely a medical specialty, one division of otorhinolaryngology

[1] The following definition was accepted by a group of nine outstanding audiologists who were consultants to the Veterans Administration: "An audiologist is one who specializes in the field of hearing, and particularly in hearing impairments. He is concerned with the assessment of hearing, and the habilitation and rehabilitation of children and adults with impairment of auditory function. He may teach in a college or university, may be concerned primarily with research, or may perform clinical activities in or direct a university, hospital, community, or governmental hearing center."

(ear, nose, and throat). The two fields—speech pathology and otology—were wedded in World War II in the so-called aural rehabilitation centers established by the armed forces for the benefit of hearing-impaired service personnel. The care and rehabilitation of these people required the closest teamwork between medical and nonmedical specialists. Some nonmedical persons recruited for work in the aural rehabilitation centers were former teachers of the deaf, but for the most part they were people whose training and experience had been in the field of speech pathology and speech correction. For years speech correctionists had assumed responsibility for working with the speech problems of hard-of-hearing children and adults. Now in the aural rehabilitation centers, they extended their responsibilities to the development of tests of hearing function, selection of hearing aids, and the development of various rehabilitative techniques which extended far beyond speech correction. Thus through the cooperative efforts of the two specialties of speech pathology and otology, a new field of specialization was created. Although there had been notable examples of individuals who devoted themselves to working with the hard of hearing before the 1940's the professional field of audiology did not exist until World War II.

As a matter of fact, the word *audiology* did not come into general use until 1945, when Raymond Carhart, a speech pathologist recruited for the Army aural rehabilitation work, and Norton Canfield, an otologist who was serving as consultant to the War Department, applied the term to the field which had been created through the joint efforts of the two fields of specialization that these men represented.[2] The identity of the person who coined the word *audiology* has been disputed by representatives of the hearing-aid industry and others. Trainor and Hargrave claim to have originated the word in 1939, and they report that as early as 1940 news items appeared using the words "audiology," "audiologist," and "audiological."[3] Whatever the true origin of the word, it is nevertheless a fact that *audiology* as a popular term dates from the time that Carhart and Canfield "coined" it, and "audiologist" has come to designate the professional rather than the commercial worker in the field. The origins of the field of audiology will be discussed more fully in Chapter 13.

If the mother and father of audiology are speech pathology and otology, there are many living relatives on both the medical and nonmedical sides of the family. Among the medical relatives are pediatrics, gerontology, psychiatry, and neurology. Pediatricians and gerontologists represent extremes in ages of patients, yet both are concerned with problems of impaired hearing as they affect the health and adjustment of their patients.

[2] George E. Shambaugh, Jr., and Raymond Carhart, "Contributions of Audiology to Fenestration Surgery," *A.M.A. Archives of Otolaryngology*, Vol. 54 (December, 1951), p. 699.

[3] M. E. Trainor and Willard Hargrave, "Audiology," *The Auricle*, Vol. 3 (May, 1963), p. 3.

Because a hearing impairment frequently does produce maladjustment, the psychiatrist, too, has an interest in audiology. Since some "auditory" disorders may involve pathology of the central nervous system, the neurologist on occasion is also vitally interested in audiology.

Among the nonmedical relatives of audiology are psychology, physics, and education. Clinical psychologists formed an important unit in the "team approach" so successfully developed in the military aural rehabilitation programs. Since the war, clinical psychologists have assumed an important role in such activities as assessing the aurally handicapped individual's potentialities, and in counseling the deaf and hard of hearing and their families. In addition, psychologists have shed light on an important and puzzling problem in audiology–the question of nonorganic or functional hearing loss in children and adults.

Two branches of the field of physics are importantly related to audiology: acoustics and electronics. Since hearing disorders represent an inability to respond normally to acoustic stimulation, the audiologist must have some knowledge of the physical properties of sound stimuli. The measurement of hearing loss requires accurate and dependable instrumentation, as does the "correction" of hearing loss by means of amplification. It is becoming increasingly important for the audiologist, regardless of his basic orientation, to develop some knowledge and understanding of electronics as it is applied to problems of diagnosing and rehabilitating those with auditory impairments. The audiologist must become, to some extent, an acoustics and electronics engineer.

Audiology is related to education particularly in matters concerning the training of deaf and hard-of-hearing children. Considerable emphasis is now being placed on training of the preschool deaf child, and we are seeing nursery schools for such children developing as part of the program of hearing centers, or as separate entities. The audiologist who works with these children must be grounded in nursery school teaching principles and methods, and must have a specialized knowledge of the training of the deaf and the hard of hearing. Rehabilitation of older children should be integrated with their regular school work, and the audiologist must cooperate closely with the classroom teacher. To work effectively with the school-age child, therefore, the audiologist should have some acquaintance with the work of the classroom teacher.

Thus we see that audiology is not a strictly delimited field but one which springs from many sources and draws upon a variety of skills and backgrounds. The "compleat" audiologist would be a combination of speech pathologist, otorhinolaryngologist, pediatrician, gerontologist, psychiatrist, psychologist, physicist, electronics engineer, and educator. This includes only the clinical aspects of the field. Actually, what might be called experimental audiology is a branch of the field which is highly important, since out of information gained experimentally come improved techniques for clinical application. In considering experimental work and research, the work of the physiologist must receive recognition. In audiology, the physiologist is concerned with problems of how we hear. On his work are based the principles of medical and surgical care of individuals with hearing impairment, and also the principles of preventive medicine, or hearing conservation. In addition to the physiologist, the experimental psychologist contributes to the field of audiology through research in the psychological processes of hearing and in the area of psycho-acoustics. And of course all the specialists mentioned above in connection with the field of clinical audiology are concerned also with research and experimentation in the areas of their principal orientation.

It can be seen, therefore, that no one individual can be expected to be the "compleat" audiologist. Every clinical audiologist, however, should have some awareness of the complexities of the field, and respect for the array of talents and backgrounds presented by his coworkers of various specialties. It is the hearing-handicapped patient who benefits from this concentration of professional interests on the field of audiology.

REFERENCES

Canfield, Norton, *Audiology, the Science of Hearing, a Developing Professional Speciality* (Springfield, Ill., Charles C Thomas, 1949).

Davis, Hallowell, and Silverman, S. Richard, eds., *Hearing and Deafness* (New York, Holt, Rinehart and Winston, 1970), Chap. 1.

2

WHAT AND HOW WE HEAR

Since audiology is concerned with the response of the human ear to auditory stimuli, it is necessary for the audiologist to know something of the physical nature of sound (the tools of his trade, so to speak) and also of the structure and functioning of the body's hearing mechanism. No attempt will be made here to go into great detail on either subject. The serious student of audiology will naturally want to pursue the study of the physics of sound and the anatomy and physiology of the ear in a more thorough way. A number of excellent books are devoted specifically to these subjects. Some of them will be mentioned at the end of this chapter.

THE PHYSICS OF HEARING

The Propagation of Sound

Sound is created when some force sets an object into vibration to the extent that molecular movement of the medium in which the object is situated occurs, and a "sound wave" is propagated. Sound is "heard" when the characteristics of the wave propagated fall within the limitations of the human ear and nervous system. The essentials for sound to be created and heard, then, are a vibrator of some sort, a force to set the vibrator into vibration, a medium to convey the wave motion originating at the vibrator, and a hearing mechanism which can receive and perceive the energy of the propagated wave.

Sound sources may be of various kinds: reeds (as in wood-wind instruments), strings (as in the piano and other stringed instruments), membranes

5

(as in drums), and columns of air (as in the pipe organ), to mention just a few. The force to set the vibrator in motion may originate in nature (as the wind causing a shutter to rattle, for example) or may be produced by human contrivance. Most sound with which audiologists are concerned is of human origin. In our modern civilization, the most important sounds for us are those communicating information, primarily the sounds of spoken language. The way in which sound may originate can be illustrated by describing how the human voice is produced. The source of the voice is the vibrating vocal folds in the larynx. By muscular action, the vocal folds are brought together, thus blocking the free air-way through the larynx. The motive power for voice is provided by air pressure built up below the vocal folds by the muscles of exhalation. When the air pressure below the larynx overcomes the muscular tension of the vocal folds, the folds are separated momentarily. When conditions of muscular tension and air pressure are almost in balance, the vocal folds are set into vibration. The original vibrations of the vocal folds are then transmitted to columns of air in the throat, mouth, and nose, which act as resonators to reinforce and selectively amplify the vibrations produced by the vocal folds.

The transmission of sound from a vibrating source to a receptor requires some kind of medium. It cannot be transmitted through a vacuum. The medium may be a gas (such as air), a fluid (such as water), or a solid (such as steel). Most sound with which we are concerned is airborne. The sound is transmitted from its source to the ear by means of movements of the molecules of air. These movements of the air particles are called a sound wave.

In the production of a sound wave, the air particles adjacent to the vibrating source are set in motion by the movements of the sound source. The moving particles next to the sound source in turn set the particles adjacent to them in motion. Thus the motion of each particle affects the position of the particle next to it, and a wave of particle movement emanates in all directions from the vibrating sound source, proceeding outward in concentric spheres at a set velocity which is determined by the temperature and density of the air. Under "standard" conditions of temperature and density as defined by engineers, this particle displacement proceeds at a velocity of about 1100 feet per second.

Actually, there are two parts to a sound wave: *compression* and *rarefaction*. The sound source "oscillates," or vibrates in simple or complex movement. A sound medium, such as air, is characterized by elasticity, that is, the particles of the medium can move in any direction in which force is applied, and when that force is removed they tend to return to their former positions. In reality, the particles oscillate also. When they are compressed, pressure is built up which forces them to "rebound" when that pressure is removed, so that the particles actually "overshoot" their former positions when compression ceases. Thus, in the compression cycle of the wave, the particles force against each other; in the rarefaction phase, they separate from each other. However, as they separate, another compression is initiated by the oscillating action of the sound source. Alternate compressions and rarefactions, then, characterize the sound wave, and each compression and rarefaction proceeds outward from the sound source at a steady velocity.

A visible illustration of this invisible phenomenon can be cited. Visualize a line of men waiting to get into a mess hall. Along comes a practical joker who gives the last man in line a shove forward. This man pushes into the man ahead of him, and so on until finally the poor fellow at the head of the line gets his head banged into the door. A wave of compression has passed down the line of men, and an interval of time has been required for the man at the head of the line to feel the effects of this compression. Now what happens? As soon as the man at the rear of the line can regain his balance, he reacts to having been pushed forward by moving back. Each man in turn regains his balance and moves back until finally the fellow at the head of the line can pull his head away from the door. Thus a wave of rarefaction has passed down the line of men. Now assume that the joker continued to shove the last man in line at regular intervals. Successive waves of compression and rarefaction passing down the line of men would be visible to the observer, and the man at the head of the line would alternately bang his head into the door and withdraw it. At any one time along the line of men, several points of compression and rarefaction would be visible. The longer the line, the more such points could be seen. In this illustration, the joker would be the sound source, the line of men the particles affected by the vibration of the sound source, and the door would be the ear receiving the vibrations.

Just as with light waves, sound waves will reflect from a non-absorbent surface and be subject to refraction. Of course there is a great deal of difference between light waves and sound waves in their velocity of propagation. Light waves travel at about 186,000 miles per second in contrast to the comparatively slow speed of sound. The difference between the velocity of light and of sound causes some interesting phenomena which all of us have observed in some form. In the days before diesel engines replaced steam locomotives, a common illustration of this difference was the observation of an approaching steam locomotive which was whistling. We could see the column of steam escaping from the whistle, sometimes several seconds before hearing the sound of the whistle, depending, of course, on how far away the train was. Another common experience is the time which frequently elapses between the observation of a streak of lightning and the sound of the thunder. We can obtain an approximate measure of the distance of the lightning from us by counting the number of seconds until we hear the thunder. If we multiply the number of seconds by 1100 feet we will have the distance.

So far we have been talking about the behavior of sound waves in air. As we mentioned previously, sound can also be propagated in liquids and in solids. In these media, the velocity of sound differs somewhat from its speed in air. In salt water of a standard temperature and density, for example, sound will travel at the rate of about 5000 feet per second; in steel the velocity of sound is about 15,000 feet per second. Thus an approaching train can be heard more quickly if an ear is placed to the rail.

Attributes of a Sound Wave

Previously we have discussed the origin and method of propagation of a sound wave. Sound has several measurable attributes that are of importance to the audiologist in his analysis of hearing impairment. The ones with which we shall be concerned are *frequency, intensity,* and *spectrum.*

Frequency. Most sounds are characterized by periodicity, that is, the sound wave consists of repetitions of compressions and rarefactions which occur at the same rate over a period of time. One successive compression and rarefaction constitute one *cycle* of a sound wave. The frequency of a sound wave is the number of cycles that occur in a second's time. The unit for expressing frequency is the *cycle per second,* abbreviated c.p.s., c/s, or most commonly cps. Thus if in a second's time a sound produces 1000 compressions and rarefactions, that sound has a frequency of 1000 cps.

Since 1960, following a recommendation of an international congress on weights and measures, the term *hertz,* abbreviated Hz, has been employed increasingly as a substitute for cycle per second. The new term honors the memory of a famous physicist, Heinrich Hertz. Thus today we usually speak of a 1000 cps tone as a 1000 Hz tone. The term *kilocycle,* abbreviated kc, means one thousand cycles per second, and so *kilohertz,* abbreviated kHz, means the same thing. We may speak of a tone as having a frequency, for example, of either 4000 Hz or of 4 kHz; the terms are used interchangeably. In keeping with the present trend, we shall refer to frequency in this book in terms of hertz instead of cycles per second.

Related to frequency is wavelength. Since sound in air travels at a fixed velocity of about 1100 feet per second, the wavelength of 1 cycle of a sound wave is equal to the frequency of the wave divided into 1100 feet. Thus, for a sound of the frequency of 1000 Hz, the wavelength is 1.1 feet. In other words, each cycle (one compression and one rarefaction) occupies the space of 1.1 feet. It can be seen that frequency and wavelength are inversely related. As the frequency of a sound increases, the wavelength must decrease, as there are then more cycles to fit into the space of 1100 feet. Thus, in formula form, $W = V/F$, where W = wavelength, V = velocity, and F = frequency. If one desires to solve for frequency instead of wavelength, the formula would be written $F = V/W$.

The human ear has certain limitations in the frequencies that it can perceive. Although there is a wide range of individual differences, it can be generalized that the young adult with normal hearing can perceive frequencies from about 20 to 20,000 Hz. We call this the *audible range* of frequencies. Moreover, the ear is not equally sensitive to all frequencies within this range. The ear is most sensitive to the frequencies from 1000 to 4000 Hz. Sounds of frequencies between 250 and 1000 Hz, and between 4000 and 8000 Hz must be made somewhat more intense, and sounds of frequencies below 250 and above 8000 Hz must be made considerably more intense in order to be perceived.

Sounds outside the frequency range of the human ear are referred to as *ultrasonic* if they are above the human limits, or *infrasonic* if they are below. Dogs appear to have sensitivity to higher frequencies than do humans. Several years ago dog whistles of ultrasonic frequency (for human beings) appeared on the market. Such whistles enable the dog owner to summon his pet without disturbing the neighborhood (except for other dogs). Dogs are frequently observed to react to train whistles and to sirens as if the sounds pained them. It is possible that the dogs are receiving very high frequencies of strong intensity, which are not even perceived by us. Ultrasonic frequencies are of interest to engineers and physicists and are being put to industrial and medical use, but as of the present time at least they do not concern the audiologist. Our concern is with audible frequencies.

The physical attribute of frequency of an audible wave is primarily responsible for the psychological sensation of *pitch*. As the frequency of a sound increases, the pitch of the sound as heard becomes higher. Scales of pitch are based on the assumption that as frequency is doubled (intensity remaining constant), pitch is raised one octave, and as frequency is halved, pitch is lowered one octave. The relationship between frequency and pitch scale is thus logarithmic to the base 2.

For scientific work, an arbitrary scale has been devised in which 256 Hz equals middle "C." In such a scale, 1 Hz would also be equal to "C." It can be seen that this scale offers mathematical conveniences. Successive octaves of "C" would be 1, 2, 4, 8, 16, 32, 64, 128, 256, 512, 1024, 2048, 4096, 8192, 16,384, 32,768, etc. Of course the first four frequencies in this series would be infrasonic, and the last frequency would be ultrasonic. The otologist's tuning forks are in octaves of "C" on the scientific scale, and until recently audiometers also were calibrated in octaves and half-octaves of "C" on the scientific scale. Lately, however, for the convenience of audiometrists and others dealing with hearing-test results, audiometers have been calibrated in round numbers of hertz instead of in octaves of "C." Thus, modern audiometers generate the following frequencies: 125, 250, 500, 750, 1000, 1500, 2000, 3000, 4000, 6000 and 8000 Hz. It is interesting to note that for musical purposes a scale in which "A" equals 440 Hz has been adopted. In the concert scale, middle "C" equals 261.6 Hz.

The term octave is misleading, since an octave has six main divisions, not eight. In other words, an octave consists of six *tones*, or twelve *semitones*. To find the number of hertz for the frequency that is one tone higher in pitch than a given frequency, multiply the lower frequency by the sixth root of two

($\sqrt[6]{2}$) which equals 1.1224. Thus the frequency that is one tone higher in pitch than 1000 Hz is 1122.4 Hz. To find the frequency of the next higher tone, multiply 1122.4 by $\sqrt[6]{2}$ (1.1224). Continuing this process yields the frequencies of successively higher tones until the result of the sixth such multiplication equals 2000 Hz.

The frequency values of semitones can be computed in similar fashion by using the twelfth root of two ($\sqrt[12]{2}$), or 1.059, as the multiplier. Since frequency is a logarithmic function, the number of hertz in an octave interval is different from octave to octave, and the same is true, of course, for tonal and semitonal intervals. Thus the octave from 500 to 1000 Hz spans a range of 500 Hz, while the octave from 4000 to 8000 Hz covers a range of 4000 Hz. Once the frequency values of tonal and semitonal intervals have been computed for one octave, they can be determined for the next higher octave by multiplying them by two, or for the next lower octave by dividing them by two.

Striking each key on a piano in succession, whether white or black, produces a series of semitones. Thus in an octave we would have the following musical designations of semitones: C, C♯, D, D♯, E, F, F♯, G, G♯, A, A♯, and B. Table 2-1 gives the semitonal values in hertz for a span of three octaves for both the scientific and concert scales.

Table 2-1. Approximate frequency values in hertz for semitones in two pitch scales*

	Scientific	Concert	Scientific	Concert	Scientific	Concert
C	128.0	130.8	256.0	261.6	512.0	523.2
C♯	135.6	138.5	271.2	277.0	542.4	554.0
D	143.6	146.8	287.2	293.6	574.4	587.2
D♯	152.0	155.5	304.0	311.0	608.0	622.0
E	160.8	164.8	321.6	329.6	643.2	659.2
F	170.4	174.6	340.8	349.2	681.6	698.4
F♯	180.4	184.9	360.8	369.8	721.6	739.6
G	191.2	196.0	382.4	392.0	764.8	784.0
G♯	202.4	207.6	404.8	415.2	809.6	830.4
A	214.4	220.0	428.8	440.0	857.6	880.0
A♯	227.2	233.0	454.4	466.0	908.8	932.0
B	240.8	247.0	481.6	494.0	963.2	988.0

*Because of rounding errors, the values of each semitone will differ depending on the starting point of the computations. The computations for the scientific scale were made for the octave 32–64 Hz and extended to the higher octaves by simple multiplication. The computations for the concert scale were made for the octave 110–220 Hz.

Intensity. The intensity of a sound wave refers to the "strength" of the particle vibration, or the rate of sound-energy transmission through a medium. A given sound source may vibrate with little or great intensity, depending upon the amount of force that sets it into vibration. Intensity is related to the square of the amplitude and the square of the frequency of the wave.

Intensity is usually measured in terms of relative pressure, using an instrument called a sound-level meter (see Chapter 9). Absolute pressure is expressed in microbars (μbars), dynes per square centimeter (dynes/cm^2), or newtons per square meter (N/m^2). Intensity may also be expressed as power flow in watts per square centimeter (watts/cm^2) or as power level in watts.

A microbar is one millionth of a bar. Standard atmospheric pressure, 14.7 pounds per square inch, is 1,013,250 μbars, or slightly more than 1 bar.[1] One newton per square meter is equal to 10 μbars, or, put another way, 1 μbar equals 0.1 N/m^2. Microbars and dynes per square centimeter are synonymous.

The normal human ear is sensitive to a wide range of intensities, from 10^{-16} watt/cm^2 (0.000,000,000,000,000,1 watt/cm^2) to 10^{-2} watt/cm^2 (0.01 watt/cm^2) expressed in units of power flow, or from 0.0002 dyne/cm^2 (2×10^{-4} dyne/cm^2) to 2000 dynes/cm^2 (2×10^3 dynes/cm^2) expressed in units of pressure. The least intensity corresponds to the minimum audible threshold of the ear, and the highest intensity represents the point at which, on the average, sound produces a sensation of pain.

Because of the difficulty of dealing with the absolute units of power or pressure, it is customary to convert units of intensity to a ratio between a given sound power or sound pressure and a standard reference power or pressure that for audiologic convenience approximates the minimum audible threshold of the normal ear. The use of a logarithmic scale to the base 10 for expressing this ratio results in a greatly simplified means of referring to intensity. The reference for *intensity level* (IL) is 10^{-16} watt/cm^2 (ten to the minus sixteen watt per square centimeter) and for *sound pressure level* (SPL) is 0.0002 dyne/cm^2 or μbar (two ten-thousandths, or triple-zero-two, dyne per square centimeter or microbar), or 20 μN/m^2 (twenty micronewtons per square meter). *Sound power level* (PWL) refers to a reference power of 10^{-12} watt (ten to the minus twelve watt). Alternate ways of abbreviating the terms intensity level, sound pressure level, and sound power level are L_I, L_P, and L_w, respectively.[2]

The ratio between two powers is computed from the formula $\log_{10} \dfrac{I_1}{I_0}$ where I_1 equals the greater power and I_0 equals the lesser power. The formula yields the number of *bels*, named for Alexander Graham Bell, between the two powers. Since the bel is too gross a unit for practical use, it is subdivided into ten parts, each of which is called a *decibel*, abbreviated dB. The formula for determining the decibel ratio between two powers then becomes $N_{dB} = 10 \log_{10} \dfrac{I_1}{I_0}$. When I_0 is the standard reference level of 10^{-16} watt/cm^2, the formula yields the intensity level of the higher power in decibels. While

[1]Arnold P. G. Peterson and Erwin E. Gross, Jr., *Handbook of Noise Measurement* (West Concord, Mass., General Radio Company, 1967), p. 4.

[2]Lewis S. Goodfriend, "Terminology, Definitions, and Usage," *Sound and Vibration*, Vol. 2 (June, 1968), p. 9.

tables are readily available to convert various ratios into their decibel equivalents, ratios that are powers of ten may be easily determined by counting the number of zeros and multiplying by ten. Thus a power ratio of 10 to 1 is an increase of 10 dB; 100 to 1 is 20 dB; and 1000 to 1 is 30 dB.

Pressure is proportional to the square root of power. The ratio between two pressures can thus be expressed by the formula $N_{dB} = 10 \log_{10} \frac{p_1{}^2}{p_0{}^2}$, where p_1 is the higher pressure and p_0 is the lower pressure. Since, with logarithms, doubling is the equivalent of squaring real numbers, the formula can be more simply written $N_{dB} = 20 \log_{10} \frac{p_1}{p_0}$. When p_0 is the standard reference level of 0.0002 dyne/cm^2, 0.0002 μbar, or 20 μN/m^2, the formula yields the sound pressure level in dB. Since the formula for pressure utilizes a multiple that is twice that used for power, the rapid method for determining the number of decibels between pressure ratios in multiples of ten is to count the number of zeros and multiply by twenty. Thus a pressure ratio of 10 to 1 is equal to an increase of 20 dB; 100 to 1, to 40 dB; and 1000 to 1, to 60 dB. Table 2-2 gives decibel equivalents of various power and pressure ratios.

Table 2-2. Ratios in decibels of power and pressure

Ratio	Power (dB)	Pressure (dB)
1	0	0
2	3.0	6.0
3	4.8	9.5
5	7.0	14.0
7	8.5	16.9
9	9.5	19.1
10	10.0	20.0
11	10.4	20.8
13	11.1	22.2
17	12.3	24.6
19	12.8	25.6
20	13.0	26.0
30	14.8	29.6
40	16.0	32.0
50	17.0	34.0
60	17.8	35.6
70	18.4	36.9
80	19.0	38.0
90	19.5	39.0
100	20.0	40.0
1000	30.0	60.0
10000	40.0	80.0
100000	50.0	100.0
1000000	60.0	120.0
10000000	70.0	140.0

One advantage of logarithms is that multiplication is accomplished by simple addition of the logarithms of the numbers to be multiplied, and division is accomplished by subtraction of the corresponding logarithms. Thus in Table 2-2 we can see that the ratio of 20 equals a dB (logarithmic) equivalent of 13.0 for power and 26.0 for pressure. Now since a ratio of 20 is the same as a ratio of 10×2, we should be able to arrive at the same dB equivalents by adding those dB values corresponding to ratios of 10 and 2. In terms of power this means adding 10.0 dB and 3.0 dB for a total of 13.0 dB, and in terms of pressure adding 20.0 dB and 6.0 dB for a total of 26.0 dB. It can be seen, therefore, that the decibel equivalents are the same regardless of how the ratio is expressed.

By multiplying the appropriate ratios and adding the corresponding dB values for these ratios, dB values can be obtained for ratios not contained in Table 2-2. For example, to determine the dB equivalents in power and pressure for a ratio of 39, add the dB values for ratios of 13 and 3, yielding values of 15.9 dB $(11.1 + 4.8)$ for a power ratio of 39 to 1, and 31.7 $(22.2 + 9.5)$ for a pressure ratio of 39 to 1. Incidentally, the reason that the pressure value is not exactly twice the power value in this example is that for purposes of simplification the dB values in Table 2-2 have been rounded to the nearest tenth of a decibel.[3]

Just as there are limitations in the frequency response of the human ear, so there is a definable range of intensities to which it will respond. The psychological sensation of loudness is closely related to intensity of the sound wave. The greater the intensity of vibration is, the louder the sound appears to the listener. It has already been mentioned that a sound pressure level of 0.0002 dyne/cm^2 corresponds closely to the least sound pressure to which the ear can respond. A sound 140 dB greater produces the sensation of pain in the average normal ear.

As was stated in the preceding section of this chapter, the ear is not equally sensitive to all frequencies. In other words, to reach the threshold of the human ear, greater intensities are required at the lower and higher end of the frequency scale than for the medium frequencies (1000 to 4000 Hz, roughly). Figure 2-1 demonstrates the limits of the ear both for frequency and for intensity. The bottom curve and the top three curves represent averages of the values found by a number of investigators. These measurements were made with subjects listening through earphones. When stimuli are presented to subjects through a loudspeaker in what is termed a *sound field*, somewhat lower sound pressure levels are obtained for minimum audible levels. The curve in Figure 2-1 marked "Average threshold (Zero of 2A Audiometer)" represents values that were assumed to be averages of "normal" hearing in the early days of audiometer manufacturing. The American National Standards Institute, formerly the American Standards Association,

[3]For clarification of the concept of the decibel and applications of the concept for solving simple problems involving increases and decreases of power and pressure, the reader is referred to a monograph entitled *The Decibel* by Jerry V. Tobias and Barry S. Elpern (Norman, Okla., 1964).

specifies the sound pressures for audiometric zero at each test frequency. These values differ somewhat from those shown in Figure 2-1. A discussion of audiometric zero will be found in Chapter 5.

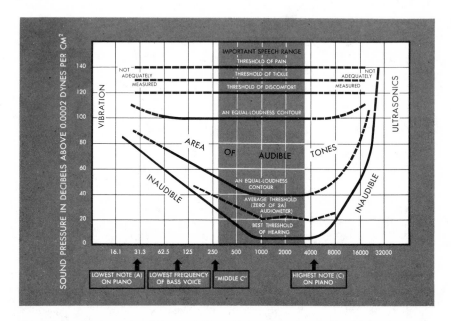

Figure 2-1.   The area of audible tones. (From Hallowell Davis, ed., *Hearing and Deafness*, 1st ed., Chap.2, Fig.3, New York, Rinehart, 1947. Reprinted by permission of the publishers.)

A term that is frequently employed in psychophysical measurement is *sensation level*. Sensation level is ". . . the pressure level of the sound in decibels above its threshold of audibility for the individual observer or for a specified group of individuals."[4] Most frequently, the term sensation level refers to the individual observer's threshold. Thus if a stimulus is presented at a level of 30 dB above an individual's threshold for that sound, we say that the sound was presented at a sensation level of 30 dB. Sensation level does not give us any information directly concerning the physical intensity of the stimulus. Before we can tell what the sound pressure level of the stimulus is, we must first know what the observer's threshold is in terms of sound pressure level.

Spectrum. The simplest form of sound is a *pure* tone, a single frequency. Such a sound can be adequately described only in terms of its frequency and intensity. Pure tones, however, are relatively rare. Most sounds in nature consist of *complex* tones, a number of frequencies existing simultaneously with

[4]*American Standard Acoustical Terminology* (S1.1—1960, New York, American National Standards Institute), p. 45.

various intensities. With appropriate instrumentation, it is possible to analyze complex tones into their component frequencies and intensities and thus obtain what has been termed a *tonal spectrum*. Oscillographic pictures demonstrate graphically the difference between a pure tone and a complex tone. These oscillographic pictures actually yield too much information about the sound and are affected by phase relationships of the component frequencies (see p. 16). It is usually more satisfactory to describe a sound by spectral analysis.

All sounds can be placed on a continuum between musical sounds and noise. Musical sounds are those which have *periodicity*—the wave form is repeated with the frequency of the *fundamental* or lowest frequency of the complex wave. We say that a musical complex wave consists of a fundamental frequency and overtones which, when their frequencies are multiples of the fundamental, are termed *harmonics*. By the process of harmonic analysis, these overtones can be identified and their relative intensity measured.

Noise may be defined psychologically as any undesired sound. In physical terms, noise is usually characterized by irregular frequencies and intensities; in other words, noise has no periodicity, no clearly defined fundamental frequency. In audiometric work, it is frequently necessary to employ a masking noise in one ear while testing the other ear. One of the best masking noises yet devised is what is called *white noise* because of its similarity to white light. White noise contains a wide band of frequencies at intervals of 1 Hz or less, at approximately the same intensity. Some audiometers employ "saw-tooth" masking, a noise composed of a complex tone usually with a fundamental frequency of 120 Hz, and including all the harmonics of this fundamental to 10,000 Hz.

With musical tones, it is not necessary to have the fundamental frequency present for the ear to identify it. The missing fundamental will be perceived provided that the harmonic structure is presented. Harmonics are multiples of the fundamental frequency. Thus, the harmonics for a fundamental frequency of 500 Hz would be 1000, 1500, 2000, 2500, 3000, etc. If a filter introduced into a communication system were to filter out all frequencies below 1000 Hz, a complex tone with the above overtone structure would still be recognized as having a fundamental frequency of 500 Hz, because that specific overtone structure could exist only for a fundamental frequency of 500 Hz.

The perception of mising fundamental frequencies simplifies considerably the problem of communication systems. The average adult male voice has a fundamental frequency between 120 and 150 Hz, and the average adult female voice has a fundamental frequency between 210 and 240 Hz; yet we usually have no difficulty in distinguishing between male and female voices over the telephone, although the telephone does not carry frequencies lower than about 300 Hz. This may be true in part because we are able to perceive the fundamental frequency which is missing from the signal coming through the receiver.

The spectrum of a sound is related to the psychological sensation of quality. We recognize the difference between a saxophone and a trumpet playing the same note because of the differences in spectra, which in turn are a function both of the complexities of vibration of the sound source and of the selective characteristics of the resonators provided for the sound source. Likewise we recognize differences among the various speech sounds because of differences in the spectra of the sounds. People's voices are recognizable, even over the telephone, because of differences in the spectra of their sounds from those of others.

Other Characteristics of Sound

Phase. Phase refers to the time relationship between two or more pure tones occurring simultaneously. In the case of pressure phase, if two tones of the same frequency and intensity are produced so that their periods of compression and rarefaction agree exactly, they will combine into a tone with twice the amplitude of either one alone. These tones are said to be "in phase." On the other hand, if the tones are separated by half a cycle, so that one wave is in compression while the other is in rarefaction, the two tones will cancel each other, and amplitude will be zero. These tones are in "opposite phase," or 180 degrees "out of phase." The cancellation effect of tones in opposite phase can be observed in some auditoriums or theaters that are of poor acoustic design. In such rooms, there are seats so located that the auditor simultaneously receives both original and reflected waves originating from the stage, but with sufficient time lag between the original and reflected waves for them to tend to cancel each other.

Phase differences account for an interesting acoustic phenomenon referred to as *beats*. If the ear receives simultaneously two tones of slightly different frequency, the sensation of beats, or pulsations, will be heard. The ear will hear as many beats per second as there are cycles of difference between the two tones in frequency. Thus if tones of 500 and 505 Hz are presented simultaneously, five beats per second will be heard. The beats result from phase differences between the two tones. The wavelength of the tone of 505 Hz is slightly less than that of the 500 Hz tone. For that reason, the periods of compression and rarefaction of the two waves occur at slightly different times. Their phase relationships are constantly changing. Five times a second, however, the two waves will be in phase for one cycle, and five times a second the waves will be 180 degrees out of phase for the space of one cycle. When they are in phase, or approaching an in-phase relationship, their amplitudes are additive, so that the ear transmits a sensation of increasing loudness. When they are out of phase, or approaching an out-of-phase relationship, the ear transmits a decreasing loudness. This swelling to a peak and diminishing to zero of the sound pressure five times a second produces the sensation of beats.

If the two frequencies are more than a few Hz apart, the beats will occur so rapidly that the ear will not be aware of them but will receive the sensation of two separate tones. If the tones are far enough apart, a *difference tone* will be perceived, equal in frequency to the difference in Hz between the two stimulus tones. Thus if tones of 1500 and 2000 Hz are presented, the ear will "hear," in addition to these two tones, a tone of 500 Hz frequency.

Another manifestation of phase differences between tones occurs in *standing waves*. When a pure-tone sound wave is introduced into a closed pipe of the same length as the wavelength of the tone, a wave is reflected back from the closed end of the pipe 180 degrees out of phase with the original wave. Thus there is a cancellation effect, and no audible sound results as with the "dead spots" in auditoriums referred to above. We shall see later how such standing waves may affect hearing-test results at certain frequencies.

Masking. When noise or sound of any kind interferes with the audibility of another sound, masking has occurred. Masking is a common auditory experience. We all know how futile it is to try to converse while a train is passing close by, and probably we have all been frustrated in movies or plays when audience noise prevents our hearing the actors' lines. Considerable research on the subject of masking has been undertaken. Much has been conducted by experimental psychologists in the laboratory, but some has been directed at practical problems of improving the audibility of speech in the presence of noise, as, for example, in military communications.

In audiometric work, it is frequently desirable to employ a masking tone or noise in one ear while the other ear is being tested, When there is a great difference in sensitivity of hearing between an individual's two ears, it is necessary to rule out the participation of the better ear while the poorer ear is being tested. This is done by the introduction of masking into the better ear. Such masking may be in the form of a pure tone (of the same frequency as the test tone), amplified "sixty-cycle hum," saw-tooth (complex) noise, white noise, or narrow-band noise. More will be said about the audiometric use of masking in later chapters.

THE HUMAN MECHANISM OF HEARING

Sound waves are received by the ear and transmitted to the brain, where meaning is attached to them. In the following sections of this chapter we shall examine the various parts of the hearing mechanism. Refer to Figure 2-2 for locating the parts of the ear described in the text.

The Outer Ear

The outer ear consists of the *pinna* or *auricle* and the *external acoustic meatus* or *canal*. Of all the parts of the ear the pinna is the most prominent and the least useful. It serves the purpose of directing sound waves into the external meatus in a more concentrated fashion than would otherwise be possible. The function of the pinna in relation to the external canal can be likened to that of cupping the hand behind the ear in a difficult listening situation.

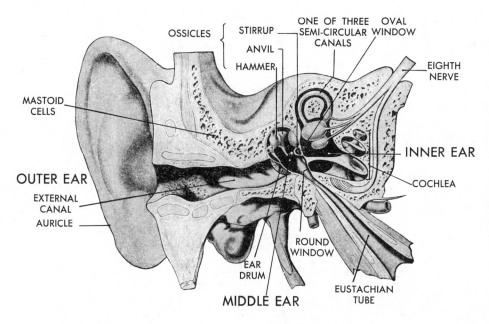

Figure 2-2. Sectional diagram of the human ear. (Reproduced by permission of the Sonotone Corporation, Elmsford, N.Y.)

The *helix* is the name given to the outer edge of the pinna which consists of folded tissue extending in almost a complete circle from just above the *tragus,* the small projection just ahead of the opening of the external meatus, to the *lobule,* which is the point at which an earring is attached. The *anthelix* is a ridge that is concentric with the helix, and the *antitragus* is the point opposite the tragus, posterior and slightly inferior to the opening of the meatus. The cavity bounded by the anthelix, the tragus, and the antitragus is called the *concha.* The opening of the external meatus is within the concha. These and other landmarks of the pinna are identified in Figure 2-3.

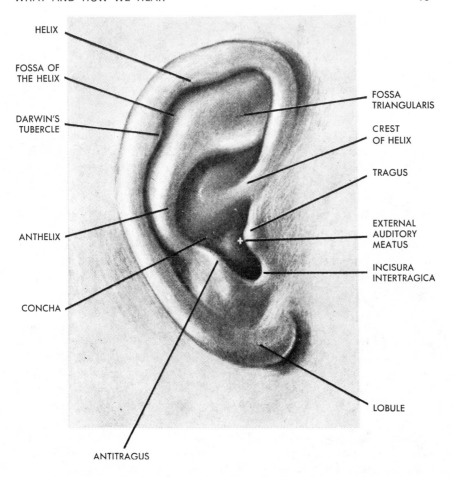

HELIX

FOSSA OF
THE HELIX

DARWIN'S
TUBERCLE

ANTHELIX

CONCHA

FOSSA
TRIANGULARIS

CREST
OF HELIX

TRAGUS

EXTERNAL
AUDITORY
MEATUS

INCISURA
INTERTRAGICA

LOBULE

ANTITRAGUS

Figure 2-3. Landmarks of the pinna. (From Francis L. Lederer and Abraham R. Hollender, *Textbook of the Ear, Nose, and Throat,* Philadelphia, F. A. Davis Company, 1947. Reproduced by permission of the publishers.)

In many animals, the pinna serves the useful purpose of providing more acute hearing and more precise sound localization. This is accomplished by the animal's moving the pinna by muscular action until it is operating most efficiently and is directed toward the source of the sound. We have all observed a dog "prick up" it ears and listen intently until it has identified the source of a faint sound. In more primitive days, when man's existence depended on the acuity of his senses, it may have been possible for him to manipulate his pinnae or "prick up" his ears. Now that accomplishment is limited to a few talented individuals who are thus able to amuse children and attain some distinction in "parlor tricks." In modern society, the pinna is almost purely ornamental, inappropriate though the word may seem, applied to something as homely as the ear!

The external meatus is a roughly cylindrical passage about a quarter of an inch in diameter and a little over an inch long. Generally, there is sufficient bend in the meatus so that it is not possible to see the eardrum membrane by simply looking into the opening of the meatus. When the otologist examines the drum membrane, he introduces a funnel-shaped instrument called a *speculum* into the canal, which has the effect of straightening the canal and bringing the membrane into view. The external meatus contains hairs and wax-producing glands, which serve to protect the drum membrane from the penetration of dirt and insects. In many people, the glands produce too much wax, or *cerumen,* with the result that the excess must be removed at regular intervals to prevent blockage of the canal.

The external meatus ends at the eardrum membrane, or *tympanic membrane,* which is the external boundary of the second part of the hearing mechanism, the middle ear. The drum membrane is a thin diaphragm which completely closes the canal.

The Middle Ear

The space between the drum membrane and the bony capsule of the inner ear is called the middle ear, or *tympanum.* Technically, the term *eardrum* is synonymous with tympanum, that is, the whole middle ear, although popularly "eardrum" refers only to the "drumhead" or membrane. In line with popular practice, "eardrum" will be used in this book to refer only to the membrane which separates the middle ear from the outer ear.

The middle ear is a cavity of between 1 and 2 cubic centimeters in volume, lined with mucous membrane which is continuous with the mucous membrane lining of the nasal cavities. In fact, the middle ear is actually an extension of the *nasopharynx* by way of the *Eustachian tube.* Connecting the eardrum and an opening in the bony wall of the inner ear is a bridge of three tiny bones which is called the *ossicular chain.* These bones, the *ossicles,* are the tiniest bones in the body. They are named the *hammer, anvil,* and *stirrup,* or *malleus, incus,* and *stapes.* The hammer, or malleus, is secured to the eardrum; the stirrup, or stapes, is set with its footplate in the opening in the inner ear which is referred to as the *oval window;* and the anvil, or incus, connects the other two bones. Figure 2-4 shows the ossicles separately with their various landmarks identified. The middle ear communicates with the air cells of the *mastoid process* of the *temporal bone.* These air cells are lined with the same mucous membrane that lines the middle ear. Two muscles are found in the middle ear: the *tensor tympani* and the *stapedius.* The tensor tympani is innervated by the Vth nerve, the trigeminal, while the stapedius is innervated by the VIIth nerve, the facial.

The eardrum is roughly circular in shape, semitransparent, slightly coned inward toward the middle ear cavity, and pearly gray in color. It completely

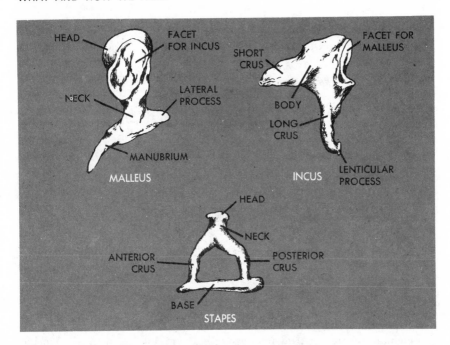

Figure 2-4. The ossicles. (From Harold M. Kaplan, *Anatomy and Physiology of Speech.* Copyright, 1960. McGraw-Hill Book Company, Inc. Used by permission.)

closes the end of the external meatus. The eardrum is kept relatively tense by the action of the tensor tympani muscle, which runs from the opening of the Eustachian tube to attach to the handle of the malleus. The eardrum consists of a large area called the *pars tensa* and a smaller area called the *pars flaccida* or Shrapnell's membrane. The pars tensa is composed of three layers of tissue. The outer layer is a continuation of the skin lining the external canal; the inner layer is a continuation of the mucous membrane lining the cavity of the middle ear; and the middle layer is connective tissue. The pars flaccida does not contain the middle layer of connective tissue. Near the center of the eardrum is its most depressed point, corresponding to the tip of the *manubrium,* the long process of the malleus. This point is referred to as the *umbo.* In Figure 2-5, the manubrium, referred to in the figure as the malleolar stria, may be seen through the eardrum, corresponding to the eleven o'clock position of an hour-hand on a clock. In a right ear, the manubrium of the malleus would be seen in the one o'clock position. The *cone of light* is seen as a reflection from the eardrum of the external light source used by an examiner looking down the external canal.

The Eustachian tube provides a means of ventilating the middle ear cavity. It serves as an air-pressure equalizer, since oxygen is constantly being absorbed.

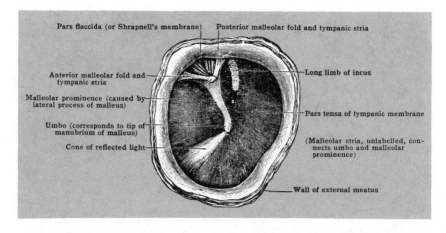

Figure 2-5. The left eardrum. (From J. Parsons Schaeffer, ed., *Morris' Human Anatomy,* tenth edition. Copyright, 1942. Blakiston Div., McGraw-Hill. Used by permission).

In addition, it enables the middle ear to compensate for changes in outside air pressure, as in crossing mountains or in flying. Without the action of the Eustachian tube to equalize air pressure in the middle ear with that outside, the eardrum would be subject to considerable stress, being forced outward when the outside pressure became less (increasing altitude) and inward when the outside pressure became greater (decreasing altitude). Normally, the Eustachian tube is in a collapsed state, so that an individual's voice and breathing sounds are not directly transmitted to the ear. It is opened only under the stress of air-pressure changes or by action of certain of the pharyngeal muscles during the act of swallowing or yawning. It is for this reason that the stewardess aboard an airliner may offer candy or gum before taking off or landing, to make the passenger use his swallowing muscles and thereby facilitate the air-pressure equalizing action of the Eustachian tube.

As has been stated, the ossicular chain forms a bridge across the cavity of the middle ear. The incus forms a link between the malleus, which is attached to the eardrum, and the stapes, which has its footplate inserted in the oval window. To the stapes is attached the stapedius muscle, which, when it contracts, tends to pull the footplate of the stapes out from the oval window. It is known that the stapedius and tensor tympani muscles have two opposed functions: first, to increase the sensitivity of the eardrum and the ossicular chain to signals of weak intensity, and, second, to serve as a "brake" to the action of the ossicular chain when the eardrum receives an unusually intense signal, and thus to protect the inner ear from receiving too much stimulation.

Just below the oval window is another connection between the middle and inner ears. This is the membrane-covered *round window.* The oval and round windows communicate with different parts of the inner ear mechanism, as we shall see in the following section.

The Inner Ear

The inner ear is more than an end-organ for hearing; it is also the sensory organ for balance. Both these important end-organs are encased in the same bony capsule, both have the same fluid systems, and both send their impulses along the same cranial nerve. Together, they are known as the inner ear, although only one of them is actually concerned with hearing. The close association of the end-organs of hearing and balance, however, has important implications for the otologist, as we shall see in the next chapter.

The balance part of the inner ear, frequently referred to as the *vestibular apparatus,* consists of the *utricle,* the *saccule,* and the three *semi-circular canals:* the anterior and posterior vertical canals, and the horizontal or lateral canal. These canals are located in planes which are at right angles to each other, and together with the utricle and the saccule they help us to maintain balance regardless of the position of the head in space.

The hearing part of the inner ear is the *cochlea,* which resembles a snail shell in appearance. The basal end of the cochlea is nearest the middle ear, the apical end is farthest from the middle ear. The cochlea and the semi-circular canals meet in a common area designated as the *vestibule.* It is in the bony wall of the vestibule that the oval window is located, and it is within the vestibule that the utricle and the saccule are found.

Sometimes the inner ear is referred to as the *labyrinth,* because of its intricate construction. The outer hard shell of the inner ear is called the bony labyrinth, and the inner, membranous portion of the apparatus is called the membranous labyrinth. The entire inner ear is filled with fluid. The membranous labyrinth is protected from the bony labyrinth by a fluid called *perilymph,* which is apparently cerebrospinal fluid supplied from the ventricles of the brain through a duct that links the cochlea with the subarachnoid space. Inside the membranous labyrinth is found another fluid called *endolymph.* The endolymphatic system is apparently entirely separate from the perilymphatic system. Whereas the perilymph cushions the membranous labyrinth throughout the inner ear, the endolymph is a closed system, with the cochlear portion and vestibular portions of the system connected by means of a narrow passage called the *ductus reuniens.* Endolymph is thought to be secreted by the stria vascularis ("area vascularis" in Figure 2-6, which shows the cochlea in cross section).

The membranous cochlea consists of a closed passage, the *cochlear duct,* or *scala media,* running the length of the two and three-quarters turns of the spiraling cochlea. The cochlear duct, occupying the central portion of the interior of the cochlea, separates the perilymphatic spaces of the cochlea into two so-called *galleries,* or *scalae:* the *scala vestibuli,* separated from the cochlear duct by the *vestibular membrane of Reissner*, and the *scala tympani*, separated from the cochlear duct by the *basilar membrane*. At the apex of the cochlea, these two perilymphatic spaces are connected by the *helicotrema*. The scala vestibuli communicates with the middle ear by means of the oval window, situated in the vestibule, and the scala tympani is connected to the middle ear by the round window.

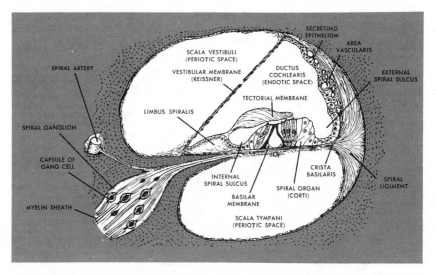

Figure 2-6. Cross section of cochlear canal. (From A. T. Rasmussen, *Outlines of Neuro-Anatomy,* 3rd ed., Dubuque, Ia., Wm. C. Brown Co. Reproduced by permission of the publishers.)

The cochlear duct, filled with endolymph, contains the sensory end organ of hearing, the *organ of Corti,* situated on the basilar membrane. The organ of Corti consists of four or five rows of hair cells, running parallel along the length of the basilar membrane: an inner row of from 3000 to 3500 hair cells, and three or four outer rows of from 9000 to 12,000 hair cells, or even more according to some authorities. From each of these hair cells project many hairs or *cilia* that make contact with the *tectorial membrane* which extends over them. The hair cells are connected in a complex fashion with some 20,000 to 30,000 nerve fibers, which run into the central core of the cochlea and there unite to form the *cochlear* branch of the VIIIth cranial, or *auditory,* nerve. The cochlear branch then joins the *vestibular* branch, coming from the semicircular canals and the utricle and saccule, and the VIIIth nerve proceeds to nuclei in the brain stem. From there, the auditory pathway extends through various nuclei to the cerebral cortex in the temporal lobes of the brain.

THE PHYSIOLOGY OF HEARING

For centuries the problem of how the hearing mechanism functions has been in dispute, and many books and articles have been written on the subject. No attempt will be made here to explain how the cochlea functions as a sound analyzer, and only brief mention will be made of the various theories of hearing. Here we shall be concerned primarily with how sound reaches the cochlea, not with what occurs electrically, chemically, and/or mechanically within the cochlea.

Hearing by Air Conduction

Normally we hear by the mechanism of air conduction, since most sounds to which we attend are air-borne, and since the mechanism of air conduction is much more sensitive than the mechanism of bone conduction. Sound waves in the air around us are directed by the pinna into the external acoustic meatus where they impinge on the eardrum. The eardrum is thus set into vibration by the movements of the air particles adjacent to it.

Since the handle of the malleus is imbedded in the eardrum, the ossicular chain is set into vibration. These three tiny bones vibrate as a unit. The in-and-out vibration of the eardrum, then, results in a rocking motion of the stapes in the oval window, which produces a pressure wave in the perilymph of the vestibule. The ossicles transform the energy collected by the eardrum into greater force and less excursion, thus matching the impedance of sound waves in air to that in fluid. When the sound stimulus striking the eardrum is extremely intense, a reflex action of the intra-aural muscles, primarily the stapedius, dampens the vibrations of the ossicular chain, apparently as a protection for the inner ear. This *acoustic reflex* occurs in both ears, even though only one ear may have received an intense signal.

Since the fluid of the inner ear is practically incompressible, there has to be some provision for the relief of the pressure produced by the inward movement of the footplate of the stapes. This relief is furnished by the round window, whose membrane reacts to the movements of the footplate of the stapes in the oval window. The interaction of the two windows is complex, but, simply described, when the footplate is pushed into the vestibule, the membrane in the round window is bulged outward toward the middle ear cavity. Without this reciprocal action of the two windows, the incompressibility of the perilymph would resist the action of the ossicular chain, which in turn would restrict the vibrations of the eardrum.

The fluid motion from the oval to the round window is transmitted through the cochlear duct. As the footplate of the stapes is pushed into the perilymph

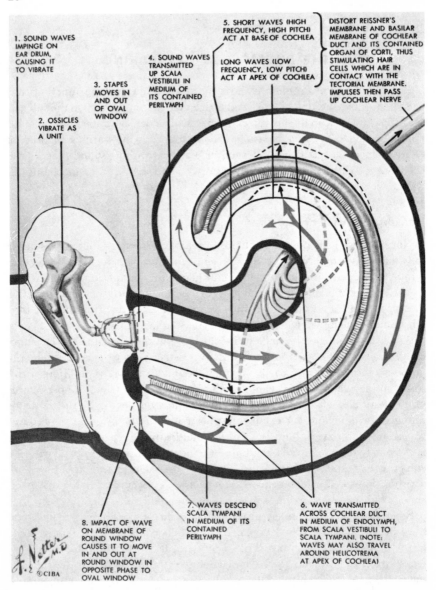

1. SOUND WAVES IMPINGE ON EAR DRUM, CAUSING IT TO VIBRATE

2. OSSICLES VIBRATE AS A UNIT

3. STAPES MOVES IN AND OUT OF OVAL WINDOW

4. SOUND WAVES TRANSMITTED UP SCALA VESTIBULI IN MEDIUM OF ITS CONTAINED PERILYMPH

5. SHORT WAVES (HIGH FREQUENCY, HIGH PITCH) ACT AT BASE OF COCHLEA

LONG WAVES (LOW FREQUENCY, LOW PITCH) ACT AT APEX OF COCHLEA

DISTORT REISSNER'S MEMBRANE AND BASILAR MEMBRANE OF COCHLEAR DUCT AND ITS CONTAINED ORGAN OF CORTI, THUS STIMULATING HAIR CELLS WHICH ARE IN CONTACT WITH THE TECTORIAL MEMBRANE. IMPULSES THEN PASS UP COCHLEAR NERVE

6. WAVE TRANSMITTED ACROSS COCHLEAR DUCT IN MEDIUM OF ENDOLYMPH, FROM SCALA VESTIBULI TO SCALA TYMPANI. (NOTE: WAVES MAY ALSO TRAVEL AROUND HELICOTREMA AT APEX OF COCHLEA)

7. WAVES DESCEND SCALA TYMPANI IN MEDIUM OF ITS CONTAINED PERILYMPH

8. IMPACT OF WAVE ON MEMBRANE OF ROUND WINDOW CAUSES IT TO MOVE IN AND OUT AT ROUND WINDOW IN OPPOSITE PHASE TO OVAL WINDOW

Figure 2-7. Pathway of sound from the eardrum through the cochlea. (From David Myers, Woodrow D. Schlosser, and Richard A. Winchester, "Otologic Diagnosis and the Treatment of Deafness," *Clinical Symposia*, 14:39, 1962, published by CIBA Pharmaceutical Company. Used by permission.)

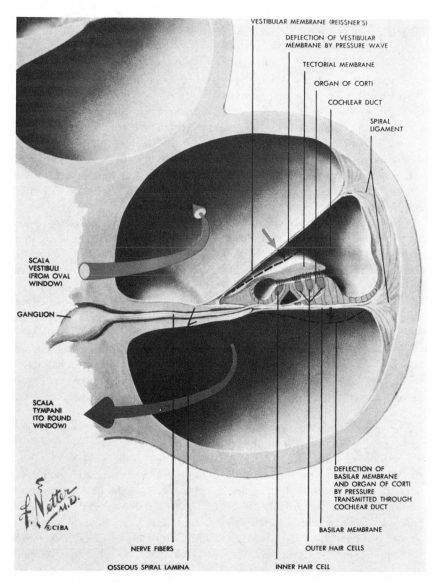

Figure 2-8.   Transmission of sound energy through the cochlear duct. (From David Myers, Woodrow D. Schlosser, and Richard A. Winchester, "Otologic Diagnosis and the Treatment of Deafness," *Clinical Symposia,* 14:39, 1962, published by CIBA Pharmaceutical Company. Used by permission.)

of the scala vestibuli, the vestibular membrane, or membrane of Reissner, is bulged into the cochlear duct, causing movement of the endolymph within the cochlear duct and movement of the basilar membrane. The cilia of the hair cells are imbedded in the gelatinous tectorial membrane, so that when the basilar membrane is displaced there is a "shearing" action on the cilia by the tectorial membrane that initiates nerve impulses. These impulses are carried by nerve fibers to the main trunk of the cochlear portion of the VIIIth nerve, and thence to the brain. Thus it is the cerebral cortex which eventually "hears" the vibrations which impinged on the eardrum. The movement of the basilar membrane is transmitted to the perilymph in the scala tympani, and the bulge produced by the inward movement of the footplate of the stapes thus reaches the round window, the membrane of which is bulged into the middle ear cavity.

Experimental studies have demonstrated that sounds of very high frequency cause movements of the basilar membrane and the hair cells of the organ of Corti at the basal end of the cochlea or, in other words, at the part of the cochlea nearest the middle ear; whereas sounds of very low frequency affect the cochlear duct at the apical end, near or at the helicotrema. In fact, work with guinea pigs has succeeded in mapping the location along the basilar membrane of the areas of sensitivity from high to low frequency, from the base to the apical end of the cochlea. Figure 2-7 illustrates the manner in which vibrations are transmitted from the eardrum to the cochlea, the transmission of energy through the cochlear duct, and the reciprocal action of the two windows that connect the middle ear with the inner ear. Figure 2-8 is an enlarged view of the transmission of energy through the cochlear duct.

The nerve fibers leading from the hair cells collect at the *spiral ganglion* and then emerge from the temporal bone through the *internal acoustic meatus,* in company with the fibers of the vestibular branch of the VIIIth nerve, and the VIIth, or facial, nerve. The neurons of the cochlear portion of the VIIIth nerve proceed to the *ventral* and *dorsal cochlear nuclei* on the ipsilateral (same) side of the upper medulla and pons of the brain stem. Next the neurons proceed to the *superior olivary complex* of the pons. Some neurons decussate (cross) through the *trapezoid body* to the contralateral (opposite) superior olivary complex. From the superior olivary complex on each side of the pons the neurons proceed in tracts called the *lateral lemnisci* to nuclei called the *inferior colliculi* at the level of the midbrain. Some additional decussation occurs at this level. The neurons then proceed to the thalamic nuclei called the *medial geniculate bodies.* From these points, *auditory radiations* spread to the cortex of the cerebrum—specifically to *Heschl's gyrus* in the temporal lobe. As we have seen, there is a crossing over of some neurons at two different levels in the ascending tracts, so that impulses originating in one cochlea eventually reach both auditory cortices. Because of this bilateral cortical

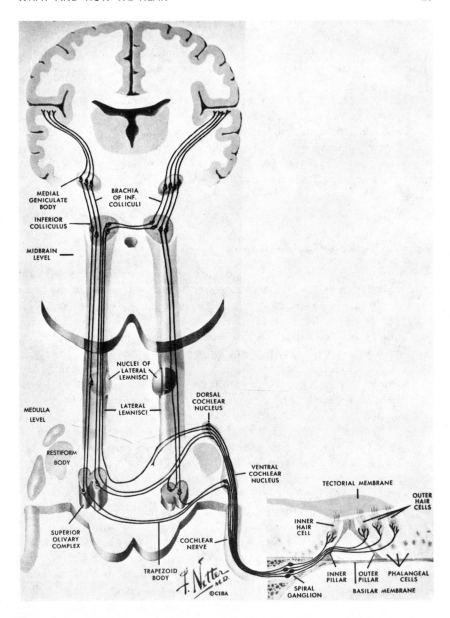

Figure 2-9.   Ascending pathways of the cochlear branch of the VIIIth nerve. (From David Myers, Woodrow D. Schlosser, and Richard A. Winchester, "Otologic Diagnosis and the Treatment of Deafness," *Clinical Symposia,* 14:39, 1962, published by CIBA Pharmaceutical Company. Used by permission.

representation of each ear, interruption of the ascending auditory tract on one side of the brain stem above the level of the cochlear nuclei, or the removal of one temporal lobe, does not result in a loss of hearing acuity in either ear. Figure 2-9 diagrams the pathways of the cochlear branch of the VIIIth nerve.

While the VIIIth nerve is primarily a sensory nerve, that is, it carries sensory information from the cochlea and the vestibular system to the brain, there are a limited number of efferent fibers—about 500—proceeding from the superior olivary complex to the cochlea. Most are crossed fibers, connecting with the cochlea of the opposite side. This descending tract is called the *olivo-cochlear* tract or Rasmussen's bundle. While its function is still not clear, the olivo-cochlear tract apparently exerts primarily an inhibitory effect on the hair cells.

Hearing by Bone Conduction

Since the inner ear is encased in bone (the *petrous* portion of the temporal bone), vibrations of this bone will cause movement of the fluid of the inner ear directly. Thus the sensation of hearing can be produced without vibrations proceeding through the eardrum and the ossicular chain. Our mechanism for transmission of sound by *bone conduction* is much less efficient than for air-conducted sound, because vibrations must be sufficiently intense to set the bones of the skull into movement before they can be heard by bone conduction. Moreover, in going through skin, flesh, and bone, sound waves are not accurately transmitted, since sounds of longer wavelength (lower frequency) are impeded less by these obstructions than are sounds of short wavelength (higher frequency). Thus our hearing by bone conduction tends to be somewhat distorted when compared with that by air conduction.

At least two modes of vibration are known to occur in bone conduction. These are known as *inertial,* or *translatory,* motion and *compressional* motion. Sounds of low frequency (roughly below 800 Hz) excite the hair cells because of the inertia of the ossicular chain. The skull apparently moves as a whole in response to low-frequency stimulation. If the ossicles lag behind the movement of the skull, vibrations are transmitted through the oval window in the same way as when air-borne vibrations set the ossicular chain in motion. A different kind of vibratory motion of the skull results from high-frequency stimulation (roughly above 1500 Hz). Instead of moving as a whole, the skull vibrates so that opposite surfaces move in an out-of-phase relationship. As the front and back of the skull move outward, the sides of the skull move inward. The effect of this skull movement is to produce a compression of the cochlea. Since the round window is the point of least resistance within the cochlea, when compression of the cochlea occurs the fluid within the cochlea causes displacement of the round window. The fluid movement within the cochlea initiates nerve impulses. Both inertial and compressional motions result from bone-conduction stimulation by frequencies between 800 and 1500 Hz.

Ordinarily, we are not conscious of hearing by bone conduction, since most sounds we are interested in are carried by air, and the air-conducting mechanism of hearing is so much more efficient than our bone-conduction mechanism. If our heads are in contact with a solid surface, however, such as the floor, the bones of the skull receive vibrations such as footsteps, and our bone-conducting mechanism is thus activated. Moreover, we tend to hear our own voices partly through the mechanism of bone conduction. This occurs because the vibrations of our vocal folds in the larynx are transmitted to the air in cavities of the head and neck, and thus also to the bones of our skull. The fluid of the inner ear is then set into motion directly. Of course we are also hearing our own voices through air conduction if we have normal outer and middle ears. The shock that many of us receive when we first hear our voices recorded is due in part to the fact that listening to our recorded voice is the first time we have heard ourselves "as others hear us," through air conduction alone.

The mechanism of bone conduction provides an alternate pathway for sound which can be utilized by people who have suffered an impairment of their air conduction, that is, an impairment of their outer or middle ear. If the inner ear is functioning normally, they can "hear," provided that sound can reach the inner ear. Such individuals usually do quite well with the amplification that an individual, wearable hearing aid furnishes. Sound can be made intense enough through amplification, delivered to either an air-conduction or bone-conduction type of receiver, to activate the bone-conducting mechanism.

Theories of Hearing

As was stated above, this book is not concerned with the controversy of how the cochlea functions in analyzing sound. The serious student of audiology will, of course, want to pursue this subject in detail. Only the briefest mention will be made here of the principal theories of hearing.

The Place Theory. This theory, originally popularized by the famous German scientist Helmholz, states that pitch perception is related to the place of maximum stimulation of the basilar membrane. Experimental evidence, as we have mentioned, indicates that the basal end of the cochlea is sensitive to high frequencies and the apical end of the cochlea is stimulated by low frequencies. The place theory holds that it is the *exact* place of stimulation of the organ of Corti along the basilar membrane which determines the pitch perceived. Helmholz proposed that structures of the cochlear duct act as resonators, much as the strings of a piano vibrate in response to particular frequencies. Later exponents of the place theory do not believe that the tuning of the cochlea is as precise as Helmholz thought. Nevertheless, the principle of the theory is the same—it is the particular region of stimulation of the basilar membrane which is responsible for the sensation of pitch.

The Frequency Theory. This theory explains pitch perception on the basis of the frequency of occurrence of impulses in the auditory nerve. Thus this theory holds that a sound stimulus of a frequency of 500 Hz would cause fibers within the auditory nerve to discharge at the rate of 500 times per second. Rutherford and more recently Boring were exponents of this theory. The development of techniques for obtaining action potentials of nerve fibers disclosed that no fiber of the auditory nerve is capable of "firing" at a rate greater than about 1000 times per second. This experimental finding meant that discrimination of high pitches could therefore not be explained on the basis of a frequency theory. Even making allowance for the synchronized action of several nerve fibers discharging at slightly different times, the frequency theory could account for pitch perceptions only of frequencies below about 5000 Hz.

The Volley Theory. This theory is a compromise between the place and frequency theories. It holds that perception of pitch for frequencies up to 5000 Hz can be explained primarily on the basis of the frequency of nerve impulses firing in "volleys," and that the primary explanation for perception of pitch for frequencies in excess of 5000 Hz is the place of greatest excitation along the basilar membrane. The volley theory is advocated principally by Wever. It is achieving popularity because it utilizes the experimental information available, which does indicate that place of stimulation within the cochlea is important, and which also shows that pitch discriminations are correlated with frequency of nerve impulses, at least for the lower frequencies of sound vibration.

The Traveling Wave Theory. No discussion of theories of hearing can ignore the contributions of Georg von Békésy, who received the Nobel prize for his many years of detailed and meticulous research in regard to the functioning of the hearing mechanism. Békésy's experimentation with cochlear models led him to formulate a theory that sound is propagated in the cochlea in the form of a traveling wave in the basilar membrane. This wave travels from the base to the apex of the cochlea. The maximum amplitude of the wave occurs at a point along the basilar membrane that corresponds to the frequency of the stimulus; that is, the point of maximum amplitude is at the point that resonates to the stimulating frequency.

The theories of hearing mentioned above are concerned primarily with the way in which the ear discriminates frequency. Intensity discrimination apparently is dependent on the number of nerve fibers activated by the stimulus, the total number of impulses per second in all fibers, and possibly the existence of certain fibers that respond only to stimuli of high intensity.

REFERENCES

Bast, Theodore H., and Anson, Barry J., *The Temporal Bone and the Ear* (Springfield, Ill., Charles C Thomas, 1949).

Bekesy, Georg von, *Experiments in Hearing* (New York, McGraw-Hill, 1960).

Davis, Hallowell, and Silverman, S. Richard, eds., *Hearing and Deafness* (New York, Holt, Rinehart and Winston, 1970), Chaps. 2 and 3.

Fletcher, Harvey, *Speech and Hearing in Communication* (New York, Van Nostrand, 1953).

Glorig, Aram, ed., *Audiometry: Principles and Practices* (Baltimore, Williams & Wilkins, 1965), Chaps. 2 and 3.

Graham, A. Bruce, ed., *Sensorineural Hearing Processes and Disorders* (Boston, Little, Brown and Company, 1967), Chaps. 1–6.

Harris, J. Donald, ed., *Forty Germinal Papers in Human Hearing* (Groton, Conn., *The Journal of Auditory Research*, 1969).

Hirsh, Ira J., *The Measurement of Hearing* (New York, McGraw-Hill, 1952).

Lederer, Francis L., and Hollender, Abraham R., *Textbook of the Ear, Nose, and Throat* (Philadelphia, Davis, 1947), Section VI.

Polyak, Stephen L., McHugh, Gladys, and Judd, Delbert K., *The Human Ear in Anatomical Transparencies* (New York, Sonotone Corp., 1946).

Rasmussen, Grant L., and Windle, William F., eds., *Neural Mechanisms of the Auditory and Vestibular Systems* (Springfield, Ill., Charles C Thomas, 1960).

Rose, Darrell E., ed., *Audiological Assessment* (Englewood Cliffs, N.J., Prentice-Hall, 1971), Chaps. 1 and 2.

Rosenblith, Walter A., ed., *Sensory Communication* (New York, Wiley and the M.I.T. Press, 1961).

Stevens, S. S., ed., *Handbook of Experimental Psychology* (New York, Wiley, 1951), Chaps. 25–28.

Stevens, S. S., and Davis, Hallowell, *Hearing* (New York, Wiley, 1938).

Stevens, S. S., Warshofsky, Fred, and the Editors of *Life*, *Sound and Hearing* (New York, *Life* Science Library, Time Incorporated, 1967).

Tobias, Jerry V., ed., *Foundations of Modern Auditory Theory*, Vol. I (New York, Academic Press, 1970).

Travis, Lee Edward, ed., *Handbook of Speech Pathology and Audiology* (New York, Appleton-Century-Crofts, 1971), Chaps. 10–12.

Wever, E. G., *Theory of Hearing* (New York, Wiley, 1949).

Wever, E. G., and Lawrence, Merle, *Physiological Acoustics* (Princeton, Princeton University Press, 1954).

Zemlin, Willard R., *Speech and Hearing Science* (Englewood Cliffs, N.J., Prentice-Hall, 1968), Chap. 6.

3

DISORDERS OF HEARING

So far we have been concerned with the functioning of the normal ear. In audiology, so much reference is made to the normal ear that some definition is in order. By "normal" ear, we mean the ear of a young adult (from 18 to 22 years of age), which has had no known pathology—no history of infection nor any kind of disorder. Actually, the phrase *normal ear* refers not to any one ear but to a hypothetical average, normal ear. As we shall see in subsequent chapters, the concept of average normal ear is frequently adopted in the calibration of equipment for testing the hearing function.

In this chapter, we shall be concerned with impairment of hearing. A disorder of hearing we shall define as any significant deviation from the behavior of the average normal ear. In later chapters we shall see how hearing impairments are measured. Here the principal types of hearing disorders and their symptoms, causes, and treatment are discussed.

CONDUCTIVE IMPAIRMENTS

Any dysfunction of the outer or middle ear in the presence of a normal inner ear is termed a *conductive* impairment of hearing. In other words, the difficulty is not with the perception of sound but with the conduction of sound to the analyzing system. Acquired hearing losses in children will most likely be of the conductive type.

Symptoms

Although it is not possible to specify with absolute accuracy the symptoms that are indicative of conductive impairment, some generalizations of symptomatology can be made. For example, it has sometimes been observed that the person with a conductive loss tends to speak in a relatively quiet voice, so that it may be difficult for others to hear him. Since by definition a person with a "pure" conductive loss has a normal inner ear, and since we tend to hear our own voices to some extent through the mechanism of bone conduction, such a person hears himself with adequate loudness at all times and, because of his air-conduction loss, may be unaware of the presence of noise about him which makes it difficult for others to hear.

Another symptom of conductive impairment is that speech discrimination is relatively unimpaired. In other words, a patient with a conductive loss understands well what he hears, provided that speech is made loud enough for him. It may be necessary, therefore, to shout at such a patient or at least to speak with more than ordinary loudness. Because he hears loud speech well, the conductively impaired patient can usually hear better in the presence of noise than can the person with normal hearing. The reason is that when it is noisy, as in a factory, for example, people with normal hearing have to speak loudly in order to hear each other above the noise, which serves as a masking device. The patient with the conductive loss is largely unaware of the noise, and he benefits from the increased loudness with which those around him are speaking. The medical term for this apparent ability of the person with a conductive loss to hear speech better in a noisy place is *paracusis willisiana (Willisii)*.

The ability of this patient to hear loud speech satisfactorily is related to another symptom of conductive impairment, namely, his ability to tolerate loud speech and other sounds of an intensity sufficient to reach the threshold of discomfort of the normal ear. The conductive impairment serves as a protection to the inner ear, giving the same effect as that of wearing an ear plug. A patient with a conductive loss of 40 dB hears a sound having an intensity of 60 dB above the normal threshold with the loudness that a person with normal hearing would perceive a sound of 20 dB intensity. The protective feature of a conductive loss does not extend to sound-pressure levels of 130 dB and higher, however. In other words, the conductively impaired patient would respond as would a person with normal hearing to these extreme intensities.

The patient with a conductive loss tends to have about the same loss of sensitivity for sounds of all frequency. Sometimes hearing is better for the higher frequencies than it is for the lower ones, and occasionally the reverse may be true, but by and large the loss pattern is "flat."

Frequently, the conductively impaired individual complains of subjective head noises which may be localized in one ear, in both ears, or may be unlocalized in the head. The otologist refers to head noises as *tinnitus*. All of us have experienced tinnitus at some time. After the shooting of a gun, our ears may "ring" for several hours. In a very quiet room, we may be conscious of hearing our pulse beat or of other physiologic noises in our head. With most of us, however, tinnitus has been of a transient nature. Many hard-of-hearing people experience tinnitus every hour of the day. It is one of the most annoying features of impaired hearing. In the case of a conductive impairment the tinnitus tends to be of relatively low frequency. An experimental study of tinnitus revealed that subjects with conductive hearing impairments matched their tinnitus to pure tones in the range from 120–1400 Hz.[1]

Etiology (Causes)

Conditions of the Outer Ear. The commonest cause of an impairment of hearing due to the improper functioning of the outer ear is a blocking or plugging of the external meatus or canal by an excess accumulation of cerumen (wax). Of course it is possible for the canal to be blocked by other substances also. Sometimes children will stuff objects such as beans or even wads of paper in the canal. The blockage will cause a conductive impairment which will persist until the object is removed. Some people produce much more cerumen than they need for the ordinary protection of the eardrum, with the result that the cerumen builds up into a plug, which effectively prevents sound waves from reaching the eardrum. The remedy is simple: remove the cerumen, and the hearing is restored to normal. Yet patients have been known to purchase hearing aids to compensate for a loss that later turns out to be due only to a blocking of the external canal. The importance of seeing a physician when a hearing loss is noticed cannot be overemphasized. Also, the importance of having a physician remove excess cerumen or other objects in the canal should be stressed. The skin lining the external canal is very sensitive and easily scratched. Probing the canal with a hairpin or any other object can result in painful lacerations of the skin with the ensuing danger of infection, to say nothing of the danger of injuring the eardrum by too deep probing. An old saying which has a lot of sense is: "Don't stick anything in your ear smaller than your elbow!"

Occasionally babies are born with missing or rudimentary pinnae and occluded canals. This condition is referred to as *agenesis* of the pinna and *atresia* of the external auditory canal. Naturally, there is a conductive loss. The remedy depends upon the extent of functioning of the inner ears, and on whether or not the middle ear mechanism is intact. If middle and inner ears are normal, it is necessary for the surgeon only to open up the occluded canals for hearing to be made functional. More often than not, however, congenital atresia is accompanied by an anomaly of the middle ear as well. Frequently the drum and ossicles are missing entirely. In such cases, surgery may still be of benefit in opening up the canal so that sound waves can reach the oval and round windows. Any such operation would presuppose a normally functioning inner ear, however.

Conditions of the Middle Ear.

1. *Otitis media.* The most common cause of conductive impairment is an inflammation or infection of the middle ear known as *otitis media*. Almost

[1] James T. Graham and Hayes A. Newby, "Acoustical Characteristics of Tinnitus," *A.M.A. Archives of Otolaryngology*, Vol. 75 (February, 1962), p. 165.

everyone sometime in his life has had otitis media in some form. Frequently it accompanies an upper respiratory infection, particularly in children. The connection between the middle ear and the nasopharynx, the Eustachian tube, provides an easy pathway for infection or inflammation to reach the ear. The common "earache" in children is usually a manifestation of otitis media.

There are various types and forms of otitis media. A convenient classification is that of considering otitis media from the effect it has on the eardrum. One form of otitis media causes the drum to be distended, or forced outward, from pressure within the ear; the other form produces retraction, or forcing inward, of the drum owing to lack of sufficient pressure in the ear.

Distention of the drum is caused by the presence of fluid in the middle ear, usually as a result of inflammation or infection in the nasopharynx. The fluid may be clear and free of bacteria, or it may be pus. If the fluid is not pus, the condition is called a *nonsuppurative*, or *nonpurulent*, type of otitis media; the presence of pus in the middle ear is referred to as a *suppurative*, or *purulent*, otitis media. In either case, the presence of fluid in the middle ear produces pressure against the inside surface of the drum, which forces it outward, producing pain and usually causing some hearing loss due to decreased mobility of the drum and ossicles and to an increased vibratory mass in the middle ear. Without prompt medical intervention, the pressure behind the drum can quickly increase to the point where the drum is ruptured spontaneously and fluid is released into the outer canal.

Otitis media of the drum-distention type may originate from a head cold, from an allergic condition, from common upper respiratory infections such as measles or mumps, or from sinusitis. In any event, the beginning of the otitis media is inflammation of the orifice of the Eustachian tube. Improper nose-blowing forces mucus into the orifice of the Eustachian tube and invites an otitis media condition. When the nostrils are pressed together in blowing the nose, pressure is built up in the nasal passage which forces mucus into the orifice of the tube. The proper way of blowing the nose is to press lightly on each nostril with the fingers without pinching the nostrils together.

Sometimes an acute case of otitis media will become chronic. With recurring infections of the middle ear, permanent damage may be done to the hearing mechanism. The most severe damage is caused by adhesions forming on the ossicles or, in extreme cases, destruction of the ossicular chain from the infectious process. Repeated ruptures of the eardrum may produce perforations which will not heal. The amount of hearing loss sustained as a consequence of the perforations depends on how much of the drum membrane is left intact and on the location of the perforations. A small perforation will cause only a slight loss in hearing acuity. A perforation in the eardrum provides an opportunity for infection to reach the middle ear by way of the outer ear. Also, a marginal perforation of the drum may result in an ingrowth of skin, forming a pseudotumor called *cholesteatoma,* which invades the middle ear and mastoid spaces. A person with a perforated drum should exercise caution in exposing his ear to possible infection. It is inadvisable, for example, for the person to go swimming or at least to swim under water. It is possible to have ear plugs made which will give some protection from the water.

Active infection in the middle ear is dangerous not only to the hearing mechanism but to life itself. Since the middle ear is connected with the air cells in the mastoid process of the temporal bone, the infection can easily spread to the mastoid region. Until the 1940's *mastoiditis* was one of the most feared and deadly conditions to which children were susceptible. A *simple mastoidectomy* (entering the mastoid process from a postauricular incision and scraping out the infected tissue) was a common operation. Now, however, the so-called miracle drugs, the antibiotics, have practically eliminated the need for this operation.

The danger to life of mastoiditis is that infection in the temporal bone will find its way to the covering of the brain, the meninges, and cause meningitis. Chronic otitis media, therefore, must always be treated with respect, for it is a potential killer.

Retraction of the drum. The middle ear receives its ventilation and its oxygen through the Eustachian tube. The tube is the pressure-regulating device for the middle ear, enabling us to undergo changes in atmospheric pressure without suffering discomfort in the ears or loss of any hearing function. A *patent* tube (one capable of conducting air to or from the middle ear) is thus necessary for our comfort and for our acuity of hearing. Blockage of the Eustachian tube will lower the air pressure within the middle ear as the oxygen is absorbed by tissue, and retraction, or forcing inward of the drum membrane, will ensue owing to the unequal pressures on the two sides of the drum. Retraction of the drum interferes with its mobility and thus with its ability to vibrate in response to sound waves striking it. A hearing loss is the result.

Not infrequently, a consequence of otitis media of the drum-retracted type is fluid collecting in the middle ear. The lack of normal pressure in the middle ear forces serum to exude from the mucous membrane. The middle ear cavity may become partially or completely filled with this fluid. If the middle ear contains both air and fluid, the otologist can see through the drum membrane a fluid line or *meniscus,* but if the middle ear cavity is completely filled with fluid there is no meniscus, and it is difficult to tell by inspection alone whether or not the middle ear contains fluid. The presence of fluid in the middle ear when the drum is retracted is a condition referred to as *serous otitis media.*

Not infrequently a serous otitis media follows an acute bout of suppurative otitis media which is treated with antibiotics. The drugs eliminate the infection but the fluid, now sterile, remains in the middle ear cavity. If it is permitted to remain, it will gradually thicken and become glue-like or *mucoid* in consistency. The thicker the fluid becomes, the more the movement of the ossicular chain is hindered, and the greater the amount of hearing loss that results. In time, adhesions may form on the ossicles, damaging or destroying them. Such a condition is referred to as *adhesive otitis media*.

The most common causes for the malfunctioning of the Eustachian tube are the growth of lymphoid tissue, commonly referred to as adenoids, around the orifice of the tube in the nasopharynx, and allergic swelling of the tubal lining. The child who is an habitual "mouth-breather" is evidencing blockage of the nasopharynx owing to enlarged adenoids and/or allergy, and may very well have some hearing loss if the adenoid growth or swollen tissue prevents normal functioning of the Eustachian tube.

Inflammation and swelling of the tissues of the nasopharynx can also cause Eustachian tube malfunctioning. It is for this reason that it is inadvisable to fly when one has a cold. If the tube cannot enable the ear to accommodate to changes in outside pressure, the eardrum will be forced outward as the plane gains altitude and inward as the plane descends. So many flyers in World War II suffered from Eustachian tube malfunctioning that the name *aerotitis* was attached to the condition. Divers, who must work under conditions of increased atmospheric pressure, will also be subject to considerable pain and distress if their Eustachian tubes are not functioning properly. Sometimes the term *barotrauma* is used to refer to middle ear difficulties resulting from exposure to abnormal atmospheric pressure.

Usually the hearing loss produced by retracted drums is temporary, and as the Eustachian tube begins to function again the drums and the hearing return to normal. In the case of excess lymphoid tissue around the orifice of the tube, however, the condition can become chronic if the lymphoid tissue is not removed. Chronic otitis media of the retracted-drum type can produce a permanent hearing loss.

2. *Otosclerosis.* This is a disease process that affects the bony capsule of the inner ear, turning the normally hard bone into spongy bone. It produces a progressive hearing loss through the fixation, or *ankylosis,* of the stapes in the oval window, owing to the invasion of the spongy bone. Actually, otosclerosis is a misnomer for this condition, since "sclerosis" means "hardening." Some authorities have proposed the term *otospongiosis* as being more descriptive of the disease process. In any event, the disease called otosclerosis apparently is hereditary, and for some unknown reason it affects the Caucasian race primarily. Women are more susceptible to the disease than men. So far no one has been able to discover what causes it. Apparently many people are otosclerotics without being aware of it, since the disease does not necessarily occur at or around the oval window. According to Walsh, otosclerosis is responsible for about one million cases of hearing loss in the United States.[2]

A diagnosis of clinical otosclerosis is made when a hearing loss of a conductive type occurs in a relatively young person (late teens or early twenties, usually) and there is no other apparent explanation for the loss. In other

[2] T. E. Walsh, "The Surgical Treatment of Hearing Loss," in Hallowell Davis, ed., *Hearing and Deafness,* 1st ed. (New York, Rinehart, 1947), Chap. 5, p. 104.

words, the eardrum is normal in appearance, and there is no history of a middle ear type of disorder. Frequently there is a history of progressive hearing loss in the family, although not necessarily so, since several generations of the family may have had otosclerosis without an effect on their hearing. Occasionally otosclerosis will be diagnosed in a child, but generally it is a disease of early adulthood. The hearing loss may progress quite rapidly, so that noticeable changes in the degree of loss occur from year to year. Often a pregnancy is blamed for a marked, sudden drop in hearing acuity in an otosclerotic woman. Although usually otosclerosis produces a conductive type of loss, because of failure of transmission of vibrations to the fluid of the inner ear, occasionally the disease invades the inner ear and causes destruction of some nerve fibers. Even though, in its initial stages, the loss produced by otosclerosis may be a purely conductive one, it is quite common for the inner ear to become involved in later stages of the disease.

Otosclerosis is almost always accompanied by an annoying tinnitus. Frequently the tinnitus will be much more disturbing to the patient than the hearing loss which he has incurred.

Treatment

Fortunately, patients with conductive hearing losses have available to them medical and surgical treatment, which usually can improve the hearing and frequently restore it completely. The simplest type of hearing loss to remedy is, of course, that occasioned by the obstruction of cerumen or a foreign object in the external meatus. Removal of the wax or foreign matter is accomplished by means of instruments and/or irrigation. If there is no other causative factor operating, the removal of the obstruction will restore the hearing.

The treatment for otitis media of the drum-distended type is usually the administration of one or more of the antibiotic drugs, in order to control the infection in the ear as well as to remove the original source of infection. If there is any danger that the drum might spontaneously rupture, the physician will make an incision in the drum to allow the middle ear to drain. This operation is called a *myringotomy*. The advantage of having a myringotomy performed is that the surgical incision is made in the best place in the drum for drainage and for quick healing to occur, whereas a spontaneous rupture may occur anywhere on the drum and may be slow to heal, with the formation of scar tissue which can impede the vibration of the drum. Also, of course, a spontaneous rupture may destroy so much of the drum that a permanent perforation results.

In chronic otitis media with drainage through a perforation and possibly with the presence of cholesteatoma, there is always the danger that the infection or the growth will reach the covering of the brain and cause meningitis or other complications. Where this danger exists, it may be necessary as a preventive measure for the otologist to perform an operation on the middle ear. The operation of choice is a *modified radical mastoidectomy*, in which an attempt is made to clear up the disease process without sacrificing any of the middle ear structures. A successful modified radical mastoidectomy does not produce additional hearing loss and may even succeed in restoring some hearing function which has been lost as a result of the disease process. Occasionally it is not possible to clear up the disease process except by removing the eardrum, the malleus, and the incus, a procedure called a *radical mastoidectomy*. Naturally, a radical mastoidectomy produces a marked hearing loss in the operated ear by destroying the sound-conducting mechanism. The operation is not designed to improve the hearing but to remove a threat to life. If the inner ear apparatus is normal, even a patient who has had a bilateral radical mastoidectomy can receive considerable benefit from a hearing aid.

Spontaneous rupture of the eardrum may result in a patient's having a perforation that will not heal. As mentioned previously in this chapter, such perforations produce some hearing impairment, the degree depending on the size and location of the perforation. Perforated drums pose a constant potential hazard to the middle ear. Fortunately, techniques have evolved that are successful in many instances in eliminating the perforation and restoring the normal vibratory function of the drum. These procedures consist of inducing healing of the drum by irritating the edges of the perforation with acid, or placing a graft over the perforation. Sometimes a thin paper patch placed over the perforation will assist in the healing of the drum, especially when the patch is used in conjunction with acid treatment of the edges of the perforation. With a patch in place, the patient's hearing is improved, although the patch, or course, is only to assist the healing process and is not intended as a prosthesis. If healing will not occur as a result of repeated acid treatments, with or without the assistance of a patch, then the skin-grafting procedure, called a *myringoplasty*, may be performed. Most patients with eardrum perforations can be helped through one of these procedures for closing the perforation. When a perforation is closed, the hearing will usually be improved.

Today a great deal of otological surgery is devoted to the preservation or improvement of function in contrast to the pre-antibiotic times when most surgery was of the life-saving variety. Naturally, where a life was at stake, little attention was paid by surgeon or patient to the preservation of hearing. The myringoplasty is one of a class of reconstructive operations called *tympanoplasty*. All the tympanoplasty procedures have as their objective the restoration of hearing through repair or reconstruction of damaged parts of the middle ear. The principle followed in tympanoplasty is that there must be reciprocal action of the oval and round windows in order for maximum movement of the cochlear fluids to occur. In the normal ear, the eardrum and ossicular chain provide a magnification of sound pressure at the oval window that is greatly in excess of any pressure exerted through the middle ear cavity on the round window. Moreover, energy that reaches the round window from the eardrum is transmitted through the air in the middle ear cavity and is in opposite phase to the vibrations reaching the oval window through the ossicular chain. If the mechanical advantage of the oval window is reduced or eliminated through an interruption in the ossicular chain, or if the phase difference between the two windows is altered because of a large perforation in the eardrum, a hearing loss results. The tympanoplasty seeks to restore the mechanical advantage of the oval window and the reciprocal action of the two windows to permit maximum fluid motion in the cochlea. According to Shambaugh, "The ideal tympanoplasty restores sound protection for the round window by constructing a closed, air-containing middle ear against the round window membrane, and restores sound pressure transformation for the oval window by connecting a large tympanic membrane or substitute membrane with the stapes footplate either via an intact ossicular chain, or the stapes alone or a substitute stapes."[3]

Treatment of otitis media of the drum-retracted type is directed toward restoring the patency of the Eustachian tubes. If the tubes have been blocked because of edematous tissue in the nasopharynx, treatment will be directed toward controlling the condition which has produced the swelling of the nasal tissue. Even after the swelling in the nasal passages has been controlled, the tube will not regain patency immediately. Frequently it will require from a week to ten days before the tube regains its normal function and the drum returns to its normal position. In the meantime, of course, any hearing loss which has been caused by the retraction of the drum will persist. The otolaryngologist may assist the tube to regain its function by means of a technique called *inflation*. Usually, in inflation the physician inserts a catheter through the nostril until its tip makes contact with the orifice of the Eustachian tube; he then forces a small amount of air through the tube into the middle ear. The air forced into the middle ear restores normal air pressure in the middle ear which permits the drum to move from its position of retraction to its normal position. There is an immediate improvement in hearing noted by the patient. Unless the Eustachian tube retains patency, however, the oxygen will soon be absorbed from the air in the middle ear, and the drum will retract again. The process of inflation may speed up the recovery of the proper functioning of the tube, however. This is a technique which should be applied sparingly, as too frequent resort to inflation may cause the eardrum to become "floppy" and lose its normal resilience. Inflation should not be employed when there is a danger of spreading infection from the nasopharynx to the middle ear.

When the drum retraction is due to the presence of excess lymphoid tissue around the orifice of the Eustachian tube in the nasopharynx. the only remedy

[3] George E. Shambaugh, Jr., *Surgery of the Ear* (Philadelphia, W. B. Saunders, 1967), p. 451.

is to remove the tissue through surgery and/or irradiation. If the tissue is profuse, an adenoidectomy is indicated. It may not be possible to remove all the tissue surgically, however, without risking the growth of scar tissue around the orifice of the tube, and this would defeat the purpose of the operation. In such cases, the offending lymphoid tissue may be eliminated by the careful use of radiation, applied usually by X ray but sometimes by direct application of a radium capsule. Because of the danger of damaging healthy tissue, however, the use of radiation in the elimination of adenoid tissue is rarely recommended.

The treatment for serous otitis media is aimed at removing the fluid in the middle ear. Usually a myringotomy will suffice, but on occasion it may be necessary to employ suction, particularly if the fluid in the middle ear has thickened, or to insert tubing through the myringotomy incision to provide continual drainage. Sometimes a myringotomy combined with inflation will serve to evacuate the fluid from the middle ear.

Surgery for otosclerosis has posed a challenge of great interest to otologists since the latter part of the nineteenth century. The first attempts at improving hearing in cases of otosclerosis were directed at mobilizing the fixated stapes. In 1890 Miot reported on a series of 200 stapes mobilization procedures which were performed in a manner similar to the technique described by Rosen in the 1950's.[4] Stapes mobilization consists of laying back the eardrum and manipulating the ossicular chain with an instrument usually at the point of the incudo-stapedial joint, until the stapes is broken free of the otosclerotic growth that surrounds it. For reasons that are not clear, the stapes mobilization operation was abandoned around the turn of the twentieth century. Shambaugh speculates that the operation may have resulted in some serious infections of the middle ear and the labyrinth that discouraged otologists from attempting operations on the ear.[5]

Also late in the nineteenth century there were some attempts to correct hearing impairment due to otosclerosis by bypassing the fixated stapes and creating a new window (*fenestra*) in the wall of the labyrinth. Early in the twentieth century, the first *fenestration* operation on the horizontal semicircular canal was performed. Gunnar Holmgren in Sweden pioneered in fenestration surgery and was the first to employ the operating microscope in ear surgery. He experienced difficulty in keeping the labyrinthine window free from bony closure, but he inspired others, notably Sourdille of France, to experiment with techniques of fenestration that finally succeeded in maintaining a mobile window. Sourdille, in the 1920's and 1930's, performed many successful fenestration operations through an operative procedure involving two or more stages. In this country, Julius Lempert, in the late 1930's and the 1940's perfected a one-stage fenestration operation that became very popular. Otologists from all over the world flocked to New York to receive instruction

[4] *Ibid.*, p. 502
[5] *Ibid.*, p. 503

in the revolutionary new technique of otological surgery that was to restore the hearing of thousands of otosclerotics to useful levels.

Briefly, the operation consists of making an endaural approach (through the external canal) to the middle ear cavity, laying aside the eardrum, and removing the head of the malleus and the incus. The middle ear cavity is enlarged so that the horizontal semicircular canal can be exposed. The surgeon then creates a window (fenestra) in the horizontal semicircular canal and covers this window with the skin flap he has cut loose in laying aside the eardrum. The purpose of the operation is to bypass the oval window which has been made inoperative through the fixation of the stapes, and to provide a new window through which sound vibrations can reach the inner ear. Since the perilymph of the semicircular canals is continuous with the peri-lymph of the cochlea, movement of the fluid in the horizontal canal will be transmitted to the end-organ of hearing. For the operation to be successful, it is necessary that the round window membrane be mobile, as two windows are essential for the transmission of sound through the incompressible fluid of the inner ear.

The fenestration operation cannot restore a patient's hearing to normal, because in the course of the operation the ossicular chain, an important part of the sound-conducting mechanism, has been broken by the elimination of the malleus and incus. Experience has shown that the maximum result obtain-able through the fenestration operation is restoration of the hearing to within 20 to 30 dB of normal. This is not to say that the operation is undesirable, however, since a residual loss of only 20 to 30 dB will seem almost like normal hearing to a patient whose preoperative loss may have been as great as 70 dB.

In 1952, while testing the mobility of the ossicular chain in a patient whom he was considering as a candidate for fenestration, Samuel Rosen, a New York otologist, "accidentally" performed a stapes mobilization that resulted in a sudden, dramatic improvement in the patient's hearing. The following year Rosen reported on the results of a number of operations in which he was successful at purposely mobilizing the stapes. Rosen's experience of "redis-covering" the principle of improving the hearing in otosclerotics by restoring the mobility of the ossicular chain resulted in a swing away from the fene-stration operation on the part of most otologists. The stapes mobilization was a simpler operation from the standpoint of the patient, and when successful it could restore hearing to normal or close to normal levels, while the fenestration operation, even at its best, left the patient with a residual hearing deficit of about 20 dB. The chances for a "successful" operative result from the fenestration procedure, however, were about eight in ten as com-pared with about five in ten for the stapes mobilization.

In 1956 a new technique of surgery for otosclerosis was reported by John Shea of Nashville, Tennessee. This technique, called *stapedectomy*, consisted in completely removing the stapes. A vein graft was used to close the oval window, and a polyethylene "strut" was inserted between the lenticular process of the incus and the vein graft. Other otologists followed Shea's lead in removing the stapes and creating a prosthetic link between the incus and the oval window, and at the present writing the stapedectomy procedure is the operation of choice for restoring hearing in cases of otosclerosis. Some otologists use a steel wire or Teflon tube in place of the polyethylene strut, and fatty tissue (from the ear lobe) or gelfoam in the oval window in place of a vein graft, but the principle of the operation is the same: the stapes in its entirety is removed and a substitute "ossicle" is inserted in its place, connecting the incus with the oval window which has been closed by means of transplanted tissue. An excellent non-technical description of the stapedectomy operation is given by Schuknecht.[6] Most surgeons perform the operation under local anesthesia. A binocular microscope provides excellent visualization of the middle ear through the ear canal, once the eardrum has been incised and elevated. It may be necessary to remove some bone from around the ear canal in order to bring the stapes into view. The stapes is removed with appropriate instruments, and the prosthesis is put in place, after which the eardrum is replaced and held in position by packing. The patient frequently will experience a dramatic improvement in his hearing while on the operating table. Later, there may be a decline in hearing until healing has taken place, a process that requires from one to two weeks. A month following the operation the hearing should be at its maximum, although there may be some slight additional gain in hearing noticed through the next six months.

As in the case of stapes mobilization, the stapedectomy procedure is, for the patient, a minor operation compared with the fenestration. The patient usually leaves the hospital the day after the operation, and rarely is there any complication such as a persistent dizziness. In contrast, the patient who has a fenestration operation must spend up to two weeks in the hospital, the operation must be performed under general anesthesia, and frequently the patient will experience severe dizziness for weeks or months following the operation. Moreover, the fenestration operation permanently alters the anatomy of the ear and imposes limitations on the patient, such as inability to go swimming, whereas stapedectomy provides a minimum of modification of the ear's anatomy, and the patient is not limited in his activities following the operation.

As is true also with stapes mobilization, the potential improvement in hearing is much greater with the stapedectomy procedure than with fenestration. If the operation is completely successful the entire conductive block can be eliminated. The operation is considered to be successful if air-conduction hearing can be restored to within 10 dB of bone-conduction hearing. According to Schuknecht, excellent results are obtained in over 90 per cent of "carefully done" stapedectomy operations which exceeds

6 Harold F. Schuknecht, "Stapedectomy Operation for Hearing Loss from Otosclerosis," *Sound,* Vol. 1 (July–August, 1962), pp. 16-21.

the percentage of success achieved with fenestration. Many patients, having experienced greatly improved hearing in the operated ear, will want the other ear operated also. If the hearing in the operated ear remains good for from six months to a year there is no reason for not operating on the other ear. To date there have been very few complications resulting from reactions to the plastic strut or the steel wire. The operation has a low rate of failure; in only two per cent of stapedectomies is there a greater loss following the operation. Ninety-five per cent of the patients who have been periodically checked have maintained their improved hearing over a three- to five-year period.[7]

None of these operations can succeed in restoring hearing that has been lost as a result of inner ear pathology; they are successful only in removing the block in the sound-conducting system. It is important, therefore, to evaluate as precisely as possible the function of the inner ear in selecting candidates for these operations. The audiologist can be of great assistance to the otologist in the selection of patients who may be expected to receive reasonable benefit from one of these operations, as we shall see in a subsequent chapter.

SENSORI-NEURAL IMPAIRMENTS

When the loss of hearing function is due to pathology in the inner ear, or along the nerve pathway from the inner ear to the brain stem, the loss is referred to as a sensori-neural impairment (also written *sensorineural* or *sensory-neural*). In this book the word has been spelled "sensori-neural" in accordance with a resolution adopted by the Committee on the Conservation of Hearing of the American Academy of Opthalmology and Otolaryngology and reported in a letter to the editor of the *Transactions of the Academy*. The resolution states:

Since the endorgan precedes the nerve functionally, this should be stressed by placing sensori before neural when speaking of hearing loss. The first part of the word should be written "sensori" instead of "sensory" because sensory is a complete word whereas sensori is not. Therefore, employment of the latter spelling tends to imply more positively that while some lesions are purely sensory and others are purely neural, a substantial fraction are probably composite. This is an important possibility to keep in mind pending the day when we can positively separate cochlear lesions from neural lesions, and these from true sensory-neural composites.

The second part of the word should be written "neural" with a hyphen separating sensori from neural. The inclusion of the hyphen helps remind us that the term is really a wastebasket term, covering some cases with pure sense organ lesions, some with pure nerve fiber lesions, and some which are composites of the two. Omission of the hyphen would tend to imply that most lesions are composite.[8]

[7] *Ibid.*, p.21.
[8] Henry L. Williams, Letter to the Editor, *Transactions of the American Academy of Ophthalmology and Otolaryngology*, Vol. 67 (March–April, 1963), p. 225.

Formerly the terms *perceptive impairment* and *nerve loss* were used in place of what we now call sensori-neural impairment. A "pure" sensori-neural impairment exists when the sound-conducting mechanism, that is, the outer and middle ear, is normal in every respect. In other words, sound is conducted properly to the fluid of the inner ear, but it cannot be analyzed or perceived normally. For purposes of analogy, the hearing mechanism can be likened to a television set, the amplifier being the middle ear, and the picture tube the inner ear. For perfect functioning, both the amplifier and picture tube must be operative. In a conductive loss it is the amplifier which is defective—it does not permit a normal signal to reach the picture tube, and naturally a normal picture or image cannot be obtained. In a sensori-neural loss, the difficulty is with the picture tube; the amplifier does a perfect job of conducting the signal to the tube, but a normal picture does not result because of the defective picture tube.

Symptoms

Just as there were certain generalizations that could be made about patients with conductive losses, so we can generalize to some extent about the symptoms exhibited by patients with sensori-neural losses. The patient with a sensori-neural impairment may speak with excessive loudness of voice in many situations where a loud voice is inappropriate. The reason is that, as we have seen, we hear our own voices to some degree through the mechanism of bone conduction. The patient with a sensori-neural loss does not have normal hearing by bone conduction, since the source of his difficulty is in the inner ear or nerve. Hence, he does not hear either his own voice or others' voices normally, and in order to achieve what to him appears to be adequate loudness he may have to talk more loudly than is necessary for others to hear him in comfort. The "shouting" type of hard-of-hearing person, therefore, is exhibiting one symptom of a sensori-neural loss. Although we may make generalizations concerning the relationship of a patient's voice level and the type of impairment he exhibits, it should be realized, of course, that individuals with sensori-neural problems do not always speak in a loud voice, nor are people with conductive losses always difficult to hear. Many patients learn to regulate their voice levels appropriately, probably because of their sensitivity to the reactions of their listeners, acquired over a long period of time.

Generally, although not always, a sensori-neural impairment causes some difficulty in speech discrimination, even at levels of loudness that are well above threshold. Although a sensori-neural loss may be severe or profound at all frequencies, the typical sensori-neural loss is characterized by better hearing for the lower frequencies than for the high frequencies. In fact, many people with sensori-neural losses may have normal or close-to-normal hearing through 500 or even 1000 Hz and then drop off rapidly on the audiogram at higher frequencies. Such people have no difficulty in hearing voices at normal intensities, since their low-frequency hearing is unimpaired. Many consonants of the English language are characterized by high frequencies and weak intensities (such as *f*, *k*, and *s*, for example). Thus a sensori-neural impairment that affects chiefly the high frequencies would result in the inability of the patient to differentiate among many words which would sound similar but contain different high-frequency consonants. For example, this patient might confuse the words *fake*, *cake*, and *sake* on the basis of hearing alone, because he does not hear the initial or final consonant sound in any of the words. A patient with sensori-neural impairment might hear all these words as *a*, that is, he would hear only the vowel sound. Because such a patient hears low frequencies well and high frequencies poorly, his is what might be termed a "confusion" deafness. He has no difficulty in hearing voices, since his low frequency hearing is good, but he does experience trouble in understanding what is said to him, because of his inability to hear many consonants. It is useless to shout at such a patient, since he can hear voices easily and he would react to shouting as would a person with normal hearing. His difficulty is in understanding, and shouting will not help, in fact it may hinder, his understanding. In speaking to a patient with sensori-neural impairment it is important to enunciate clearly and not to speak too rapidly. One should not exaggerate the sounds of speech but simply speak carefully and clearly. Many older patients with high-frequency-type sensori-neural losses complain that the present generation does not speak as carefully and precisely as people did when they were young. Although this may be true, it is probable that the difference is not in how people speak now and how they spoke then, but rather in how well the patient's hearing functioned in the past compared with its present functioning.

The negative reaction of patients with sensori-neural impairment to shouting is related to another characteristic of sensori-neural loss, at least of sensori-neural loss due to malfunctioning of the inner ear. This is the rapid increase of the sensation of loudness once the patient's threshold of hearing has been crossed. As we have seen previously, a conductive impairment acts to reduce the intensity of all sounds reaching the inner ear by the same amount, regardless of the strength of the sound wave (that is, up to the point of its reaching the patient's threshold of discomfort). The situation with some patients who have sensori-neural impairment is different; once a sound is intense enough to be perceived, an increase in intensity causes a disproportionate increase in the sensation of loudness. Thus such a patient, with a loss of 40 dB, can just barely detect the presence of a sound with an intensity of 40 dB above the normal threshold but may hear a sound of 45 dB intensity with a loudness greater than a normal-hearing person would hear a sound of 5 dB. Further increases in the intensity of the stimulus would result in more rapid increases in the patient's sensation of loudness, so that he might perceive a sound of 60 dB intensity above the normal threshold with the same loudness as a normal ear would perceive a sound of that intensity. Thus, over a range of 20 dB in intensity of the stimulus, in this example, the patient's loudness perception has increased as much as the normal ear's in going from zero to 60 dB. This rapid increase in the sensation of loudness once threshold has been reached is referred to as *recruitment,* or the *recruitment factor,* sometimes abbreviated as RF. Recruitment of loudness is thought to be characteristic of sensori-neural impairment due to cochlear involvement. According to some clinicians, recruitment does not exist in cases of sensori-neural impairment resulting from lesions of the VIIIth nerve.[9] Because of recruitment, and because of the speech-sound discrimination difficulty associated with this type of sensori-neural impairment, these patients do not hear well in noisy surroundings, in contrast to patients with conductive impairment.

Figure 3-1 illustrates the growth of loudness with increasing intensity in the normal ear, in the non-recruiting impaired ear, in recruiting ears, and in an ear that exhibits the opposite of recruitment—*decruitment.* In both the normal and the non-recruiting impaired ears, the growth of loudness is proportional to the increase of intensity. In the recruiting ears, the sensation

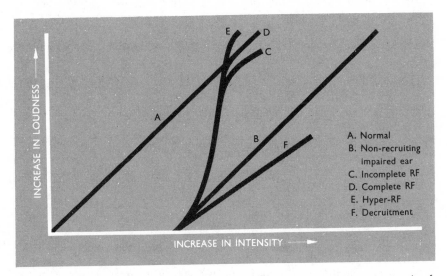

A. Normal
B. Non-recruiting impaired ear
C. Incomplete RF
D. Complete RF
E. Hyper-RF
F. Decruitment

Figure 3-1. Three degrees of loudness recruitment compared with the growth of loudness in the normal ear and in the non-recruiting impaired ear.

[9]L. G. Eby and H. L. Williams, "Recruitment of Loudness in the Differential Diagnosis of End-Organ and Nerve Fiber Deafness," *Laryngoscope,* Vol. 61 (1951), pp. 400-414.

M. R. Dix, C. S. Hallpike, and J. D. Hood, "Observations upon the Loudness Recruitment Phenomenon with Especial Reference to the Differential Diagnosis of Disorders of the Internal Ear and VIIIth Nerve," *Journal of Laryngology and Otology,* Vol. 62 (November, 1948), pp. 671-686.

of loudness increases out of proportion with increases in intensity. Three degrees of recruitment are illustrated in Figure 3-1. Complete recruitment consists of the impaired ear's catching up with the normal ear's sensation of loudness at some intensity above the impaired ear's threshold. In incomplete recruitment, the impaired ear's sensation of loudness increases disproportionately but never reaches the level of the normal ear's sensation of loudness. And hyper-recruitment occurs when a given intensity evokes a sensation of loudness that exceeds a normal ear's sensation of loudness for that intensity of the stimulus. Decruitment refers to a disproportionately slow increase in loudness with increasing intensity. It has been reported in association with a neural or *retrocochlear* impairment in contrast with recruitment, which is associated with a cochlear type of sensori-neural impairment. Tests for determining the presence and degree of recruitment will be described in Chapter 7.

Sensori-neural impairment may be accompanied by a distortion in the sensation of pitch called *diplacusis*. In binaural diplacusis, the two ears respond to a given frequency in different ways. There may be simply a noticeable pitch difference between the ears, or one ear may perceive a pure tone normally, while the other perceives it as noise or something other than a pure tone. If a single stimulus produces two different sensations in the same ear, we call it monaural diplacusis.

The patient with sensori-neural impairment is usually subject to tinnitus of a somewhat different sort from that associated with conductive impairment. Generally, the patient with sensori-neural impairment reports a constant "ringing" or "buzzing" noise, which may be localized in either ear or may not be localized. In the experimental study of tinnitus referred to previously, it was found that patients with sensori-neural impairment matched their tinnitus to pure tones covering a wide frequency range, from 155–7800 Hz[10]. In general, the pitch of tinnitus tends to be higher in sensori-neural impairment than in conductive impairment. Patients have reported getting up in the night to answer the telephone or the doorbell, only to find that the noise was "in their heads."

Etiology

Most babies born with impaired hearing have sensori-neural impairments, with the principal exception of congenital atresia, referred to above in the section on conductive impairments. Sensori-neural impairments may also be acquired at any time during life.

Congenital Causes. Some cases of congenital sensori-neural loss may be ascribed to heredity, a defect in the genes. Not much is known about the causes of hereditary deafness. It has been observed, however, that where both parents are congenitally deaf for unexplained reasons, they are likely to have

[10]Graham and Newby, *op. cit.*

children with congenital deafness. This is one important reason against segregating the deaf educationally, since the segregation tends to perpetuate and multiply hereditary deafness. Occasionally deaf infants will be born to parents whose hearing is normal and whose pedigrees disclose no instances of deafness. In such cases it can only be presumed that each parent carried a mutant gene for deafness, or that the infant's hearing was damaged in the course of the pregnancy. When more than one deaf child is born to normal-hearing parents, however, the chances are high that the deafness is on an hereditary basis.

Many times congenital deafness can be explained in terms of damage to the embryo *in utero*. It is known, for example, that when the mother incurs certain diseases in pregnancy, usually but not always during the first three months of pregnancy, the embryo is subject to injury of various sorts, including impairment of the hearing. German measles (rubella) is one of the most insidious diseases in its effects on the embryo. It may produce such anomalies, singly or in combination, as deafness or some lesser degree of hearing impairment, blindness, heart defects, cerebral palsy, and mental deficiency. Other diseases incurred by the mother during pregnancy may have harmful effects on the embryo or fetus—influenza, for example—but more is known about the effect of rubella than is known about the effect of any other disease.

Acquired Causes. Sensori-neural impairments may be acquired at any time during life. The causative agent may be disease, injury, toxic effect of drugs, or simply the inexorable process of growing older. By far the most common cause of sensori-neural hearing impairment is the aging process. As the human organism grows older, sensory processes tend to deteriorate. In hearing, sensitivity for higher frequencies gradually diminishes with increasing years. The study of large samples of the population demonstrates that the process starts at about the age of twenty and becomes increasingly noticeable with each succeeding decade. This progressive loss of hearing owing to increasing age is called *presbycusis*. With medical science extending man's life span more and more, problems of hearing loss due to presbycusis are increasing. Not all old people are hard-of-hearing, but the curves based on surveys of thousands of people show the mean hearing loss increasing and extending into lower frequencies with each succeeding decade of life after age twenty. Surveys differ in the mean or median hearing-level values reported for various ages because of differences in sampling, differences in the age groupings reported, and perhaps also differences in test environment and testing techniques. Table 3–1 presents information from one study of hearing levels (audiometric levels) of a select sample of male and female ears of various ages. Females tend to have better hearing than males except at frequencies below 1000 Hz in the older age groups. Recently, as we shall see in Chapter 9, evidence has been presented that in populations protected from

Table 3-1. Median hearing levels by age groups and sex of both ears of selected subjects (N = 1247) "who passed the rigid screening criteria related to otological disorders and extent of noise exposure." These hearing levels in dB re ISO-1964 audiometric zero were computed from sound pressure levels presented by John F. Corso, "Age and Sex Differences in Pure-Tone Thresholds," *A.M.A. Archives of Otolaryngology,* Vol 77 (April, 1963), pp. 398-399.

		Frequencies in Hz								
Age	Sex	250	500	1000	1500	2000	3000	4000	6000	8000
18–24	M	1.3	0.2	–0.5	0.1	–1.8	3.8	2.0	20.8	13.5
	F	–0.3	–1.0	–0.2	–0.8	–3.7	–0.2	0.7	13.0	8.3
26–32	M	0.5	0.9	0.2	–0.5	–1.5	4.2	4.1	26.0	20.5
	F	0.2	0.9	–0.3	0.4	–1.2	–0.8	–0.6	13.7	12.1
34–40	M	–1.3	0.1	0.4	0.5	–0.1	5.8	10.4	27.4	24.8
	F	0.0	0.0	–0.3	0.9	–0.2	0.7	2.6	17.5	16.5
43–49	M	–0.7	3.4	–1.0	8.0	5.5	17.6	23.0	37.5	26.5
	F	–0.3	2.1	–0.6	4.8	2.9	3.8	6.8	25.4	16.3
51–57	M	2.0	3.9	4.4	5.1	6.1	16.9	17.8	33.7	32.5
	F	4.5	5.8	6.2	6.0	9.0	10.8	12.7	27.2	24.5
59–65	M	8.1	5.9	7.1	10.3	14.4	28.6	39.8	52.3	47.7
	F	10.4	8.0	5.3	8.1	9.2	13.2	16.9	34.5	32.3

the noises and other stresses of modern civilization the effects on the hearing that can be attributed to aging per se may be rather negligible. It is difficult if not impossible to separate the long-term effects on hearing of our exposure to modern civilization from the effects of the aging process. The hearing levels reported in Table 3–1 should represent reasonably good estimates of the effects of aging on male and female ears in our culture, since individuals with known otological problems or history of exposure to noise were excluded from the sample. While presbycusis is listed here as a sensori-neural impairment, there is evidence that aging also affects the structures in the middle ear. The very elderly may have a substantial conductive component of their presbycusis.[11]

The diseases that may cause sensori-neural hearing impairment include measles, mumps, scarlet fever, diphtheria, whooping cough, influenza, and any of the unnamed virus infections. Such diseases may also cause conductive impairments through otitis media originating in an infection of the nasal passages. When these diseases produce a sensori-neural impairment, it is due to the toxic effect of the disease process on the sensitive nerve endings in the cochlea. Infections of the cerebrospinal fluid, such as occur in cases of meningitis, also cause sensori-neural impairments from cochlear damage. Tumorous growths in the region of the pathway of the VIIIth nerve between the cochlea and the brain stem may cause sensori-neural loss through pressure exerted on the nerve trunk. The most common tumor is an *acoustic neurinoma,* which apparently originates in the cells of the sheath of Schwann covering

[11] Hallowell Davis, "Abnormal Hearing and Deafness," in Hallowell Davis and S. Richard Silverman, eds., *Hearing and Deafness* (New York, Holt, Rinehart and Winston, 1970), pp. 110-112.

the VIIIth nerve. Typically the tumor grows within the internal acoustic meatus, compressing both the VIIth (facial) and VIIIth nerves. As the tumor expands other cranial nerves may be affected. While cases of bilateral acoustic nerve tumors have been reported, typically only one side is affected and the hearing impairment and tinnitus that usually are the first symptoms of the tumor are unilateral.

Special mention should be made of *Ménière's disease or syndrome* as a cause of sensori-neural impairment, as this is a condition confined to the inner ear. The symptoms of Ménière's disease are a combination of tinnitus, vertigo (dizziness), and hearing loss. The immediate cause of these symptoms is apparently an increased fluid pressure within the membranous labyrinth, so that Ménière's disease is also referred to as *endolymphatic hydrops*. The cause of the increased fluid pressure is not known, but it is thought to be related to vascular changes in the inner ear which in turn may be caused by allergy. Ménière's disease usually consists of "attacks" of vertigo, accompanied by nausea, and of tinnitus and deafness which temporarily are quite severe, followed by periods of remission of symptoms. In extreme cases, the patient may be incapacitated for weeks at a time. The hearing loss fluctuates with the other symptoms, although a certain amount of permanent damage apparently occurs when the attack lasts more than a few days. The patient with Ménière's typically is affected primarily in one ear, and the hearing loss in this ear is characterized by severe recruitment. In fact, the affected ear generally builds up loudness so rapidly once threshold is reached that the sensation of loudness in that ear exceeds the sensation of loudness in the better ear for a stimulus of fixed intensity or, in other words, the affected ear exhibits "hyper-recruitment." The serious student of audiology will want to pursue the study of Ménière's disease in detail , as this is a condition affecting hearing in which the audiologist plays a particularly important role in assisting the otologist in a diagnosis. The various otological journals contain a wealth of information in reports of research and clinical experience, and entire books have been devoted to a discussion of Ménière's disease.[12]

Related to Ménière's disease in its symptomatology is sudden, severe hearing loss in which the patient overnight may lose almost all the hearing in one or both ears. Tinnitus is almost always present and there may or may not be an accompanying vertigo. Such sudden losses are thought to be due to an interruption of the blood supply to the cochlea, probably a spasm of the cochlear artery. If the condition persists more than a few hours, the cochlea suffers irreparable damage and the hearing loss becomes permanent.

Although it is rare in occurrence, sensori-neural loss due to mechanical injury of the inner ear is possible. Thus, in the case of a fracture of the temporal bone, the inner ear may be damaged, producing a sensori-neural hearing impairment on that side. Automobile accidents and wartime injuries

[12]Henry L. Williams, *Ménière's Disease* (Springfield, Ill., Charles C Thomas, 1952).

contribute their bit to producing sensori-neural impairments of this character.

Trauma of a different sort is responsible for the occurrence of many cases of sensori-neural impairment. Exposure to intense noise can cause permanent damage to the hair cells in the cochlea. Actually, the term *acoustic trauma* is reserved for cases of damage to cochlear structures—and frequently also to middle-ear structures—resulting from a single exposure to a very intense noise, such as a blast or explosion. Much more common is the gradual, progressive loss of sensitivity resulting from years of exposure to noxious levels of sound, called *noise-induced hearing impairment*. People differ considerably in their ability to withstand intense noise. Our modern industrial civilization is a noisy one. In many vocations, noise-induced hearing loss is an accepted occupational hazard. "Boilermaker's ear" is a time-honored syndrome among otologists. Because of the intense noise in a boiler factory, it was taken for granted that sooner or later all the workers in such a vocation would develop some sensori-neural loss. In modern times, there are many occupations in which the worker is subject to an extremely noisy environment, and the whole question of industrial compensation for hearing loss is receiving concentrated attention from employers, labor organizations, and the legal and medical professions.

Military service, with its attendant exposure to noises of great intensity, is responsible for producing many cases of sensori-neural hearing impairment. People with delicate ears, that is, ears that are easily susceptible to damage from noise, may incur permanent damage to their hearing from even brief exposures to gunfire or to aircraft-engine noise. Now that we are in the jet and rocket age, the problems of noise-induced hearing loss in military and civil aviation are rapidly multiplying. The entire matter of the effect of noise on hearing is justifiably receiving the attention of various experts, so that (1) methods of reducing or controlling the noise may be discovered, (2) ways to protect the worker's ears effectively from the noise may be found, and (3) techniques of discovering which individuals are most susceptible to loss of hearing from noise exposure may be devised and utilized in order to govern the proper placement of workers in industry or in the military service. Chapter 9 covers in detail the problems of industrial noise control and noise-induced hearing impairment.

Typically, noise exposure causes reduction in sensitivity for the higher frequencies first, presumably because the basal end of the basilar membrane is stimulated by traveling waves of all frequencies and thus receives more "wear and tear" than the more apical parts of the cochlea. The region of the basilar membrane corresponding to frequencies of 3000 to 6000 Hz seems to be the most susceptible to injury from noise exposure. In fact, it is so common to see audiograms showing the greatest amount of impairment in this area that a "4000-Hz dip" is taken to be an indication of damage through exposure to noise (see Figure 5-9, Chapter 5). Although the point of greatest impairment may be localized at or around the 4000-Hz level, loss due to noise exposure will extend below and above this point, if the person with noise-susceptible ears incurs exposures to noise over a period of years. Most noise-induced hearing impairment results from continued exposure to wide-band noise of high intensity. When the noxious stimulus is a pure tone, or a narrow-band noise approaching a pure tone, the greatest loss will usually be found for frequencies that are from a half-octave to an octave higher than the frequency of the stimulus. Ward explains the susceptibility of the ear to impairment in the region of 4000 Hz on the basis that the ear is most sensitive to the frequencies from 1000 to 4000 Hz. The aural reflex (stapedius reflex) reduces the intensity of stimuli below 2000 Hz but not of stimuli above 2000 Hz. Therefore, stimuli between 2000 and 4000 Hz reach the cochlea at full strength, and the maximum loss of sensitivity occurs from a half-octave to an octave higher than the frequency of the stimulus.[13]

Brief exposures to intense noise can produce a temporary hearing loss or threshold shift, and after a period of rest the ear will regain its former sensitivity. We have all experienced temporary threshold shift. A good example is the decrease of auditory sensitivity for several hours after completing a flight in a noisy airplane. The effect of exposure to noise is cumulative, however. If we were to fly in this noisy plane every day, we would find that our hearing would not recover completely after each flight, or in other words that we were acquiring a permanent hearing loss. It is not uncommon to find veteran airline pilots whose hearing is markedly diminished as the result of the accumulation of their many years of exposure to the noise of aircraft engines. Pilots whose experience is exclusively with jet aircraft may fare better, because their craft travel so fast that the engine noise is largely left behind. The ground crew around jet aircraft are more likely to incur noise-induced hearing impairment.

Just as ears differ in their susceptibility to damage through exposure to noise, so also do they differ in their reaction to drugs that may have a toxic effect on the inner ear. In the past, quinine was responsible for producing sensori-neural impairment, as it was a popular agent in the treatment of malaria and even the common cold. With the control of malaria, and the development of other drugs for treating malaria, quinine is no longer extensively used. Today the drugs that are chiefly responsible for causing sensori-neural hearing loss are *streptomycin*, or, more properly, *dihydro-streptomycin*, which has a toxic effect on the cochlea, *neomycin*, and *kanamycin*. Generally, the effect of these drugs on the hearing is profound, although their effect is of course related to the dosage. Since physicians are well aware of the danger to the hearing from these drugs, large doses are prescribed only when urgent as a life-saving measure. When the saving of life is involved, sacrifice of the hearing assumes a secondary importance.

[13]W. Dixon Ward, "Adaptation and Fatigue," in A. Bruce Graham, ed., *Sensorineural Hearing Processes and Disorders* (Boston, Little, Brown, 1967), p. 117; "Effects of Noise on Hearing Thresholds," in W. Dixon Ward and James E. Fricke, eds., *Noise as a Public Health Hazard* (Washington, The American Speech and Hearing Association, 1969), p. 44.

Treatment

In contrast to conductive impairments, which are frequently susceptible to medical or surgical treatment, sensori-neural hearing loss generally cannot be helped through treatment, with the exception of the loss due to Ménière's disease and sudden, severe deafness due to an interruption of the blood supply to the cochlea. In the special case of Ménière's, the hearing loss, as well as the other symptoms, is subject to remissions. In the case of sudden, severe hearing loss, the prompt administration of a vasodilator, perhaps in combination with an anticoagulant, will sometimes result in a dramatic restoration of hearing. From time to time there have been reports in the literature concerning the beneficial effects of vitamin therapy in improving the hearing, but the consensus of medical opinion is that sensori-neural impairment is irreversible. Once the nerve fibers in the cochlea or in the VIIIth nerve are destroyed, there is no regeneration, and since the cochlear portion of the VIIIth nerve is specific to the sensation of hearing, no other pathway for sound is possible.

Thus medical care of patients with sensori-neural impairment (with the exception of Ménière's disease and vascular disturbances, of course) is limited to the prevention of further loss. If the causative factor of the loss is noise exposure, the physician can only advise that the patient try in the future to avoid exposure to noise or protect his ears with "ear defenders" or with muffs. Probably the physician will also advise the patient to beware of promiscuous drug usage, since ears that are susceptible to damage from noise may also be easily affected by drug intake. About the only other tack that the physician can take with patients who have sensori-neural impairments is to advise proper nutrition, rest, and personal hygiene, so that the patient's general resistance will be at an optimum level.

In the case of sensori-neural loss due to Ménière's disease, various treatments are feasible. The hearing loss is not specifically treated—rather, the treatment is directed at the whole syndrome. In extreme cases, a labyrinthotomy, or destruction of the membranous labyrinth, may be performed in order to alleviate the symptoms of vertigo. Such a procedure is rarely followed unless the hearing loss is so profound that the patient would not be further handicapped through the destruction of the inner ear. Relief from vertigo without destruction of the hearing has been reported through the use of ultrasonic vibrations applied to the horizontal semicircular canal. Section of the VIIIth nerve may also be performed as a "last-ditch" treatment for Ménière's.

When the sensori-neural loss is due to destruction of nerve fibers through the pressure of a tumor, naturally, where it is safe to do so, the tumor would be removed surgically. This operation would usually not restore any hearing function that has been lost, however.

OTHER HEARING DISORDERS

So far in this chapter we have been concerned with the symptoms, etiology, and treatment of the two principal types of organic hearing disorders: conductive and sensori-neural losses. Now brief mention will be made of other kinds of auditory disturbances.

Mixed Impairments

In the preceding sections of this chapter, conductive and sensori-neural losses were discussed as separate entities. In other words, only "pure" conductive and "pure" sensori-neural losses were considered. Actually, there are many instances of patients exhibiting symptoms of both types of loss. An elderly patient with presbycusis may also have some conductive loss because of otitis media, for example, or an otosclerotic may have some secondary nerve involvement. Such cases, demonstrating some degree of both types of hearing loss, are referred to as "mixed" impairments. Defined in audiometric terms, a patient with a mixed impairment shows some loss by bone conduction but a greater loss by air conduction. In Chapter 5, sample audiograms of the various types of hearing loss will be given.

Central Deafness

Sensori-neural impairments refer to losses that occur because of improper functioning of the inner ear or damage to the VIIIth nerve between the inner ear and the brain stem. Once the nerve fibers enter the brain stem, they proceed by various pathways to the temporal lobes of the cerebral cortex. Any interference with these pathways from the brain stem to and including the cortex produces a *central* auditory disorder. The cause of the impairment may be a brain tumor or abscess, vascular changes in the brain, or brain damage resulting from trauma or from *kernicterus* associated with *erythroblastosis fetalis.*

Erythroblastosis fetalis is a congenital hemolytic disease that results from blood-group incompatibilities of the mother and fetus. One such incompatibility is that concerned with the *Rh factor*. In the 1940's, scientists discovered that human blood could be sub-classified from the major blood groups (A, B, AB, and O) as either positive or negative in regard to the presence or abscence of a substance referred to as the Rh factor. This factor is present in the blood in about 85 per cent of the white population, who would therefore be classified as Rh positive. The remainder of the population would be classified as Rh negative. When Rh positive blood is mixed with Rh negative blood, antibodies are formed which attack the red blood cells of the Rh positive blood. Thus Rh positive and Rh negative blood are said to be incompatible. Antibodies are created when a person with Rh negative blood is transfused with blood that is Rh positive, or when the Rh positive blood of a fetus crosses the placenta in the course of the pregnancy of a woman whose blood is Rh negative. When a child is conceived by an Rh negative mother and an Rh positive father, the fetus may be Rh positive. If so, antibodies are created in the mother's bloodstream which in turn destroy the Rh positive cells in the blood of the fetus (erythroblastosis). Generally the first child born of Rh-incompatible parents will not be harmed, as the antibodies in the mother's blood are not created in sufficient number to affect the child's blood. After the first pregnancy, however, the antibodies may be present in sufficient number to cause trouble to any child with Rh positive blood.

If extensive fetal damage occurs, the result may be a miscarriage or a stillbirth. If the physician is alerted to the existence of the Rh incompatibility, however, it is possible to save the lives of many of these babies and even to prevent serious brain damage from occurring by completely transfusing the baby's blood within a few hours of birth. Repeated complete exchange transfusions may be necessary to prevent *kernicterus*, which is the pathologic process that results in the jaundicing of nuclei in the brain. This process begins at birth as a result of the destruction of the infant's red blood cells and subsequent deposition of blood pigments in the brain stem. Without exchange transfusions, the kernicterus may cause cerebral palsy (usually of the athetoid type), mental deficiency, and/or an auditory disturbance. Children with auditory disorders due to erythroblastosis and kernicterus may give the appearance of being deaf, and audiologic testing may demonstrate various degrees of what would seem to be sensori-neural impairment. The evidence is contradictory, however, as to whether or not such children have peripheral or central impairments of hearing.[14]

The evidence from post-mortem studies of kernicteric athetoids is also contradictory. The preponderance of such evidence, however, seems to point to normal cochleas but to abnormalities within the ventral and dorsal cochlear nuclei in the brain stem which as early as 1949 led Goodhill to suggest the term "nuclear deafness" as appropriate with erythroblastotic children.[15] Carhart theorized that lesions in the cochlear nuclei could produce audiometric results suggestive of peripheral sensori-neural involvements of cochlear origin and thus lead to misdiagnoses.[16] To confound the

[14]Victor Goodhill, Peter Cohen, Helen Hannigan, Jack Rosen, and Helmer Myklebust, "The Rh Child: Deaf or 'Aphasic'?" *Journal of Speech and Hearing Disorders,* Vol. 21 (December, 1956), pp. 407-425.

Robert W. Blakely, "Erythroblastosis and Perceptive Hearing Loss: Responses of Athetoids to Tests of Cochlear Function," *Journal of Speech and Hearing Research,* Vol. 2 (March, 1959), pp. 5-15.

Richard M. Flower, Richard Viehweg, and William F. Ruzicka, "The Communicative Disorders of Children with Kernicteric Athetosis: 1. Auditory Disorders," *Journal of Speech and Hearing Disorders,* Vol. 31 (February, 1966), pp. 41-59.

[15]Victor Goodhill, "Auditory Pathway Lesions Resulting from Rh Incompatibility," Chap. 14 in Freeman McConnell and Paul H. Ward, eds., *Deafness in Childhood* (Nashville, Tennessee, Vanderbilt University Press, 1967), pp. 215-228.

[16]Raymond Carhart, "Audiologic Tests: Questions and Speculations," Chap. 15, *ibid.*

diagnostic problem further, the possibility exists that a particular kernicteric child may in fact have a peripheral hearing impairment from causes unrelated to erythroblastosis.

Central deafness is similar in its symptom picture to *auditory agnosia,* a form of *receptive aphasia.* Aphasia, which is a disturbance in symbolic functioning, results from a lesion in the "dominant" hemisphere of the brain, the left hemisphere in all but a few individuals. Aphasia may be of the *expressive* type, the *receptive* type, or a mixture of the two. In the expressive type, the patient is unable to express himself through language, usually in either the spoken or the written form. In receptive aphasia, the difficulty is in comprehending language as it is heard or read. Auditory agnosia refers to the inability to recognize sound. In other words, the patient can "hear" but does not understand what he hears.

Central deafness is thus not a hearing-loss problem in the sense in which we have been applying the term *hearing loss* in this chapter. Because it is a neurological disorder, it falls within the domain of the neurologist and the neuropsychiatrist rather than that of the otologist. The audiologist, however, is interested in central deafness, because part of the audiologist's job is to differentiate hearing loss of the conductive and sensori-neural type from central deafness or aphasia. When brain injury exists from the time of birth or occurs at an age before the use of language would have developed, central deafness is difficult to distinguish from impairment of the peripheral hearing mechanism, that is, the middle ear, the inner ear, or the VIIIth nerve.

Functional or Nonorganic Hearing Loss

Another condition of auditory disturbance not due to an impairment of the peripheral hearing mechanism is *functional* or *nonorganic* hearing loss, sometimes referred to as *psychogenic* hearing loss. In other words, the cause of the auditory disorder is psychological rather than organic. Frequently, under emotional stress an individual unconsciously develops a "hearing loss" as a protective device or as an escape from what is to him an intolerable situation. The terms *hysterical deafness* and *conversion deafness* serve to describe such a condition. A patient with hysterical deafness is not trying to "fool" anybody. He himself is convinced that he has a genuine hearing loss. Sometimes the patient may have a mild-to-moderate degree of actual organic impairment but behaves as if his hearing were profoundly impaired. This patient would be described as having a "functional overlay" on a true hearing loss.

Both the otologist and the audiologist are concerned with the job of differentiating true organic loss from functional loss. In children who have never developed language, differential diagnosis presents special problems. The treatment of functional hearing loss of the hysterical or conversion type is in the province of psychiatry, however, since the assumed loss is a symptom of an underlying psychological disturbance. Demonstration to a patient that he actually can hear destroys his defenses without solving his problems, and it can be expected that the patient will develop other psychogenic disturbances in place of the hearing loss of which he has been deprived. These disturbances may take the form of blindness, inability to vocalize (aphonia), or paralysis of one or more limbs. It must be emphasized that all such psychogenic manifestations are on an unconscious level. The patient himself is convinced that the disorder is geniune.

An entirely different sort of assumed hearing loss occurs in the case of the *malingerer*, who adopts the role of deafness or hearing impairment consciously and deliberately for purposes of his own. Usually these purposes are concerned with financial reimbursement for "injury" incurred on the job, or while a member of the armed forces. The motive then is purely pecuniary, and the "patient" is well aware of the true state of his hearing. Sometimes a hearing loss will be assumed by an individual in order to be relieved of an onerous duty. This form of "goldbricking" is employed on occasion by servicemen in order to get out of the front lines and into a hospital, or perhaps in order to obtain a medical discharge.

In Chapter 7, the problems of differential diagnosis of genuine hearing loss and functional or nonorganic hearing loss will be discussed in detail.

REFERENCES

Davis, Hallowell, and Silverman, S. Richard, eds., *Hearing and Deafness* (New York, Holt, Rinehart and Winston, 1970), Chaps. 4, 5, and 6.

Graham, A. Bruce, ed., *Sensorineural Hearing Processes and Disorders* (Boston, Little, Brown and Company, 1967).

Lederer, Francis L., and Hollender, Abraham R., *Textbook of the Ear, Nose, and Throat* (Philadelphia, Davis, 1947), Sections VI and VII.

Pool, J. Lawrence, and Pava, Arthur A., *Acoustic Nerve Tumors* (Springfield, Illinois, Charles C Thomas, 1957).

Sataloff, Joseph, *Hearing Loss* (Philadelphia, J. B. Lippincott Company, 1966).

Schuknecht, Harold F., ed., *Otosclerosis* (Boston, Little, Brown and Company, 1962).

Shambaugh, George E., Jr., *Surgery of the Ear* (Philadelphia, W. B. Saunders Co., 1967).

Travis, Lee Edward, ed., *Handbook of Speech Pathology and Audiology* (New York, Appleton-Century-Crofts, 1971), Chap. 12.

Ward, W. Dixon, and Fricke, James E., eds., *Noise as a Public Health Hazard* (Washington, American Speech and Hearing Association, 1969).

4

THE DEVELOPMENT OF HEARING
TESTS

Hearing impairment is a matter of *degree* of loss and also of *pattern* of loss. When a patient complains to the otologist that his hearing is defective, the physician needs to know certain things about the patient's hearing loss—information which, together with the patient's medical history and the results of the physical examination, will enable the otologist to make a diagnosis of the type of hearing impairment that the patient has and to give him some basis for estimating the possible effect on the loss of treating the patient, medically or surgically. To perform these functions of diagnosis and prognosis the otologist needs to know: (1) How much hearing loss is there in the low-, middle-, and high-frequency ranges of the ear? (2) How does the patient's air-conduction hearing compare with his bone-conduction hearing? (3) How seriously is this patient handicapped by his hearing loss?

To provide the answers to these questions, otologists have devised various tests of patients' hearing, ranging from the crude watch-tick and coin-click tests to the extensive quantitative measurements made possible by the development of pure-tone and speech audiometers. Between these extremes fall such time-honored tests (among otologists) as the spoken- and whispered-voice test, and the various tuning-fork tests. Even with today's modern audiometric instrumentation available, many otologists prefer to diagnose and "measure" hearing loss by means of voice and tuning-fork tests. Perhaps the reason for this preference is that measurement of the hearing function with modern test equipment requires technical skill on the part of the tester and more time than most otologists can spend with their patients, whereas the voice and the tuning-fork tests are administered by the otologist himself and in a brief space of time.

Because the audiologist frequently will receive reports from otologists referring to the results of nonaudiometric hearing tests, and also because our modern audiometric tests are merely refinements of some of these earlier tests, we shall now briefly examine the so-called noninstrumental tests of hearing.

WATCH-TICK AND COIN-CLICK TESTS

These tests would usually be administered by a general practitioner rather than by an otologist. The technique of administration is simple. The physician holds his watch next to the patient's ear and asks the patient to inform him when he ceases to hear the tick as the doctor moves the watch away. From previous experience, the physician knows the distance at which the person with normal hearing can just barely detect the tick. Hearing loss is expressed in terms of a fraction, of which the distance in inches that the patient can hear the watch tick is the numerator and the distance the normal ear can hear the tick is the denominator. Thus if the patient ceases to hear the tick at a distance of 12 inches, whereas the normal ear can hear it to a distance of 30 inches, the patient's hearing loss in the ear under test would be described as 12/30 (30/30 being normal). To administer such a test to a patient with any amount of hearing loss, the physician must possess a fairly noisy watch. Most modern watches are so quiet that even an acute ear could not hear them ticking at distances of more than 4 to 6 inches. Naturally, the physician obtains only the crudest information about his patient's hearing function from the watch-tick test.

The coin-click test consists of the physician's dropping a large coin, usually a half-dollar, on a hard surface. The patient is instructed to report whether he hears the coin "ring" or only a dull thud. If he hears the coin ring as it strikes the hard surface, his high-frequency hearing acuity is normal. If he hears only a thud, he is presumed to have a high-frequency hearing loss. This test yields no information as to which frequencies are affected or the extent of the loss. Also, it cannot be used successfully in monaural testing (testing one ear separately). Even with considerable clinical experience, therefore, the results of the coin-click test are difficult to interpret meaningfully. Both the watch-tick and the coin-click tests are a step better than nothing in evaluating hearing loss. Neither one is used to any extent today.

CONVERSATIONAL VOICE TEST

When it is employed by an experienced examiner aware of its limitations, the conversational voice test is useful in detecting gross deviations from normal hearing. Unfortunately, this test has been applied extensively as a means of quantifying hearing sensitivity for speech, particularly by the armed forces. In World War II, the conversational voice test was given as part of the routine physical examination procedure at induction and separation centers, just as the Snellen chart was used to measure visual acuity. If, at a distance of 20 feet, we can identify letters on the Snellen chart that "normal" eyes can identify at that distance, we are said to have 20/20 vision. In the same manner, it was assumed that, if we were able to identify spoken words at a prescribed distance, our hearing was normal. The conversational voice test was administered at a distance of 20 feet in the Army and 15 feet in the Navy. "Normal" hearing was represented by a test score of 20/20 or 15/15. Whereas in visual testing a standard chart was employed in every induction or separation center, in hearing testing there was no attempt to control the speech stimuli provided either as to intensity or as to specific words. In visual testing, it is necessary only to light the chart properly and measure off distances on the floor; it does not matter in what kind of room the test is administered. In hearing testing, the size, shape, and acoustic characteristics of a room influence the manner in which the voice is heard at some distance from the speaker. Naturally, it was not feasible for the armed forces to construct "standard" rooms for hearing testing in every induction and separation center, so that the conversational voice test was not given under the same physical conditions in various places. Although the manner of scoring the conversational voice test suggests that hearing might be measured with the same degree of precision as vision, actually there is no comparison in the control of testing conditions between the two tests.

In administering the conversational voice test, the patient is placed at the prescribed distance from the examiner so that first one ear and then the other is directed toward the examiner. The patient plugs the ear not under test with his index finger. He is instructed to repeat the words he hears the examiner speaking. Then, in a "normal" level of voice, the examiner speaks some numbers, simple words, and simple phrases. If the patient is unable to repeat these, the examiner moves toward the patient until he is able to repeat what the examiner is saying. A score of 10/20 means that the examiner had to move to a distance of 10 feet from the patient before he was able to repeat what the "normal" ear is supposed to hear at 20 feet.

In the armed forces, the responsibility for administering the conversational voice test was usually vested in a medical corpsman who may have had only a vague conception of how the test should be administered. Different examiners made their own interpretation of what was meant by a "normal" level of conversational voice. As a result of this slipshod method of "measuring" the hearing, many men with impaired hearing were inducted into the service with a clean bill of health. If, at the time of their discharge, these men requested a careful audiometric examination which disclosed a hearing loss, the armed services had no evidence that the loss had not occurred during the claimant's period of service. The Veterans Administration today is paying hundreds of thousands of dollars annually in compensation to veterans whose hearing loss antedates their entrance into the service, because by the crude methods of hearing testing at the time of their induction their hearing was considered to be normal. Fortunately, the situation has changed, so that today most inductees or recruits are given audiometric tests. In many cases their hearing is checked with "automatic" audiometers (discussed in Chapter 9).

TUNING-FORK TESTS

In otology, the classic method of measuring, or more properly describing, hearing loss is by noting the patient's responses to vibrating tuning forks. Forks of various frequencies are selected for administering the standard tests. These frequencies are octaves of "C" on the scientific scale, from 128 Hz through 8192 Hz. The most common fork tests are the Rinne, Weber, Bing, and the Schwabach, named after their nineteenth century German originators.

The Rinne Test

The purpose of this test is to differentiate between conductive and sensori-neural hearing loss and thus assist the otologist in a diagnosis of the type of hearing impairment that a particular patient exhibits. To perform the test, the otologist sets a tuning fork into vibration (by pinching, then releasing the tines with his fingers, or by striking the fork with a soft mallet) and holds it close to the patient's external ear. When the patient reports that he can no longer hear the sound produced by the fork, the otologist quickly places the handle of the vibrating fork against the patient's mastoid process and asks if the patient can again hear the fork. If the patient replies affirmatively, the result of the test is said to be a *Rinne negative*, which is indicative of a conductive-type lesion. If the patient hears the fork longer by air conduction than by bone conduction, the result is labeled a *Rinne positive* and indicates a sensori-neural loss. A Rinne test on a normal ear will yield a positive result also, since normally our hearing is more sensitive by air conduction than by bone conduction.

The method of administering the Rinne test may be just the reverse of that described above. That is, the examiner may begin by pressing the handle of the fork against the patient's mastoid and then shift the fork to the external ear. Or the test may be performed first by one method and then the other in order to validate the result obtained. Standard procedure calls for the use of three forks in performing the Rinne test: forks with frequencies of 128, 256, and 512 Hz. Most otologists will want to test at 1024 and 2048 Hz as well, since hearing for speech depends to a considerable extent upon frequencies higher than 512 Hz. Instead of expressing the results in terms of positive or negative, some otologists prefer to say that air conduction is greater than bone conduction (in the case of a positive Rinne), or that bone conduction is greater than air conduction (in the case of a negative Rinne).

There are limitations to the use of the Rinne, of which the otologist must be aware. In the first place, before a negative Rinne can be obtained, the patient must have exhibited more than a slight conductive loss. Since normally the ear is much more sensitive to air-borne sounds, a slight conductive impairment will not overcome the normal differential between air and bone conduction, and the test result will be a positive Rinne, even though the patient's impairment is actually of the conductive type. Another limitation involves the testing of a patient who has a severe sensori-neural impairment in one ear, the other ear having normal, or close to normal, bone conduction. Then the Rinne test result will be negative (bone conduction better than air conduction) on the severely impaired ear which actually has a sensori-neural loss. The result might lead the otologist to diagnose a conductive loss, which, of course, would be grossly wrong. What produces this misleading test result is the participation of the ear with normal bone conduction when the handle of the fork is pressed against the mastoid of the poorer ear. When the fork is placed on the mastoid, the bones of the skull are set into vibration, and the fluid in both inner ears is agitated. If the nerve endings in only one cochlea are insensitive to the vibrations in the fluid, the sound will be heard by the other, normal cochlea. The patient with a unilateral loss who states that he hears the fork longer by bone conduction than by air conduction, therefore, might actually be responding to the bone-conducted vibrations in his better ear. To safeguard against making a false diagnosis in this situation, the otologist must prevent the participation of the better ear by introducing a masking noise to the better ear, a masking noise of sufficient intensity to make it impossible for the better ear to hear the bone-conducted sound produced by the handle of the fork pressing against the mastoid of the opposite ear. With a unilateral hearing loss, however, the otologist can check the results of the Rinne against the results of the next test to be described, the Weber.

In passing, it is interesting to note that while the originator of this test was of German nationality, many authors in the past have written his name as if it were French, Rinné. As a matter of fact it appeared this way in the first edition of this book. The author is grateful to Dr. Walter Heck for correcting this error.[1]

The Weber Test

This test also has as its purpose the differentiation between conductive and sensori-neural hearing impairment. The Weber, however, is used only in cases of unilateral loss or in losses characterized by better hearing in one ear. It is a test of lateralization, that is, a test to see to which of the ears the tone

[1] Walter E. Heck, "Dr. A. Rinne," *Laryngoscope,* Vol. 72 (May, 1962), pp. 647-652.

is referred, or lateralized, when the handle of the fork is placed on the midline of the skull. If, when the fork is placed on the midline, the patient reports that he hears the tone in his *poorer* ear, a conductive impairment is indicated. If he hears the tone in his *better* ear, the impairment is a sensori-neural one. If there is no difference in sensitivity between the ears, the tone will be heard equally in the two ears. The tone refers to the poorer ear in cases of conductive impairment because of the *occlusion effect*. This can be demonstrated with a normal-hearing individual by instructing him to close each external canal alternatively with finger pressure on the tragus while the vibrating fork is held on the midline of the skull. The tone will "shift" back and forth, always lateralizing to the ear that is occluded. A conductive impairment acts in the same way to occlude the passage of air-conducted sound, and thus the tone appears to be heard only in the ear having the greater occlusion, that is, the greater conductive impairment. In the case of unequally functioning inner ears, as would be true in unilateral sensori-neural impairment, the fork tone is referred to the side having the better cochlea, since this is a test of bone-conduction functioning. Caution must be exercised in evaluating the patient's responses to the Weber test. Unless the patient is informed that he might hear the tone in his poorer ear, he is likely to respond consistently that he hears the tone in his better ear, because it is not logical to the patient that he could ever hear better in his poorer ear. His judgment thus belies the evidence of his senses.

The Bing Test

The Weber test is useful in cases of unilateral impairment, or where there is more than a slight difference in sensitivity between the ears. The Bing test, which also is based on the occlusion effect, can be used in cases of bilateral impairment to distinguish between conductive and sensori-neural loss. The vibrating fork is placed on the mastoid as it is in the Rinne test. When the patient reports that the tone has become inaudible, the examiner immediately closes the external canal by light finger pressure on the tragus while the still vibrating fork is left in place. If the patient reports that the tone again becomes audible, it is evident that occluding the ear was responsible for enhancing the ear's sensitivity for the bone-conducted sound. Thus it can be presumed that there is no conductive impairment, or at least that there is some sensori-neural involvement. If the tone is not heard again when the canal is closed, the ear has a conductive impairment that is already effectively occluding the passage of air-conducted sound. When "secondary perception" occurs, the result is termed a *Bing positive* and is indicative of a sensori-neural impairment. Of course a normal ear will also yield a Bing positive result, just as a normal ear yields a Rinne positive. If there is no secondary perception of the tone when the ear canal is closed, the result is a *Bing negative* and is indicative of a conductive impairment for the reason stated above.

The Bing test provides valuable information to the audiologist in pure-tone audiometry when performed with the bone-conduction vibrator of the audiometer instead of a tuning fork.

The Schwabach Test

The Rinne, Weber, and Bing tests are qualitative tests of hearing, that is, they give information as to what type of impairment the patient has. The Schwabach is a quantitative test; in other words, it attempts to tell how much impairment a patient has. Like the Weber and the Bing, the Schwabach is a test of bone conduction. In performing the test, the examiner places the handle of a vibrating tuning fork on the mastoid of the patient and tells the patient to notify him when he ceases to hear the tone. As soon as the patient reports that the tone is inaudible, the examiner places the handle of the fork on his own mastoid and counts the number of seconds he continues to hear the fork vibrate. Of course this method of testing presumes that the examiner has normal hearing. The results of the tests are expressed in terms of the time that the patient's hearing is diminished in comparison to the examiner's for each fork. Thus, if the examiner can hear the tone for ten seconds longer than the patient can, the test result is expressed as "diminished ten." Since this is a test of bone-conduction acuity, it can be seen that the Schwabach measures the amount of sensori-neural loss present. Even with such "quantification" as the Schwabach provides, however, the test result is difficult to interpret in terms of the amount of the patient's loss, since units of time rather than loudness serve to express the loss. Nevertheless an experienced clinician can make effective use of this test to judge the severity of sensori-neural impairment.

THE PURE-TONE AUDIOMETER

Tuning-fork tests provide information concerning a patient's hearing at discrete frequencies, but, as we have seen, these tests are useful primarily for providing a qualitative description of a patient's loss. The next logical development in hearing tests was to design an instrument which would yield quantitative as well as qualitative information about a patient's hearing. Such an instrument is the pure-tone audiometer. Although some experimentation was conducted in the late nineteenth century with "electrical" hearing-testing devices, the prototype of the modern, vacuum-tube audiometer was not developed until the 1920's.

The audiometer is an instrument for electronically generating tones of essential "purity" such as those produced by the tuning fork. The intensity of these tones is accurately controlled by an *attenuator*, which is usually calibrated in 5-dB steps, although some audiometers are calibrated in steps of 1 or 2 dB. Zero dB hearing level at each frequency is theoretically the lowest intensity at which the average normal ear can detect the presence of the test tone 50 per cent of the time. Hearing "loss" is thus expressed as the number of dB in excess of this zero point that the intensity of the tone must be increased in order for the impaired ear just barely to detect its presence. The test tones produced by the audiometer are delivered to the patient's ear through an earphone for air-conduction tests, and through a bone-conduction vibrator for tests of inner ear functioning. Comparison of a patient's hearing sensitivity by air and by bone yields information of diagnostic significance, as does the Rinne tuning-fork test, with the added advantage of measuring the amount of loss in dB by each method of testing. The audiometer provides a more accurate type of Schwabach test, since it measures bone-conduction loss in dB rather than in units of time. Therefore the audiometer performs both the Rinne and Schwabach tests, but in an improved manner. The Weber and Bing tests can also be administered with the audiometer, by means of the bone-conduction vibrator instead of a tuning fork, although there would be little point in performing an audiometric Weber test for routine diagnostic purposes, as the hearing loss in each ear can be accurately measured with the audiometer both by air and by bone. The audiometric Weber test for determining the need for masking will be discussed in the next chapter.

For many years, audiometers were designed to generate the same frequencies as those of tuning forks: octaves and mid-octaves of "C" on the scientific scale. More recently, upon the recommendation of various scientific associations, audiometer manufacturers have standardized their instruments on a scale based on even thousands of hertz. Thus the modern audiometer may contain all the following test frequencies: 125, 250, 500, 750, 1000, 1500, 2000, 3000, 4000, 6000, and 8000 Hz.

So far, in our discussion of intensity in this book, we have been referring to sound pressure levels, that is, the intensity in relation to a specified physical reference level, usually a pressure of 0.0002 dyne/cm^2. Another way to speak of intensity is by referring to the threshold of the "average normal ear" as a reference. The sound pressure level required to make any frequency barely audible to the average normal ear is called zero *hearing level*. Audiometers are calibrated to national and international standards, based on studies of normal-hearing subjects, that specify the sound pressure levels for zero hearing level — or audiometric zero — at each frequency. The intensity of any frequency can thus be specified in terms of its hearing level in dB, which means, of course, how much greater its sound pressure level is than the sound pressure level for audiometric zero. The hearing level required to reach the threshold of an impaired ear is the *hearing loss* or *threshold hearing level* for that ear. Some audiologists prefer the term *hearing-threshold level*,[2] but since any audiometric value is a hearing level regardless of whether one is referring to threshold or to infra- or supra-threshold levels, there would

[2] Hallowell Davis, "Acoustics and Psychoacoustics," in Hallowell Davis and S. Richard Silverman, eds., *Hearing and Deafness* (New York, Holt, Rinehart and Winston, 1970), p. 27.

seem to be an advantage in keeping the words "hearing" and "level" together in referring to any audiometric reading. Thus in this book, the term "threshold hearing level" will be used interchangeably with "threshold" and "hearing loss."

As was seen in Figure 2–1 (Chapter 2), the sound pressure level for audiometric zero is not the same for all frequencies. The human ear is more sensitive to the frequencies in the range from 1000 through 4000 Hz than it is to lower and higher frequencies. The audiometer is compensated for this uneven response curve of the ear, so that the same zero-dB setting on the hearing-level control applies to every frequency. Because of the uneven response of the ear, higher sound pressure levels are required to reach audiometric zero for the frequencies below 500 and above 4000 Hz. Since only so much amplification is available in the audiometer, there is less intensity available above audiometric zero at the extreme low and high frequencies than there is at the middle frequencies. The maximum hearing level available in most pure-tone audiometers is 110 dB. At the frequencies below 500 Hz and above 4000 Hz, the maximum hearing level available is less than this maximum, for the reasons just discussed. Since zero hearing level represents a statistical average of threshold levels of normal ears, and some ears would have better than average normal hearing, the hearing-level dial on some audiometers provides for the measurement of up to 10 dB better than average normal hearing at all frequencies. A minus sign precedes the designation of a level that is lower than zero dB hearing level.

In addition to the frequency and intensity controls, an audiometer includes an interrupter switch, which enables the operator to turn the test tone on or off immediately and noiselessly; a masking circuit, so that the ear not under test can be prevented from participating; and a selector switch for directing the test signal to the right earphone, the left earphone, or the bone-conduction vibrator. In addition, some audiometers include a voice circuit, which enables the operator to amplify his voice for the patient, making communication possible in cases of extreme loss, and also providing for the administration of certain speech audiometric tests; and a patient-signaling device, usually a cord and push button connected with a small lamp on the face of the audiometer, so that the patient can indicate silently when he is hearing the test tone. The operation of the pure-tone audiometer will be explained in detail in the next chapter.

THE SPEECH AUDIOMETER

Just as the pure-tone audiometer represents an extension and quantification of tuning-fork tests, so also the modern speech audiometer has developed from the early crude conversational voice test. Speech audiometry, as it is practiced today, had its inception during World War II in the military aural rehabilitation centers. It is interesting to note that the test materials for speech audiometry were developed originally under government contract by the Harvard Psycho-Acoustic Laboratory for the purpose of comparing the efficiency of various communications systems in transmitting speech.[3] For this purpose, subjects with normal hearing were tested. Differences among communications systems in efficiency of speech transmission were represented by differences in test scores made by the same subject as he shifted his listening from one system to another. Someone with clinical orientation soon saw that, if the test materials were valuable in differentiating among communications systems used with normal ears, they should also be useful in differentiating normal from impaired hearing by means of a single communications system.

Speech audiometry should be performed in a two-room facility with the patient in a room that is reasonably sound-isolated and the examiner in a separate control room. A two-way communications system provides for introducing the test materials to the patient and conveying his responses to the tester. Ideally, the speech audiometer should provide inputs from a microphone, for live-voice testing; from a turn-table and a tape recorder, for recorded speech tests; and from a white-noise generator, for masking purposes. The level of the test materials going into the amplifier is monitored by means of volume controls and one or more volume indicator meters. The output of the amplifier is directed through an attenuation system to one or both of a pair of earphones, or to one or two loudspeakers. The attenuation system provides for control of the output in 1- or 2-dB steps over a range of hearing levels from zero or –10 dB (that is, 10 dB better than the average normal threshold) to 100 or 110 dB. With such equipment, the following measures can be obtained monaurally and binaurally: (1) speech-reception threshold, (2) most comfortable listening level, (3) tolerance for loud speech, and (4) articulation, or word discrimination, ability. These measures, and procedures for obtaining them, will be explained in Chapter 6.

REFERENCES

Bunch, C. C., *Clinical Audiometry* (St. Louis, Mosby, 1943)

Davis, Hallowell, and Silverman, S. Richard, eds., *Hearing and Deafness* (New York, Holt, Rinehart and Winston, 1970), Chap. 7.

Feldmann, Harald, "A History of Audiology," *Translations of the Beltone Institute for Hearing Research*, No. 22 (January, 1970).

Glorig, Aram, ed., *Audiometry: Principles and Practices* (Baltimore, Williams & Wilkins, 1965), Chap. 1.

O'Neill, John J., and Oyer, Herbert J., *Applied Audiometry* (New York, Dodd, Mead & Co., 1966), Chap. 3.

Watson, L. A., and Tolan, T., *Hearing Tests and Hearing Instruments* (Baltimore, Williams & Wilkins, 1949).

[3] J. P. Egan, *Articulation Testing Methods*, OSRD Rept, #3802 (Harvard University, Psycho-Acoustic Laboratory, 1944).

5

TESTING THE HEARING FUNCTION:
PURE-TONE AUDIOMETRY

EQUIPMENT REQUIRED

There are several pure-tone audiometers available commercially. These vary from simple portable models designed for school-testing to elaborate "research"-type audiometers, with which it is possible to administer all kinds of special, advanced tests, in addition to the standard measures. To conduct the routine tests of pure-tone audiometry, it is necessary only to have an instrument that provides for air-conduction and bone-conduction testing and for introducing masking. Of course, any instrument must be properly calibrated. Methods of checking on the calibration of an audiometer will be given later.

Pure-tone audiometers are of two main types: discrete frequency and sweep frequency. The former provides tones only at octave and mid-octave steps as the frequency dial is turned; the latter type provides a tone that is continuously variable in frequency. Most audiometers in use today are of the discrete-frequency type. The hearing level dial on audiometers is graduated in steps of 5 dB, and in most audiometers intensity changes of 5 dB only are possible. There is a trend today for audiometer manufacturers to provide intensity controls in 1- or 2-dB steps, although it is doubtful that the results of routine hearing tests will ever be presented in steps of less than 5 dB.

Regardless of the make and type of pure-tone audiometer, certain necessary controls will be common to all instruments, and the audiometrist must learn to operate them in order to give hearing tests. These basic controls are:

1. Power switch
2. Frequency selector

3. Hearing-level control (attenuator)

4. Output selector (bone, right, left)

5. Interrupter switch

6. Switch and attenuator for masking noise

As stated in the preceding chapter, audiometers do not produce the same maximum hearing level for all frequencies. On the frequency-selector dial of most audiometers, a small number printed under the frequency designation indicates the maximum hearing level that is available for the specific frequency. Thus the figure 90 which appears beneath the frequency 250 means that 90 dB is the maximum hearing level that the audiometer will produce at the frequency of 250 Hz. If no small digits appear beneath the frequency designation, the maximum hearing level of 110 dB shown on the hearing-level dial is available for that frequency. With most audiometers, this maximum is available for the frequencies of 500 through 6000 Hz.

On most audiometers, the interrupter switch is able to work in either of two ways: (1) when depressed it turns the tone on, or (2) when depressed it turns the tone off. Some audiometrists prefer to have the interrupter function in one way, and some in the other. The interrupter switch is spring-loaded, so it returns to its on or off position, whichever the case may be, whenever the examiner releases it.

The design and arrangements of an audiometer's basic controls will differ from instrument to instrument. Figure 5-1 shows a typical arrangement.

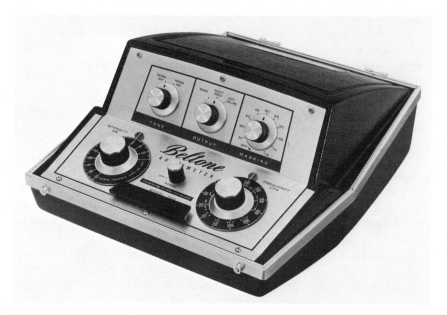

Figure 5-1.   A portable pure-tone audiometer. (Reproduced by permission of Beltone Electronics Corporation, Chicago, Illinois.)

In order to obtain valid hearing-testing results, there must be some control over the conditions under which the testing is performed. Ideally, all testing should be performed in a sound-isolated room in which ambient noise is at a minimum. Good sound-isolated rooms are expensive to construct. Some portable sound-treated rooms are on the market at less than it would cost to construct comparable facilities. Actually, however, unless it is intended to conduct research studies involving precise measurement of normal ears, it is not necessary to have an expensive, highly isolated room. For purposes of ordinary hearing testing to differentiate between normal and impaired ears, a room that provides a reduction in outside noise of about 40 dB will be adequate, provided, of course, that the room is not situated in a particularly noisy location. As a matter of fact, most of the testing done in the public schools must perforce be performed in rooms that are not specially treated, and, unless the surroundings are unusually noisy, sufficiently accurate results can be obtained to differentiate those children who have hearing losses from those whose hearing is essentially normal. Of course, any follow-up testing of those discovered to have losses should be performed under better testing conditions than is found in the average school, in order to obtain accurate threshold measurements. Refer to Chapter 9 for suggested maximum octave-band levels of ambient noise within test rooms where hearing levels as low as zero dB are to be measured.

AIR-CONDUCTION TESTING

Before detailing the step-by-step procedure in administering a hearing test, it is well to point out that the audiometer is not a magical instrument which can be connected to a patient and yield automatically the exact amount of hearing loss that patient has at each frequency. In the hands of an experienced clinician, the audiometer is a useful tool for obtaining measures of the extent and type of hearing loss. The point is that the audiometer is a *tool*, and as such it can be operated skillfully by the craftsman or clumsily and ineffectively by the amateur. The results of a hearing test must always be evaluated in terms of the individual who performed the test. There is an unfortunate tendency for some physicians and educators to accept audiograms at face value, without regard for the conditions under which the tests were administered or by whom. The audiogram is not a photograph of an individual's hearing loss; it is the best estimate by the audiometrist of the state of the patient's hearing, based on his observation of the patient's behavior in the testing situation. Because patients differ considerably in their reactions in test situations, it is not possible to prescribe in detail the steps that should be followed invariably in obtaining an audiogram. In hearing testing, as in almost every human activity, there is no substitute for experience. The experienced clinician will adapt his testing techniques to suit the situation instead of following a set procedure that makes no allowance for individual differences from patient to patient. The beginner, however, must follow a rather rigid procedure if the results that he obtains are to be at all reliable. It is urged, therefore, that those who are just beginning their hearing-testing experience follow the steps set forth below in every case until they develop sufficient skill through experience to introduce their own modifications and improvisations. With this word of caution, then, let us proceed to the step-by-step procedure to be applied in administering a pure-tone audiometric test by air conduction.

1. Plug in the audiometer, if it is the type that operates on "house current." Most audiometers are designed to operate on 60-cycle alternating current of 110 volts, although some may be operated on 220 volts as well. Just be sure that, for the instrument being operated, the electric supply is proper.

2. Turn on the audiometer's power switch, making certain that the instrument actually does receive power by seeing that the dials light up or, if it is a vacuum-tube instrument, that the tubes begin to glow. Allow the audiometer to "warm up" for at least ten minutes before proceeding. Even with audiometers that contain transistors instead of vacuum tubes, it is good practice to allow the electronic components to stabilize for several minutes before starting the test.

3. If the earphones and the patient's signal cord are not already plugged into the audiometer, plug them in, seeing to it that they go in the proper jacks and are in the jacks all the way, making good contact.

4. Set the frequency control at 1000 Hz and the hearing-level control at 40 dB. Put on the earphones and listen to the tone as you switch from one ear to the other. When you are satisfied that the tone is present in equal strength in each earphone, listen to the tone as you gradually turn the hearing-level control toward zero-dB hearing level. If you have normal hearing, you should be able to hear the tone at near zero-dB hearing level. The purpose of this check is to verify that the audiometer and earphones are performing properly, and that the levels of sound in the phones are approximately as indicated on the hearing-level dial.

5. If you plan to have the patient use the signal cord and light in the course of the test, give them a trial to make sure they are working.

6. You are now ready to test with the audiometer, and it is time to instruct the patient, who should be sitting and facing you in such a position that he cannot see the controls of the audiometer. Some examiners prefer to have the patient seated so his back is toward the examiner. The disadvantage of this arrangement is that you cannot observe the facial expressions of the patient which frequently are helpful in evaluating the patient's responses. In some installations, the patient may be seated in a test room alone while you are in an adjacent control room with the audiometer, watching the patient through an observation window.

In these instructions, and subsequently in this chapter, we shall assume that the patient is an adult or an older child. Special problems of testing young children will be dealt with in Chapter 7. The following instructions should be considered only as a guide. The words, and the manner of giving the instructions, may, of course, be varied to fit the situation.

We are now going to test your hearing. I am going to place an earphone over each ear, but we shall test only one ear at a time. The object of the test is to find the point where you can just barely detect the presence of the tone. We shall start each time with the tone off. Then I shall gradually introduce the tone until you can just hear it. As soon as you first hear the tone, signal me. Then I'll make the tone louder so you can hear it well. I shall next make the tone softer until you signal me that you can no longer hear it. Then I'll make it louder and softer and turn it on and off while you tell me whether or not you can hear the tone each time, until I am satisfied that we have the point where you can just detect the presence of the tone. Then we'll shift to a different tone and start the process all over. You can signal that you hear the tone by pressing the button on the end of this cord, which will cause a light on the audiometer to turn on. Keep the button depressed as long as you hear the tone at all. When you no longer hear the tone, do not push the button. Do you hear any better with one ear than with the other? If so, we'll test the better ear first; if not, we'll begin with the right ear. Are you ready? Signal when you hear the tone by pushing the button, and hold it down until you cease to hear the tone. Here we go. . . .

Note that the instructions to the patient are given *before* the earphones are placed on the patient's head. The examiner should if necessary raise his voice when speaking to the patient and of course should articulate clearly. It is advisable for the examiner to follow a routine of always putting the earphones on patients in the same way; for example, red (or gray) phone on the right ear, and blue (or black) phone on the left ear. Such habits tend to prevent errors in recording test results for the respective ears. It should be pointed out here that it is not necessary to utilize the patient's signal button and light if this system should, for any reason, seem inadvisable. Sometimes it is difficult for the patient to concentrate on listening and at the same time co-ordinate his muscles to push and release the button at the right moment. Other methods of signaling are permissible, such as having the patient raise a finger when he hears the tone and lower the finger when he no longer hears it. Or the patient can be instructed to say "Yes" when he hears the tone. The tester can soon discover whether or not the push button presents a mental or physical hazard for the patient and shift to an easier type of response, if necessary. The advantage of the signal light is that it permits no equivocal reponses: the light is either on or off. If the patient is signaling by raising and lowering a finger, he may, when uncertain that he is hearing the tone, have the finger only partially raised. The examiner, therefore, has a problem in interpreting the response. Nevertheless, many audiologists prefer to utilize the finger-raising response.

7. As indicated in the instructions, test the better ear first, if the patient reports that there is a difference in sensitivity between the two ears. The reason for this procedure is to alert the audiometrist to the need for masking the better ear if the difference in sensitivity between the ears should be so great as to make it possible that the better ear will participate in the test of the poorer ear. Whenever the apparent thresholds of the two ears differ by 40 dB or more, you should suspect that the thresholds obtained for the poorer ear may actually be a "shadow curve" of the better ear's hearing. In that event, what happens is that, before the tone can be made loud enough to be heard by the poorer ear, it is heard by the ear not under test, probably in large part by transmission through the bones of the skull by means of bone conduction. Thus it is advisable to test the better ear first, so that as soon as the test of the poorer ear begins you can tell whether there is sufficient difference between the ears to make masking necessary. More will be said later about masking. If the patient reports that there is no difference between the ears, it is suggested that the right ear be tested first. The reason for this suggestion is merely to establish a routine, since there are fewer chances for error in conducting the test and recording the results if the same procedure is followed in test after test.

8. It is advisable to begin a test at the frequency of 1000 Hz, since this frequency is near the center of the most sensitive area of the human ear. Also it has been demonstrated to have a good test-retest reliability.

9. Throughout this description of testing, it is assumed that the tone is inaudible except when the interrupter switch is depressed. The procedure to follow in testing at 1000 Hz, and at all succeeding frequencies, is to start with the hearing-level control at its minimum reading—either −10 dB or zero dB, depending on the particular instrument you are using—depress the interrupter switch, and gradually increase the intensity until the patient signals that he hears the tone. Increase the intensity of the tone beyond this point by about 20 dB in order to give the patient an opportunity to hear the tone well. If there is evidence that the patient is abnormally sensitive to above-threshold intensities, increase the tone by only 5 to 10 dB, as an increase of 20 dB may make the tone uncomfortably loud.

10. Now decrease the intensity of the tone in a steady counter-clockwise movement of the hearing-level control until the patient signals that he can no longer hear the tone. Note mentally what the reading of the hearing-level dial is at this point.

11. Immediately reverse the direction of rotation of the hearing level control, increasing intensity of the tone until the patient signals that he hears it again. Make a mental note of this hearing-level dial reading. You now have "bracketed" the patient's threshold within 10 to 15 dB by sweeping across it first in a descending fashion and then in an ascending manner.

12. At this point, you have stopped as soon as the patient signaled that he heard the tone. Now cut off the tone completely by releasing the interrupter. The patient should immediately signal that he does not hear the tone. While

the interrupter switch is off, decrease the setting on the hearing-level dial by 10 dB. Depress the interrupter, and see whether or not the patient signals that he hears the tone. If the patient does not hear the tone, skip the next step and proceed to step 14.

13. If the patient signals that he hears the tone again, release the interrupter switch and lower the intensity by another 10 dB. This time, when you depress the interrupter, the patient should not hear the tone, provided that steps 10 and 11 have been performed properly.

14. With the tone off again, this time *increase* the intensity by 5 dB, and then depress the interrupter. If the patient does not hear the tone, repeat this step until he does signal that he hears the tone.

15. When the patient signals that he hears the tone, release the interrupter briefly and decrease the intensity by 10 dB. The patient should signal that he does not hear the tone. If the patient signals that he hears the tone, repeat this step until he no longer hears it.

16. Increase the intensity by 5 dB and depress the interrupter briefly. If the patient does not respond, increase the intensity by 5 dB again and depress the interrupter. Continue in this manner until the patient responds. As soon as he responds, drop the intensity by 10 dB again and repeat the procedure of presenting brief bursts of tone at 5-dB steps of increasing intensity until the patient responds. Each time he responds, decrease the intensity and repeat this procedure, until the patient has responded at least four times. For audiometric purposes, the patient's threshold is defined as the lowest hearing level at which he responds correctly to the presence of the tone at least 50 per cent of the time. Suppose, for example, that in step 14 the minimum hearing level at which the patient responds is 40 dB. In step 15 you present the tone at 30 dB and the patient does not respond. In step 16 you present the tone at 35 dB and the patient responds. You decrease the intensity to 25 dB and there is no response. Again, as you present the tone in 5-dB steps of increasing intensity the patient does not respond until the level of 40 dB is reached. Once more you decrease the intensity by 10 dB and then increase it in 5-dB steps, and the patient first responds at 35 dB. He has now responded twice at a minimum level of 40 dB and twice at 35 dB. You record his threshold as being 35 dB, since this is the minimum hearing level at which he responded correctly to the presence of the tone for at least 50 per cent of the trials. When there is doubt that the patient is responding appropriately 50 per cent of the time, the tester should record the next higher 5-dB step as the patient's threshold. If no consistent picture emerges from steps 14, 15, and 16, you had better start all over with step 9. The patient may have become confused as to what he is to listen for, and it may be necessary for you to give him a good "listen" before trying it again. In a later section of this chapter there will be further discussion of the term *threshold*.

17. Assuming that you have succeeded in getting a consistent threshold picture at 1000 Hz, change the frequency control to 500 Hz and start again at step 9. Next test at 250 Hz, and then (if time permits) at 125 Hz, although

very few audiologists believe there is any advantage to testing frequencies lower than 250 Hz. Allow the patient to "rest" while you record the threshold hearing level at each frequency.

18. Having obtained thresholds for the frequencies below 1000 Hz, test again at 1000 Hz. Pay no attention to the previous threshold obtained at this frequency until you have completed the steps necessary to obtain another threshold measurement. Then compare the second with the first threshold obtained. If they agree exactly, or differ by no more than 5 dB in either direction, you can be satisfied that the reliability of your test is adequate. You should then proceed to obtain threshold measurements for frequencies above 1000 Hz. If, on the other hand, there is a difference of 10 dB or more between your first and second threshold measurements at 1000 Hz, the reliability of the test is in doubt, and it would be advisable to repeat from the beginning, even to restating your instructions to the patient.

19. Ordinarily, one would test only the even octaves above and below 1000 Hz, except that frequently 6000 Hz would be the highest frequency tested. If the loss pattern at the octave intervals is uneven, it may be desirable to obtain thresholds at other mid-octave intervals: 750, 1500, and 3000 Hz. It is necessary to consider the patient's fatigue, however, in the testing situation. As the patient tires, the reliability and validity of your test suffer. It would be better to obtain accurate measures of the patient's hearing at the even-octave intervals than to have a complete test of all frequencies with questionable accuracy. Then, too, it is always possible to perform additional testing on the patient after an interval of rest or even on another day.

20. Special caution must be exercised in testing a patient at 8000 Hz, to make sure that his threshold is not influenced by standing waves. It will be recalled from Chapter 2 that, when a pure tone is introduced into a closed pipe of the same length as the wavelength of the tone, the reflected wave from the closed end of the pipe produces a cancellation effect. The cancellation results because the original tone and the reflected tone are 180 degrees out of phase. The wave is said to be "standing" because particle movement in the medium is at a standstill. The wavelength of a tone of 8000 Hz frequency is about one and one-half inches. When the diaphragm of an audiometer earphone is approximately one and a half inches from the eardrum, a standing wave might result, because the external canal and eardrum may be likened to a closed pipe. The cancellation effect of the standing wave thus minimizes the vibration of the eardrum. In other words, the patient may not respond to the test tone because of the standing wave rather than from a hearing loss at this frequency. If a patient presents an apparent hearing loss at 8000 Hz, a slight adjustment of the earphone away from the ear may cause the patient to respond at lower hearing levels. Moving the earphone breaks up the standing wave by altering the distance from the earphone diaphragm to the eardrum. Because of the problem of standing waves and also because audiometer earphones are least stable at very high frequencies, many audiologists

prefer not to test at 8000 Hz. Actually, the threshold at 8000 Hz contributes little to the clinical picture.

21. After completing the measurements on the first ear, switch the output selector to the opposite earphone and proceed in the same manner to obtain threshold hearing levels on the other ear.

22. If the threshold hearing levels of the second ear tested appear to differ by 40 dB or more from those of the first ear, you should repeat the test while masking the better ear in order to rule out its participation. Since in "cross-hearing" the non-test ear is apparently stimulated largely through the mechanism of bone conduction,[1] there may be occasions when the need for masking in air-conduction testing is not apparent until after bone-conduction threshold hearing levels have been determined. According to Studebaker, the need for masking is determined by comparing the air-conduction thresholds of the test ear with the bone-conduction thresholds of the contralateral (nontest) ear. Studebaker's rule is to use masking whenever differences between air-conduction threshold hearing levels of the test ear and bone-conduction threshold hearing levels of the contralateral ear equal or exceed 35 dB at 250 Hz, 40 to 45 dB at 500, 1000, or 2000 Hz, or 50 dB at 4000 Hz.[2] Thus, to cite an example, the difference between the ears in air-conduction threshold hearing levels may be only 25 to 30 dB—a magnitude of difference that ordinarily would cause no concern as to cross-hearing. Yet the difference between the air-conduction thresholds of the poorer ear and the bone-conduction thresholds of the better ear may be on the order of 45 to 50 dB. In such a circumstance, the air-conduction threshold hearing levels of the poorer ear should be measured again while the better ear is masked.

23. If masking is indicated, it is best to explain to the patient that you are going to introduce a noise to his better ear, so that you can obtain a more accurate measure of the hearing loss in his poorer ear. Caution the patient not to be distracted by the masking noise but to concentrate on listening for the tone and to signal as before when he hears it. Then turn on the masking switch of the audiometer. The selection of the intensity setting on the masking control dial may present a problem. There is no one setting that would be appropriate for all instances of masking. Moreover, it is seldom clear just what intensity values are indicated by the graduations on the masking control— sound pressure levels, hearing levels, or "effective masking" levels. While formulas for determining the proper levels of masking have been worked out,[3] they cannot be applied unless the examiner performs considerable experimentation with a given audiometer to develop information as to the effectiveness of various dial settings in masking tones in normal ears. The

[1] Josef Zwislocki, "Acoustic Attenuation Between the Ears," *Journal of the Acoustical Society of America,* Vol. 25 (July, 1953), pp. 752-759.

[2] Gerald A. Studebaker, "Clinical Masking of Air- and Bone-Conducted Stimuli," *Journal of Speech and Hearing Disorders,* Vol. 29 (February, 1964), p. 24.

[3] *Ibid.,* p. 29.

problem is to use sufficient masking intensity to prevent the masked ear from hearing the test tone, but not so much intensity that the masking noise affects the sensitivity of the test ear (overmasking). Overmasking is not likely to occur in air-conduction testing, since the *interaural attenuation*—the barrier to sound transmission from one ear to the other—in air-conduction testing, plus the amount of hearing loss in the ear under test, combine to protect the test ear from overmasking even at maximum intensity settings of the masking control on most audiometers. To be certain, however, you should experiment by obtaining thresholds in the ear under test while various levels of masking are tried on the contralateral ear. The technique of selecting the correct masking level through experimentation is discussed in the next section of this chapter. In bone-conduction testing, the selection of the "correct" intensity of masking is more critical.

24. If a choice of masking noises is available, it is best to use complex noise—consisting of a fundamental frequency of about 120 Hz and numerous harmonics—for masking at frequencies below 1000 Hz, and white noise for masking the frequencies of 1000 Hz and higher. In white noise there is more energy available at higher frequencies because of its uniform spectrum. If you have access to a narrow-band masker, which is furnished by some audiometer manufacturers as an accessory, this will provide the most efficient masking of all. For each test frequency a segment of noise with its maximum energy centered on the test frequency makes possible the masking of each frequency with a lesser amount of sound energy than is required with a wide-band masker. Thus, in addition to being more efficient, narrow-band masking is more comfortable for the patient.

25. Avoid spending a great deal of time on the test. The beginner usually makes the mistake of spending too much time on each frequency, in an effort to guarantee that he is obtaining the best possible threshold for the patient. Actually, the tester is probably unconsciously postponing the time when he must make the decision as to what the threshold hearing level is, because of lack of confidence in his testing ability. By prolonging the test, however, he is only defeating his purpose of striving for accuracy, since patients tire quickly in the testing situation, especially when they have to listen for any length of time to tones that are close to threshold levels. It is preferable, therefore, in the interest of testing accuracy, to proceed through a test rather quickly. For the average patient, no more than ten to fifteen minutes should be required to obtain air-conduction measurements for both ears.

26. Make sure, in operating the interrupter, that you do not fall into "rhythm patterns" that the patient can follow, even though he may not hear the test tone. The pattern of tonal presentations should be irregular, that is, one time the interrupter switch may be off for several seconds, and the next time it may be depressed almost immediately after it has been released. In any event, the patient should not be able to predict what the length of time of the next interruption will be.

27. Some ears *adapt* rapidly to a tone, that is, a tone becomes inaudible in a very short time. The purpose in seeking threshold by means of short bursts of tone is to avoid producing adaptation which, of course, would result in erroneous threshold determinations. It is best to limit the bursts of tone presented to durations of no more than one to two seconds. The silent intervals between tonal presentations permit recovery from any adaptation that might occur. Information as to the validity of a patient's responses is obtained by noticing how promptly he becomes aware of the presence of the tone, and also how promptly he indicates that the tone is inaudible. Some audiometers provide for automatic pulsing of the tone, so that every time the interrupter is depressed the tone goes "beep-beep-beep . . ." for as long as the interrupter is held down. For many patients the pulsed tone is easier to hear at near threshold levels. Of course the examiner can pulse a tone manually as well. On some audiometers there is provision for warbling a tone, that is, modulating its frequency over a range of several Hz. A warbled tone is easier to distinguish than a tone of fixed frequency, especially for the patient who confuses a test stimulus with his tinnitus. Sometimes a patient will continue to signal that he hears the tone after you have released the interrupter. On the other hand, he may signal that he hears the tone for only a fraction of the time that it is presented, that is, he may push the button and release it immediately before you have released the interrupter. If the patient's responses are inconsistent in either of these ways, it may be necessary to repeat the instructions to the patient that he is to signal as soon as he detects the presence of the tone and keep signaling as long as the tone is present. Even with the repetition of these instructions, there will be some patients whose responses pose a problem in interpretation for the tester. In such cases, the tester must exercise his best judgment in determining threshold and should note on the audiogram that the patient's responses were not consistent.

28. The method of threshold determination recommended here is based on the suggestions of Carhart and Jerger that determining threshold by an ascending method, that is, proceeding from inaudibility to audibility, is preferable to using a descending technique (proceeding from supra-threshold levels to inaudibility) or a combination of ascending and descending procedures.[4] Carhart and Jerger urge that all audiologists follow the same method for determining threshold so that test results will not be influenced by differences in test procedure. They suggest that the ascending technique, originally ascribed to Hughson and Westlake,[5] be used in preference to other techniques because of its long history and general acceptability to otologists and audiologists.

4 Raymond Carhart and James F. Jerger, "Preferred Method for Clinical Determination of Pure-Tone Thresholds," *Journal of Speech and Hearing Disorders*, Vol. 24 (November, 1959), pp. 330-345.
5 Walter Hughson and Harold Westlake, "Manual for Program Outline for Rehabilitation of Aural Casualties Both Military and Civilian," *Transactions of the American Academy of Ophthalmology and Otolaryngology Supplement*, Vol. 48 (1944), pp. 1-15,.

BONE-CONDUCTION TESTING

After the air-conduction tests, it is standard practice to administer bone-conduction tests on each ear. Of course, if the air-conduction tests disclose no hearing loss, it would be useless to subject the patient to bone-conduction tests, for you know already that his hearing is normal. The purpose of bone-conduction testing is to determine whether the loss detected in air-conduction testing is due to conductive or sensori-neural factors, or perhaps to a combination of the two. If the bone-conduction thresholds obtained are essentially normal, the loss is of the conductive type. On the other hand, if the bone-conduction measurements show losses that are equal to those obtained by air-conduction testing, the loss is of the sensori-neural type. If there is some loss by bone, but not as much as by air, the loss is a mixed one.

Bone-conduction testing is performed with a small hearing-aid type bone-conduction vibrator that is attached to a fabric-covered metal headband. The traditional method of testing bone conduction is to place the vibrator on the mastoid process of the temporal bone behind the pinna of the ear to be tested. More recently, new techniques of testing bone conduction have been suggested. These will be discussed at the conclusion of this section. The method to be described here in detail is the one involving mastoid placement of the vibrator, since at the present writing it is the procedure most commonly in use.

Some authorities recommend that masking be utilized routinely in every bone-conduction test in order to prevent the opposite ear from participating in the test. Whereas a difference in sensitivity of 40 to 50 dB between the ears by air conduction is necessary before the tone will be transferred to the opposite ear, a bone-conducted sound may be heard by the opposite ear if the difference is as slight as 10 to 15 dB, or even in some cases when there is no apparent difference between the ears in bone-conduction sensitivity. In other words, the interaural attenuation in bone-conduction testing varies from zero dB at 250 and 500 Hz to a maximum of 15 dB at 4000 Hz with values between zero and 15 db at 1000 and 2000 Hz. In both air- and bone-conduction testing, the opposite ear is stimulated through the mechanism of bone conduction. An air-conduction earphone, however, is not as efficient a transducer for bone conduction as is a vibrator that has been specifically designed for this purpose. Hence, in air-conduction testing, the interaural attenuation greatly exceeds that existing in bone-conduction testing.

Although, where there is doubt, masking should be used in bone-conduction testing, it is not always necessary to mask. In fact, sometimes it is sufficient to test only one ear. If a patient presents a bilateral loss pattern by air conduction and an unmasked bone-conduction test of one ear reveals threshold hearing levels that are approximately the same as those obtained by air conduction, it is unnecessary to test the bone conduction of the other ear. Because of the minimal interaural attenuation involved, you know that the bone-conduction threshold hearing levels of the other ear could not vary from those of the first ear tested by more than zero to 15 dB. On the other hand, if the initial bone-conduction threshold hearing levels indicate that there is a significant air-bone gap, that is, better hearing by bone conduction than by air conduction, it will be necessary to test the bone conduction of both ears, using masking at least on the "better" ear by bone conduction and perhaps on both ears. Even though there are equal air-conduction threshold hearing levels in each ear, the bone-conduction sensitivity of the two ears may be markedly different. The unmasked bone-conduction results reflect the ear with the more sensitive bone conduction, regardless of where the vibrator is placed.

The audiometric Weber test can be helpful in determining the need for masking.[6] Place the bone-conduction vibrator on the midline of the forehead and gradually increase the intensity of the tone until the patient reports that he can just barely hear it. Increase the intensity by 10 to 15 dB and then ask him if he hears the tone in one ear or the other, or if it seems to be equally loud in each ear, that is, unlocalized. If he reports that the tone lateralizes to one ear, masking should be delivered to that ear while the contralateral ear is tested by bone conduction. If he reports no lateralization at any frequency, probably the ears are equal in bone-conduction sensitivity. If the Weber test results are inconclusive or inconsistent, the examiner should employ contralateral masking when testing each ear, although in retrospect it may be determined that the unmasked bone-conduction threshold hearing levels were in fact valid. Incidentally, it should be mentioned that any use of masking—either in air-conduction or in bone-conduction testing—even at such low levels of intensity that overmasking is impossible will result in shifting the threshold of the test ear by 5 dB at each frequency. This phenomenon is called "central masking," because it apparently is a function of the central nervous system.[7] The examiner should subtract 5 dB from bone-conduction threshold hearing levels obtained with contralateral masking as a correction for central masking.

As stated earlier, various formulas for determining the "correct" amount of masking have been developed, but none has received universal acceptance. The following procedure is suggested as an empirical method that can be applied regardless of how the masking noise is calibrated on a particular audiometer. It is an adaptation of the "plateau" method suggested by Hood[8] and described in detail by Studebaker.[9] The examiner must arbitrarily select a given level of masking with which to begin the testing. For example, suppose that he selects a setting of 60 dB on the masking control dial, regard-

6 D. M. Markle, E. P. Fowler, Jr., and H. Molouquet, "The Audiometric Weber Test as a Means for Determining the Need for and the Type of Masking," *Annals of Otology, Rhinology, and Laryngology*, Vol. 61 (September, 1952), pp. 888-900.

7 Studebaker, *op. cit.*, p. 24.

8 J. D. Hood, "The Principles and Practice of Bone Conduction Audiometry," *Laryngoscope*, Vol. 70 (1960), pp. 1211-1228.

9 Studebaker, *op. cit.*, pp. 29-33.

less of what actual intensity value that setting may be. The examiner then proceeds to obtain a bone-conduction threshold hearing level of the ear under test while that level of masking is applied to the opposite ear. He should then increase the level of the masking noise by 10 dB and again obtain a threshold on the ear under test. If the threshold hearing levels are the same regardless of whether the masking control is set at 60 or at 70 dB, he can be assured that the level of the masking noise is not interfering with the ear under test. If, on the other hand, the threshold hearing level in the ear under test should increase by 10 dB when 70 dB of masking is applied, there may be two explanations: (1) the contralateral ear was insufficiently masked with 60 dB of masking, so that the threshold obtained with that amount of contralateral masking was underestimating the amount of loss present; or (2) the increase in the level of the masking noise caused an interference with the ear under test, and the threshold obtained with 70 dB of masking was an overestimation of the amount of loss. To determine which explanation is correct, it is necessary for the examiner to continue increasing the level of the masking noise and to obtain a threshold of the ear under test at each 10-dB increase in masking. If the threshold in the ear being tested increases proportionately with the increases in level of the masking noise, the examiner knows that the masking noise is too intense, and was too intense at the point where the threshold began to increase in proportion to increases in the masking level. When the proper level of masking is attained, an increase or decrease of 10 dB in the masking noise will not affect the threshold of the ear under test. In other words, the "plateau" will have been reached and the bone-conduction threshold of the ear under test should remain stable over a range of at least 20 dB in masking noise. It is the examiner's responsibility, through experimentation, to locate the level of the masking noise within this range. This experimentation must be conducted at each frequency to be tested by bone conduction, as the same level of masking may not be suitable for all the frequencies tested.

In bone-conduction testing, it is important that the room noise be at a minimum, especially if the patient's air-conduction loss is slight. In a normal ear, it is almost impossible to obtain zero-dB bone-conduction threshold hearing levels except in the very quietest of soundproof rooms, since any sounds heard by air conduction serve to mask the bone-conducted tones. It may not be feasible, therefore, to check the calibration of the bone-conduction vibrator on a normal ear. Rather, it should be checked on ears known to have pure sensori-neural losses, by comparing the obtained air- and bone-conduction threshold hearing levels. With such patients, the differences between the thresholds obtained by air and by bone should average out to zero.

In routine testing, whenever substantially greater losses are obtained by bone conduction than by air conduction, the examiner should suspect the level of room noise, the calibration of the vibrator, or the validity of the patient's responses. Theoretically, it is not possible for a patient to have greater losses by bone than by air. There are many variables operating in bone conduction, however, which may combine to give a confusing picture of the patient's bone-conduction sensitivity. In addition to the factors of room noise and vibrator calibration, the thickness of the skin and tissue covering the mastoid bone and the degree of *pneumatization* of the mastoid itself affect the sensitivity of the individual to bone-conducted sound. The type of bone in the mastoid and the thickness of its covering are factors obviously beyond the control of the examiner. Since bone-conduction vibrators must be calibrated for the "average" mastoid, one must expect variations both above and below the average. The examiner, therefore, should not be concerned if, with a given patient, bone-conduction threshold hearing levels are obtained that are greater than air-conduction threshold hearing levels by no more than 10 to 15 dB. The examiner should bear in mind also that with a particular patient, bone-conduction thresholds that are better than air-conduction thresholds by 10 to 15 dB do not necessarily mean that there is an actual air-bone gap signifying some conductive component.[10]

Bone-conduction vibrators are more limited in their sound-transmission characteristics than are air-conduction earphones. For this reason, it is not possible to test by bone conduction all frequencies tested by air. Generally, audiometer manufacturers recommend bone-conduction testing only from 250 through 4000 Hz. Many examiners will check bone conduction only at 500, 1000, 2000, and 4000 Hz. At 250 Hz, the patient may respond to the vibrations of the vibrator without actually hearing the tone. For this reason, bone-conduction testing at 250 Hz may produce misleading results.

Audiometers are calibrated differently for air-conduction and bone-conduction testing. More power must be delivered to the bone-conduction vibrator than to the air-conduction earphone in order to reach the threshold of the normal ear. Consequently, bone-conduction hearing levels are measured only up to 65 or 70 dB. Usually a notation will be found on the hearing-level control of an audiometer indicating the maximum hearing level for bone conduction at each frequency.

The step-by-step procedures in bone-conduction testing are similar to those detailed above for air-conduction testing.

1. Explain to the patient that now you are going to check his hearing by bone conduction, that is, determine how well he hears sounds conducted through the mastoid bone. Explain that the sounds he hears will be the same as those he has been tested with already, and that he can signal to you in the same manner in which he has been signaling.

2. Theoretically, the better ear should be tested first, as in air-conduction testing. It is difficult if not impossible for a patient to tell which ear is the better by bone conduction. It is possible that the ear that is poorer by air conduction may be better by bone conduction, as in a unilateral conductive impairment, for example. Therefore, in order to determine which is the better ear by bone conduction, it may be desirable to perform the audiometric

[10] Gerald A. Studebaker, "Intertest Variability and the Air-Bone Gap," *Journal of Speech and Hearing Disorders,* Vol. 32 (February, 1967), pp. 82-86.

Weber test, as mentioned previously. If neither ear is "better," it makes no difference which is tested first.

3. Place the bone-conduction vibrator carefully, so that it is making good, solid contact with the mastoid bone. Avoid having the vibrator touch the pinna. It may be necessary for you to experiment with the placement of the vibrator while the patient listens to a test tone, until you are sure that the vibrator is properly placed for maximum sensitivity of the patient.

4. If you are not employing masking during the bone-conduction testing, do *not* cover the opposite ear with an air-conduction earphone. To do so would create a moderate degree of air-conduction loss in the opposite ear, and might cause the tone produced by the vibrator to refer to the covered ear, just as a Weber tuning-fork test causes the tone to refer to the ear that has the greater conductive loss. In Europe it is customary to perform bone-conduction tests with both ears occluded. The thresholds thus obtained are called *absolute* bone-conduction thresholds, as contrasted with *relative* bone-conduction thresholds obtained with the ears uncovered. With normal ears, the difference between absolute and relative bone conduction (the "occlusion effect") exceeds 20 dB at 250 and 500 Hz, amounts to about 15 dB at 1000 Hz, and is negligible (less than 5 dB) at 2000 and 4000 Hz.[11] In this country it is customary to obtain relative bone-conduction measurements. Therefore, both ears should be uncovered during bone-conduction tests, unless, of course, masking of the opposite ear is being employed.

5. Follow the same routine of testing as was suggested for the air-conduction test: test first at 1000 Hz; sweep up, down, and up again in intensity, bracketing the threshold; then find the threshold point by means of the interrupter and by changing the intensity of the tone in the manner suggested in air-conduction testing. Next, test the frequency or frequencies below 1000 Hz, recheck 1000 Hz, and then test the frequencies above 1000 Hz. After testing one ear, switch the bone-conduction vibrator to the other mastoid and repeat the test procedure. If masking is required, determine the correct amount through experimentation, as described earlier in this section.

6. Tell the patient that he may have the sensation of hearing the test tone in the ear not being tested, and that if this occurs he should inform you. Sometimes, even when maximum masking is employed, the patient will insist that he hears the tone in the ear not being tested. Theoretically, he should not be able to hear the tone on the ear which is being masked, provided, of course, that the masking has an appropriate spectrum and is sufficiently intense. No one can say for certain, however, that the patient is not reporting what is actually happening. In such circumstances, the only thing that the examiner can do is to record the obtained results of the test, with the notation that even with maximum masking the patient reported that he heard the tone in the ear not under test.

Some audiometers are equipped so that bone-conduction testing may be

11 Scott N. Reger, "Pure-Tone Audiometry," in Aram Glorig, ed., *Audiometry: Principles and Practices* (Baltimore, Williams & Wilkins, 1965), p. 128.

performed in a different fashion. It was Rainville who first suggested a method of bone-conduction testing that was designed to avoid the problems of lateralization of the bone-conducted signal to the contralateral ear and the difficulties of masking in bone-conduction testing.[12] Rainville suggested that bone-conduction hearing level could be determined by comparing the amount of masking required to mask a pure-tone signal delivered at threshold through an air-conduction earphone when (1) a white noise was delivered through the same air-conduction earphone as the signal, and (2) the masking noise was delivered through a bone-conduction vibrator on the mastoid of the ear receiving the pure-tone signal.

Following Rainville's lead, investigators in this country developed tests in which the masking noise was introduced through the bone-conduction vibrator while the pure-tone signals were delivered through an air-conduction earphone. Jerger and Tillman called their test SAL (for sensori-neural acuity level),[13] while Lightfoot[14] called his test M-R for Modified-Rainville. Both of these methods are similar. There are two main differences between the SAL and M-R tests and the Rainville method: the SAL and M-R tests utilize the middle of the forehead for vibrator placement, and they determine bone-conduction hearing levels by comparing threshold shifts produced by the bone-conducted masking noise in normal-hearing subjects and in patients. In terms of popularity, the SAL test is the preferred method of assessing bone-conduction hearing with the masking noise delivered to the bone-conduction vibrator, so it will be described here.

The SAL test requires a standard pure-tone audiometer, a noise generator, and a bone-conduction vibrator. The bone-conduction vibrator, connected to the noise generator, is placed on the patient's forehead, and the headset containing the two air-conduction earphones connected to the audiometer is placed on the patient's head. The first step is to obtain the patient's air-conduction thresholds in each ear without any noise delivered to the bone-conduction vibrator. While the whole range of audiometric frequencies can be tested, Jerger and Tillman suggest that the frequencies between 250 and 4000 Hz are the most useful for purposes of the SAL test.[15] Next the air-conduction measurements are repeated with the noise turned on. Then what Jerger and Tillman term the "sensorineural loss" at each frequency in each ear is determined by subtracting the threshold shift produced by the noise from the amount of shift normal-hearing individuals experience under these conditions. In obtaining their norms, Jerger and Tillman sought a noise intensity that would result in threshold shifts of approximately 50 dB for

[12] M. J. Rainville, "New Method of Masking for the Determination of Bone Conduction Curves," *Translations of the Beltone Institute for Hearing Research*, No. 11 (July, 1959).

[13] James Jerger and Tom Tillman, "A New Method for the Clinical Determination of Sensorineural Acuity Level (SAL)" *A.M.A. Archives of Otolaryngology*, Vol. 71 (June, 1960), pp. 948-955.

[14] Charles Lightfoot, "The M-R Test of Bone-Conduction Hearing," *Laryngoscope*, Vol. 70 (November, 1960), pp. 1552-1559.

[15] Jerger and Tillman, *op. cit.*, p. 950.

the frequencies from 1000 through 4000 Hz. They determined experimentally that when the noise level resulted in a signal strength of 2 volts across the vibrator the desirable amount of threshold shift occurred in normal ears. According to their norms, this signal strength of the noise resulted in air-conduction threshold shifts of 20 dB at 250 Hz, 45 dB at 500 Hz and 50 dB at 1000, 2000, and 4000 Hz. These, then, are the norms from which the threshold shifts obtained with patients at a noise level of 2 volts at the vibrator are subtracted to determine sensori-neural loss (bone-conduction threshold hearing levels). Testing an experimental group of patients with pure sensori-neural hearing losses, Jerger and Tillman determined that the SAL technique is at least as good as conventional bone-conduction audiometry in measuring sensori-neural loss. The principal advantage of the SAL technique over conventional bone-conduction audiometry is that the method eliminates the problem of whether or not to mask the contralateral ear and how much masking to use. Both inner ears are stimulated with the vibrator at the midline of the skull, and the ears are isolated by the amount of difference in sensitivity required before an air-conducted signal will cross over from the test ear to the opposite ear (40 to 60 dB). Because masking in conventional bone-conduction audiometry presents problems to so many clinicians, the SAL test offers many advantages for clinical use.

In the years following the description of the SAL technique by Jerger and Tillman, a number of articles appeared, some praising and some criticizing the method. Even Tillman concluded that "the SAL test cannot be viewed as an adequate substitute for properly applied bone-conduction tests."[16] In an effort to resolve the questions concerning the clinical utility of the SAL test, Jerger and Jerger undertook a "systematic evaluation" of the test that concluded that the original recommended procedure for SAL audiometry produced results that were valid and equivalent to bone-conduction results obtained with both conductive and sensori-neural losses, provided that the conditions for both methods were comparable. Since the SAL technique requires the occlusion of the test ear with an earphone, the results of the SAL test should be compared with conventional bone-conduction thresholds obtained with the test ear occluded, or in other words, with absolute rather than with relative bone-conduction thresholds. If SAL results are compared with relative bone-conduction thresholds, then there will be disagreements between the two methods in some instances.[17]

One modification of conventional bone-conduction testing that is gaining increasing acceptance is the use of forehead placement of the bone-conduction vibrator. Since both cochleas are stimulated with almost equal loudness when the vibrator is placed on either mastoid, it seems logical to place

16 Tom W. Tillman, *A Critical View of the SAL Test*, Technical Documentary Report No. SAM-TDR-62-96 (August, 1962), School of Aerospace Medicine, Brooks Air Force Base, Texas, p. 2.

17 James Jerger and Susan Jerger, "Critical Evaluation of SAL Audiometry," *Journal of Speech and Hearing Research*, Vol. 8 (June, 1965), pp. 103-127.

the vibrator midway between the ears and eliminate the involvement of the nontest ear through the use of masking, particularly since the frontal bone provides a better surface for the vibrator than the rounded mastoid process. Moreover, the vibrator can be left in place while testing both ears. The disadvantage to forehead placement is that more signal intensity is required to obtain bone-conduction hearing levels at the forehead, so that the range of hearing levels that can be measured is more limited at the forehead than at the mastoid. Several investigators have reported differences between forehead and mastoid bone-conduction threshold hearing levels obtained with normal ears. The means of the differences obtained in six studies as reported by Dirks, Malmquist, and Bower are shown in Table 5-1.[18] The values in Table 5-1 represent zero-dB hearing level at each frequency for forehead placement when the test ear is not occluded and appropriate masking is applied to the nontest ear. Martin presents a strong case for the routine clinical use of forehead placement of the vibrator and occlusion of both ears with air-conduction earphones. He points out that the occlusion effect compensates for the loss of sensitivity resulting from forehead placement, thus making available the full range of bone-conduction hearing levels present in the traditional mastoid placement of the vibrator.[19]

Table 5-1. Differences in dB between thresholds of normal ears obtained by forehead and by mastoid placement of the bone-conduction vibrator.

		Frequency (Hz)		
250	500	1000	2000	4000
14.6	14.3	9.2	9.5	5.5

Studebaker[20] and Dirks and Malmquist[21] report that in testing ears with various conductive impairments lower (better) bone-conduction hearing levels on the average can be obtained with forehead placement of the vibrator than with mastoid placement. Dirks and Malmquist divided their conductively impaired group into subgroups according to surgically confirmed middle-ear pathology and compared bone-conduction hearing levels obtained with forehead placement and with mastoid placement in each subgroup. Their results suggest that the differences in bone-conduction sensitivity by the two methods of testing may have diagnostic significance in differentiating the locus of pathology in conductive impairments.

Before leaving the subject of bone-conduction testing with all its complexities of masking, cross-hearing, interaural attenuation, and occlusion

[18] Donald D. Dirks, Carol W. Malmquist, and Deborah R. Bower, "Toward the Specification of Normal Bone-Conduction Threshold," *Journal of the Acoustical Society of America,* Vol. 43 (June, 1968), p. 1241.

[19] Frederick N. Martin, "Evidence for the Use of Occluded Forehead Bone Conduction," *Journal of Speech and Hearing Disorders,* Vol. 34 (August, 1969), pp. 260-266.

[20] Gerald A. Studebaker, "Placement of Vibrator in Bone-Conduction Testing," *Journal of Speech and Hearing Research,* Vol. 5 (December, 1962), pp. 321-331.

[21] Donald D. Dirks and Carolyn M. Malmquist, "Comparison of Frontal and Mastoid Bone-Conduction Thresholds in Various Conductive Lesions," *Journal of Speech and Hearing Research,* Vol. 12 (December, 1969), pp. 725-746.

effect, some mention should be made of the influence exerted by the earphone and its cushion on audiometric results. Interaural attenuation or its reciprocal—the level at which cross-hearing occurs—is dependent on the area of the head making contact with the earphone cushion. The greater the area of contact, the lower the amount of interaural attenuation and the lower the level at which cross-hearing occurs.[22] The occlusion effect is dependent on the volume of air trapped under the cushion. The greater the volume the lesser the occlusion of the ear and the lesser the occlusion effect.[23]

The earphone most commonly employed in audiometry today is the Telephonics TDH-39 mounted in an MX41/AR cushion. Such an earphone and cushion combination is called a *supra-aural* phone, because it fits over the ear. The area of the cushion making contact with the head is relatively large, and the volume of air under the cushion is relatively small. The earphone and cushion effectively occlude the ear, and we know that the interaural attenuation they provide is on the order of 40 to 60 dB.

Interaural attenuation can be substantially increased by using an insert phone, which is a hearing-aid type receiver attached to an earpiece that inserts in the meatus. Such a phone is useful for introducing masking to the nontest ear, since the chances of overmasking are reduced owing to its superior isolation characteristics.

To eliminate or substantially reduce the occlusion effect, an earphone-cushion combination that encloses a large volume of air—on the order of 1500 to 2000 cc—is desirable. Perhaps the most popular such combination is the Pedersen, which has a small loudspeaker mounted in a spherical enclosure. Since the enclosure goes around the ear instead of over it, the Pedersen is called a *circumaural* earphone. When Jerger and Jerger wished to compare SAL results with relative bone-conduction thresholds, they used Pedersen earphones to obtain unmasked and masked air-conduction thresholds.[24]

At present, the use of insert receivers and circumaural earphones is restricted largely to audiological research activities. The standard earphone mounted in an MX41/AR cushion is not likely to be replaced for routine clinical uses.

MAINTENANCE OF THE AUDIOMETER

The accuracy of testing depends upon the proper functioning of the audiometric equipment, as well as upon the skill of the audiometrist and the adequacy of the testing room. Audiometers must be calibrated at regular intervals to insure that the frequency and hearing-level outputs are actually

---

[22] Zwislocki, *op. cit.*, p. 755.

[23] Ralph F. Naunton, "The Measurement of Hearing by Bone Conduction," in James Jerger, ed. *Modern Developments in Audiology* (New York, Academic Press, 1963), p. 21.

[24] Jerger and Jerger *op. cit.*, pp. 105-106.

as indicated on the controls. Manufacturers recommend that audiometers which are given hard usage be sent to the factory for calibration and cleaning every year. Actually, it is not necessary to send the audiometer to the factory until it is apparent that the instrument is not in calibration and unless it is not feasible to apply corrections to measurements that are in error. The audiometer can be cleaned by any radio serviceman. The most important part to clean is the attenuator. When the contacts of the attenuator are dirty, static is produced in the earphone when the hearing-level control is rotated back and forth. This static is annoying to the patient and may even be mistaken by the patient for the stimulus to which he should respond.

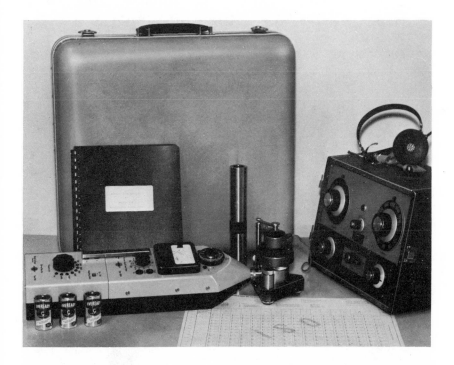

Figure 5-2. Checking the intensity calibration of an audiometer with an artificial ear. (Reproduced by permission of B & K Instruments, Inc., Cleveland, Ohio.)

Intensity calibration is accomplished by varying the resistance in the output circuits of the audiometer's oscillators (pure-tone generators) so that the desired output at the earphone is obtained in a 6 cc coupler and read off the dial on an *artificial ear*. An artificial ear couples the earphone from the audiometer with a precision-made condenser microphone of known characteristics. The coupler is so constructed that its volume approximates the volume of the external canal and middle ear plus the air between the earphone diaphragm and the opening of the canal.[25] The microphone output is led to a sound-level meter. The audiometer being calibrated is set at a prescribed hearing level for a particular frequency, and the oscillator for that frequency is adjusted until the output, as determined by the reading on the sound-level meter, agrees with the specified value for that frequency and hearing-level dial setting. Figures 5-2 and 5-3 illustrate one type of artificial ear.

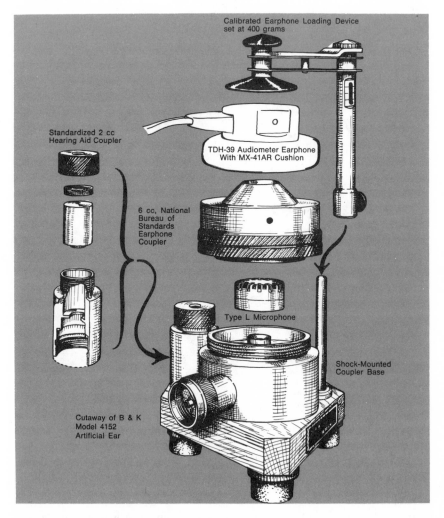

Figure 5-3.   Details of the artificial ear attachment for the sound-level meter. (Reproduced by permission of B & K Instruments, Inc., Cleveland, Ohio.)

[25] Hallowell Davis, "Audiometry: Pure Tone and Simple Speech Tests," in Hallowell Davis and S. Richard Silverman, eds., *Hearing and Deafness* (New York, Holt, Rinehart and Winston, 1970), p. 192.

The American National Standards Institute of New York City (ANSI) publishes standards for manufacturers of various kinds of measuring equipment, including audiometers. ANSI was formerly known as the American Standards Association (ASA) and for a brief period as the United States of America Standards Institute (USASI). In a 1951 publication (Z24.5–1951) the association specified the sound pressure level for audiometric zero at each octave interval on the audiometer, based on the results of hearing tests conducted during a health survey by the U.S. Public Health Service in 1935–36.[26] These levels, employed by audiometer manufacturers in this country until 1964, were known both as the "American standard" and the "ASA–1951 standard" for audiometric zero. Subsequent hearing surveys of large populations conducted at state and world's fairs tended to confirm the adequacy of the Beasley findings as representing "average normal hearing."[27]

Studies that were performed under better-controlled testing conditions, however, in this country and abroad, indicated that average "normal" hearing might be as much as 10 to 15 dB "better" than the ASA–1951 standards for audiometric zero. Many European countries adopted sound pressure levels for audiometric zero that differed from our American standards. For several years, scientists from various countries met under the aegis of the International Standards Organization (ISO) in an effort to agree on the sound pressure levels to define audiometric zero, or, in other words, to write an international standard for audiometer calibration. Finally this task was accomplished in 1964. The American representatives to the International Standards Organization recommended that the international standards be adopted in this country beginning January 1, 1965. Many scientific associations, including the American Speech and Hearing Association, endorsed the new standards—referred to as ISO–1964 standards—and agreed to implement them immediately.

Between 1964 and 1969 there was much confusion in the audiological world regarding audiometer calibration and audiometric data. It was necessary for manufacturers to indicate to which standards their products were calibrated and for audiologists, otologists, and others reporting test results to specify whether their results were based on ASA–1951 or ISO–1964 standards. Many audiogram forms used in this period contained both an ASA–1951 ordinate and an ISO–1964 ordinate, so the recorded hearing levels could be referred to the ordinate of choice. Some audiogram forms contained instructions as to the number of decibels to add or subtract to correct one standard to the other. Fortunately, the confusion should now be ended, since the American National Standards Institute has published a

26 Willis C. Beasley, *National Health Survey (1935–36), Preliminary Reports, Hearing Study Series, Bulletins 1-7* (Washington, D.C., U.S. Public Health Service, 1938).

27 J. Donald Harris, "Steps Toward an International Audiometric Zero," in "Identification Audiometry," *Journal of Speech and Hearing Disorders,* Monograph Supplement 9 (September, 1961), p. 66.

revised set of standards that replaces the ASA–1951 standards with the ISO–1964 recommendations, so now this country is officially "in step" with the other countries of the world that have accepted the ISO–1964 levels.[28] Table 5-2 contains the new standards and, for comparison's sake, the old American standards and the differences between the new and the old.

Table 5-2. Sound pressure levels in dB re 0.0002 dyne/cm² for audiometric zero according to present and former American standards. Adapted from Fred W. Kranz, "Audiometer Principles and History," *Sound*, Vol. 2 (March–April, 1963), p. 31, and reproduced by permission. Values are rounded to the nearest $\frac{1}{2}$ dB.

Frequency Hz	Present American Standard (ANSI–1969, same as ISO–1964)	Former American Standard (ASA–1951)	Differences
125	45.5	54.5	9.0
250	24.5	39.5	15.0
500	11.0	25.0	14.0
1000	6.5	16.5	10.0
1500	6.5		
2000	8.5	17.0	8.5
3000	7.5		
4000	9.0	15.0	6.0
6000	8.0		
8000	9.5	21.0	11.5

The calibration of an audiometer and its earphones can be checked at any time by means of the artificial ear, comparing the obtained meter readings with those which are specified for correct calibration. Portable artificial ears are on the market, so that in many cities the calibration of audiometers can be checked without the necessity of sending the audiometer to the factory. Some hearing centers possess their own artificial ears and regularly check the calibration of their audiometers. If an audiometer is discovered to be out of calibration, a correction chart must be prepared, the audiometer must be recalibrated by a qualified technician, or it must be sent to a factory-authorized repair station for recalibration.

The results of the calibration check made on an audiometer should be recorded on a form such as that shown in Figure 5-4. Checks are made at each frequency at the attenuator (hearing-level control) setting prescribed by the manufacturer of the artificial ear. The instruction book that accompanies the artificial ear will specify the meter readings that should be obtained at each frequency for the particular earphone and cushion being tested. This value should be recorded on the chart for each frequency, so that obtained readings can be compared with specified values

[28] "American National Standard Specifications for Audiometers" (ANSI S3.6–1969, New York, American National Standards Institute, Inc., 1970).

AUDIOMETER CALIBRATION

Date: July 23, 1970
Calibration Unit: B & K
Calibrated by: E. Jones

Audiometer: Beltone 10-D, #20324
Earphone: TDH-39
Cushion: MX41/AR

EARPHONE OUTPUT CHECK AT 70-dB HEARING LEVEL

Test Frequency	Normal Calibration Level ANSI-1969 for TDH-39	Left Earphone			Right Earphone		
		Measured Level	Error	Correction	Measured Level	Error	Correction
125	115.0	114.2	-0.8	0	114.0	-1.0	0
250	95.5	95.7	+0.2	0	95.5	0.0	0
500	81.5	82.8	+1.3	0	81.8	+0.3	0
1000	77.0	78.8	+1.8	0	79.0	+2.0	0
1500	76.5	77.0	+0.5	0	76.4	-0.1	0
2000	79.0	78.4	-0.6	0	78.8	-0.2	0
3000	80.0	80.2	+0.2	0	81.0	+1.0	0
4000	79.5	80.2	+0.7	0	81.2	+1.7	0
6000	85.5	82.6	-2.9	-5	84.8	-0.7	0
8000	83.0	84.1	+1.1	0	85.9	+2.9	+5

Figure 5-4. Recording the results of a calibration check.

and the error at each frequency can be computed. Usually calibration checks are made at each frequency at a hearing-level dial setting of 70 dB in order to avoid any possible interference from room noise or internal noise from the artificial ear. The specified artificial ear meter reading at each frequency will not be exactly 70 plus the ANSI–1969 SPL value in most cases, however, because the earphones furnished with audiometers differ in their response characteristics from the Western Electric 705-A earphone specified in the ANSI–1969 standard. Reference threshold values for various makes of commercially available earphones are based on loudness-balance studies of those particular earphones with the Western Electric 705-A and are given in an appendix to the published ANSI–1969 standard.[29]

Once the error is determined at each frequency, a correction chart can be prepared, showing corrections to apply to hearing-level dial readings, so that the thresholds to be recorded will be correct to the nearest 5-dB step. In order to correct the audiometer hearing-level dial readings to the nearest 5-dB step the correction is applied in the same direction as the error; that is, if there is an error of − 6.3 dB at a particular frequency, meaning that the earphone output is 6.3 dB less than it should be at that hearing-level dial setting, the appropriate correction would be to subtract 5 dB from an obtained hearing level before recording the threshold on the audiogram. A correction chart should be secured to the face of the audiometer, so that anyone using the instrument will know what corrections must be made before recording thresholds. A calibration check must be made on each earphone, and if the audiometer being checked is a two-channel instrument, each earphone must be checked with each channel.

With some artificial ears it is possible to run checks on the linearity of the attenuator. An attenuator check consists of measuring the changes in voltage that occur in the earphone circuit or the changes in sound level pressure that occur in the coupler when the hearing-level control is rotated. If the attenuator is functioning properly, the meter on the artificial ear should show exactly 5 dB of change in voltage or sound pressure level when the hearing-level control is shifted one 5-dB step. The attenuator should be checked over its entire range. The calibration check of the audiometer output at each frequency yields an error value that may apply only at the hearing level at which the check was conducted, usually 70 dB. If there is an attenuator problem, the correction computed on the basis of the output check may not be at all appropriate for other attenuator settings at that frequency. If the attenuator is found to be seriously in error, that is, if some of the intensity steps should be found to differ by more than 2.5 dB from the 5 dB they should be, the audiometer should be returned to the factory for repair or replacement of the attenuator.

It is possible for an audiometrist to keep check on the calibration of his equipment even though he does not have access to an artificial ear. Every

[29] *Ibid.*, p. 21.

audiometrist should constantly be aware of the possibility that his audiometer may not be functioning properly. Before giving a test, he should check his own responses to the frequency of 1000 Hz as he decreases intensity until he reaches his threshold. Every few days he should check his responses to all the test frequencies. Since the audiometrist presumably knows his own hearing-level pattern, he can thus spot gross deviations in audiometer output.

Another method of checking the calibration of an audiometer requires a second audiometer that is known to be in calibration. The procedure here is for the audiometrist to set the calibrated audiometer at a given frequency and hearing level, set the other audiometer at the same frequency, and then, without looking at the dial setting, adjust the hearing-level control until his ear tells him that the loudness of the tones produced by the two audio-meters is approximately equal. He then checks the hearing-level dial setting on the audiometer he has been adjusting. If the dial setting is different from that of the calibrated audiometer, a correction is indicated. For example, suppose the audiometrist sets the calibrated instrument at 2000 Hz and a hearing level of 70 dB. He then sets the other audiometer at 2000 Hz and, without watching the dial setting, adjusts the hearing-level control until he judges that the loudness of the tone in the earphone is the same as the loudness of the tone in the earphone of the calibrated instrument. He makes this loudness balance judgment by listening alternatively to the earphones from the two audiometers, using only one ear in the process. Let us say in this illustration that he finds the audiometer being checked agrees in loudness with the calibrated audiometer at 2000 Hz when the hearing-level control is set at 75 dB. There is thus a 5-dB difference in output at this frequency. On the correction chart, the audiometrist would indicate that, at 2000 Hz, 5 dB should be subtracted from the indicated hearing level. The same procedure would be followed for all frequencies—balancing the loudness of output of the two audiometers, with the calibrated instrument, of course, being the standard.

It should be noted that in the loudness balance method of calibration the direction of the correction is apparently opposite that of the error, in contrast to checks with an artificial ear where the sign of the correction is the same as the sign of the error. Actually there is no difference in principle between the two methods. In the example just cited, it was necessary to set the hearing-level control of the audiometer being checked to 75 dB to match the loudness of the calibrated audiometer at 70 dB. In other words, the output level of the audiometer being checked was too low at a dial reading of 70 dB. The error measured with an artificial ear would be a minus one, calling for a correction to be subtracted from an obtained hearing level before recording a threshold on an audiogram.

An audiometer may get out of calibration because of changing character-istics of some electronic components: tubes, transistors, resistors, or condensers, or, as is more likely, the earphones may be damaged through dropping or rough handling, so that they do not respond as they did when the instrument was last calibrated. The earphones are the weakest link in the audiometric chain, and they should always be handled with care. When the audiometer comes from the manufacturer, it has been calibrated to the particular earphones that accompany it. It is not possible to substitute other phones without jeopardizing the calibration, since the factory has selected phones that are closely matched in output at all frequencies. From time to time loudness balance checks should be made with the two earphones, to make sure that they are producing the same output at a given hearing-level setting at all frequencies. If significant differences are found between the two earphones, it is better to send the audiometer to the factory or to an authorized repair service for recalibration with new earphones than to attempt to correct for the errors in either earphone.

Checking on the calibration of the audiometer for bone-conduction testing is more difficult than checking the air-conduction calibration. Attempts have been made to develop an *artificial mastoid,* so that instrumental checks of bone-conduction vibrator output can be made in a comparable fashion to the artificial ear measurements of the output of air-conduction earphones. Weiss described the development of an artificial mastoid for the Beltone Company which is now being produced commercially.[30] A working group of the International Standard Organization is engaged in developing standards for calibrating bone-conduction vibrators. Until these standards are published, those concerned with the specification of audiometric zero for bone conduction may be guided by the recommendations of the Standards Committee of the Hearing Aid Industry Conference (HAIC). These recommendations specify the root-mean-square (rms) force levels in dB re 1.0 dyne for audiometric zero at each frequency as measured with the Beltone Model 5 artificial mastoid when the vibrator is used on the subject's mastoid and the nontest ear is appropriately masked.[31] The "HAIC Interim Bone Calibration" is based on data accumulated from several laboratories in this country. Studies of "normal" bone conduction performed since the publication of the HAIC interim standard show reasonably good agreement with the recommended artificial mastoid values.[32]

Since relatively few clinics have access to artificial mastoids, audiometrists must keep check themselves on the calibration of their bone-conduction vibrators. The best way is to have available two or three patients who are

[30] Erwin Weiss, "An Air Damped Artificial Mastoid," *Journal of the Acoustical Society of America,* Vol. 32 (December, 1960), pp. 1582-1588.

[31] S. F. Lybarger, "Interim Bone Conduction Thresholds for Audiometry," *Journal of Speech and Hearing Research,* Vol. 9 (December, 1966), pp. 483-487.

[32] Peter B. Weston, Roy W. Gengel, and Ira J. Hirsh,"Effects of Vibrator Types and Their Placement on Bone-Conduction Threshold Measurements," *Journal of the Acoustical Society of America,* Vol. 41 (April, 1967), pp. 788-792.

Wayne O. Olsen, "Comparison of Studies on Bone Conduction Thresholds and the HAIC Interim Standard for Bone Conduction Audiometry," *Journal of Speech and Hearing Disorders,* Vol. 34 (February, 1969), pp. 54-57.

known to have pure sensori-neural losses of mild to moderate degree. By definition, then, their bone-conduction hearing levels should exactly equal their air-conduction hearing levels. If the audiometrist is confident that his audiometer is properly calibrated for air-conduction testing, or if he can correct for any known errors in output, he need only compare air- and bone-conduction threshold hearing levels on a few patients with sensori-neural impairment to check on the output of the bone-conduction vibrator. Because of differences in patients' responses to bone-conducted sounds, owing to the differences in conductivity of skin and bone among different individuals, the threshold hearing levels by air and by bone should be averaged for the patients cooperating in the study and the averages should be compared rather than comparing the individual measures of air and bone for each patient. Thus, if at 500 Hz the average air-conduction hearing level for the patients was 25 dB and the average bone-conduction hearing level was 30 dB, the audiometrist would conclude that the bone-conduction vibrator was producing a signal at this frequency which was 5 dB too weak. On his correction chart, he would indicate that 5 dB should be subtracted from the obtained bone-conduction hearing level at 500 Hz. Naturally, the success of this method of checking the calibration of the bone-conduction vibrator depends upon the availability of some patients who are definitely known to have pure sensori-neural losses. If there is any doubt as to whether their losses are purely sensori-neural, the method should not be adopted. Also, more accurate results can be obtained with eight or ten patients instead of only two or three, since the effect of random errors should be canceled out.

While in calibration procedures the primary concern of the audiologist is with the output level of the audiometer at each frequency, it is advisable to determine periodically that each frequency is within the allowable frequency limits specified by the American National Standards Institute.[33] Since frequency-measuring equipment is not always available, the audiologist may have to depend on the manufacturer for frequency-calibration service.

Some audiometrists have the mistaken notion that they should always turn off the power to the audiometer as soon as they have completed a test, apparently on the assumption that the longer the power is on the more wear the audiometer parts receive or in an attempt to conserve electricity. Actually, the wear on the audiometer parts occurs from turning the instrument on and off, and the amount of electricity that the audiometer consumes is minimal. When the audiometer is first turned on, power surges through the tubes and the other electronic components, and it is at this time that "weak" parts will fail. If more than one test is to be given during the day, it is better to leave the audiometer turned on throughout the day than it is to turn the instrument on and off for each test. In some television stations, the electronic equipment is kept turned on twenty-four hours a day, because the engineers realize that the components will last longer this way. Of course in a TV station, an

[33] ANSI S3.6–1969, *op. cit.*

engineer would be on duty at all hours. It is preferable to turn audiometric equipment off at the end of each day, however, because of the danger of fire when no one is around.

THE AUDIOGRAM

Hearing-test results are recorded in the form of a graph which is called an *audiogram*. The audiogram has two dimensions: frequency along the abscissa, and intensity along the ordinate. The patient's hearing level, or threshold, at each frequency tested is plotted on the audiogram for each ear separately both by air conduction and by bone conduction. Symbols are standardized to indicate the threshold points for each ear at the appropriate 5-dB step, separate symbols being used for air-conduction and bone-conduction thresholds. Also, different colors have been selected to differentiate between the ears, red denoting the right ear and blue or black the left.

Figure 5-5 shows a typical audiogram form with a listing and explanation of the symbols. At the top of the audiogram form, there is space for recording pertinent information obtained from the patient and comments bearing on the testing situation. On the right side of this audiogram form space is provided for recording the results of speech audiometric tests. The abbreviations here stand for terms that will be discussed in the next chapter.

The symbols O and X are used to plot the air-conduction threshold points at each frequency for the right and left ears, respectively. Arrows pointing to the right and left indicate bone-conduction threshold hearing levels for the right and left ears, respectively. The term *threshold* has occurred many times in this book thus far without having been defined. In psychological and physiological work in the field of sensation, threshold is defined as the intensity of stimulus required just barely to elicit a sensation in whatever sensory modality is being studied. A subject's threshold at a particular time can be measured in the laboratory with a high degree of precision. In hearing, a subject's threshold would be expressed in terms of fractions of a decibel. Sensory thresholds are not absolutes, that is, they do not remain constant, but tend to fluctuate somewhat as a function of the subject's physical, emotional, and mental state. Nevertheless, at a given moment, the threshold can be established rather precisely.

In clinical hearing testing, in contrast to laboratory measurements, gross increments of sound intensity are employed, generally in steps of 5 dB. The patient's threshold is defined as the lowest level at which he can detect the presence of the test tone at least 50 per cent of the time. If the intensity is decreased by another 5 dB, the patient will no longer be able to hear the tone. Actually, his true threshold may be as much as $4\frac{1}{2}$ dB less than that obtained, but, since the audiometer indicates gross steps of intensity, only gross thresholds may be measured—gross, that is, by laboratory standards.

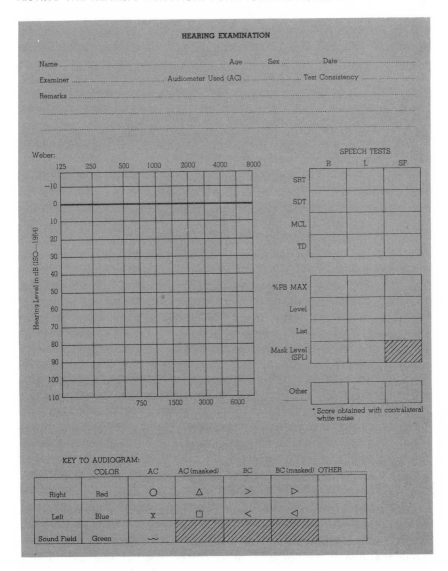

Figure 5-5.   A typical audiogram form.

In audiometric work, the terms *above* and *below* threshold, and *raised* and *lowered* threshold are frequently confused. The confusion arises from the fact that, the lower a patient's audiogram curve appears on the graph, the greater the amount of hearing loss he has. We tend to think of the terms *above, below, raised* and *lowered,* therefore, in relation to the position of the patient's curve of hearing sensitivity on the audiogram. Actually, this is just the reverse of the way the terms should be applied. Let's say that a certain amount of intensity is required to reach a patient's threshold at a certain frequency. If we have an intensity less than this amount, that tone is *below* the patient's threshold—it is not sufficiently intense for him to hear it. If we then increase the intensity beyond the point at which the patient can just barely hear it, we have gone *above* the patient's threshold. If one patient has less hearing loss than another, we say that his threshold for sound is *lower,* that is, he can respond to a lower intensity of sound. By the same token, if a patient's hearing is improved by an operative procedure, or by wearing a hearing aid, we speak of the improvement in his hearing as a *lowering* of his threshold—he can now respond to sounds of less intensity than he formerly could. Contrariwise, if his hearing becomes worse, his threshold is *raised*—a greater amount of intensity is now required for him to respond. We must always remember, then, that the terms *above, below, raise,* and *lower,* when applied to thresholds, have no reference to the position of the audiogram curve, since a *lowered* threshold actually means a *higher* position of the curve on the audiogram.

Customarily, the O's and X's which mark the points of threshold hearing level across the audiogram would be connected by solid lines of the appropriate color, red for the O's and blue or black for the X's. Thus, at a glance, the contour of the hearing loss by air conduction can be seen for each ear. Usually the bone-conduction threshold levels are not connected by lines, although some audiometrists prefer to connect them by dashed lines, which contrast with the solid lines connecting the air-conduction threshold hearing levels. If masking is used during the test, appropriate symbols serve to indicate that fact. The symbols to indicate that masking was employed are the triangle for the right ear and the square for the left ear, for air conduction, and triangles pointing to left or right for bone conduction. Sometimes it is desirable to record thresholds obtained both without and with masking, and then all the symbols would be needed. If the patient does not respond by air conduction to the maximum hearing level at a given frequency, an arrow should be drawn pointing downward at that hearing level—to the right of the frequency ordinate for the right ear, and to the left for the left ear. To indicate no response by bone conduction, the downward arrow should originate with the appropriate bone-conduction symbol at the maximum hearing level for that frequency, or, more simply, the examiner can say, "No response by bone conduction" in the "Remarks" portion of the audiogram.

It should be mentioned here that there is not universal agreement concerning the symbols to represent bone-conduction results. Some feel that the arrows should be reversed from the way they appear in the sample audiogram in Figure 5-5. Their logic is that the arrow represents the pinna of the patient and that, as the patient sits facing you, his right pinna is to your left; therefore, an arrow pointing to the *left* should represent his bone-conduction hearing in the *right* ear. Others agree with this reasoning but say that, instead of arrows, brackets would be preferable to represent bone conduction, so that [to the left of the ordinate for a given frequency would represent the bone-conduction threshold for the right ear, and] to the right of the ordinate would represent bone conduction for the left ear. To avoid confusion, the audiometrist must mark clearly on the audiogram the meaning of the symbols that he has adopted.

Because of the diversity of symbols for bone conduction, and also to some extent for masked air conduction, Martin and Kopra sent a questionnaire to 250 audiologists requesting reports on the symbols they preferred. Two hundred fourteen questionnaires were returned—a good indication of the degree of interest in the subject. The most popular symbols for masked air conduction and for unmasked bone conduction were the ones that appeared in the previous editions of this book and shown in Figure 5-5. Opinions were more equally divided on the symbols for masked bone conduction. While the most popular choice for masked bone-conduction symbols were filled-in triangles pointing to the right and left for the right and left ears, respectively, the authors recommended that open triangles pointing to the right for the right ear and to the left for the left ear be used because they were simpler to draw. Since 206 of the 214 respondents to the questionnaire indicated their willingness to standardize symbols based on the results of the study, perhaps the future will bring greater agreement on audiometric symbols than has been true to date.[34]

Fortunately, there has been good agreement for years among otologists and audiologists as to how air-conduction thresholds should be recorded on the audiogram. Some clinicians, however, prefer forms that have separate audiograms for the left and right ears, appearing side by side. A separate audiogram for each ear does eliminate the confusion that may arise from recording two air-conduction thresholds and two bone-conduction thresholds at the same hearing level. Most audiometrists, however, prefer to record all information on a single audiogram. In the next section of this chapter, sample audiograms will illustrate different types and degrees of hearing loss, and the reader can see how the various symbols are employed. Naturally, in this book, it will not be possible to show the color differences, which would make the audiograms more readable.

---

[34] Frederick N. Martin and Lennart L. Kopra, "Symbols in Pure-Tone Audiometry," *Asha,* Vol. 12 (April, 1970), pp. 182-185.

For some purposes, it is preferable to record hearing levels in numbers rather than on an audiogram form. If, for example, one is keeping a cumulative record of hearing tests on a particular patient, the use of such a form as that shown in Figure 5-6 makes it possible to determine at a glance how hearing levels might have changed from test to test. In Chapters 6 and 7 examples of the test form used by the Veterans Administration will be shown. On this form all threshold hearing levels are recorded in numbers.

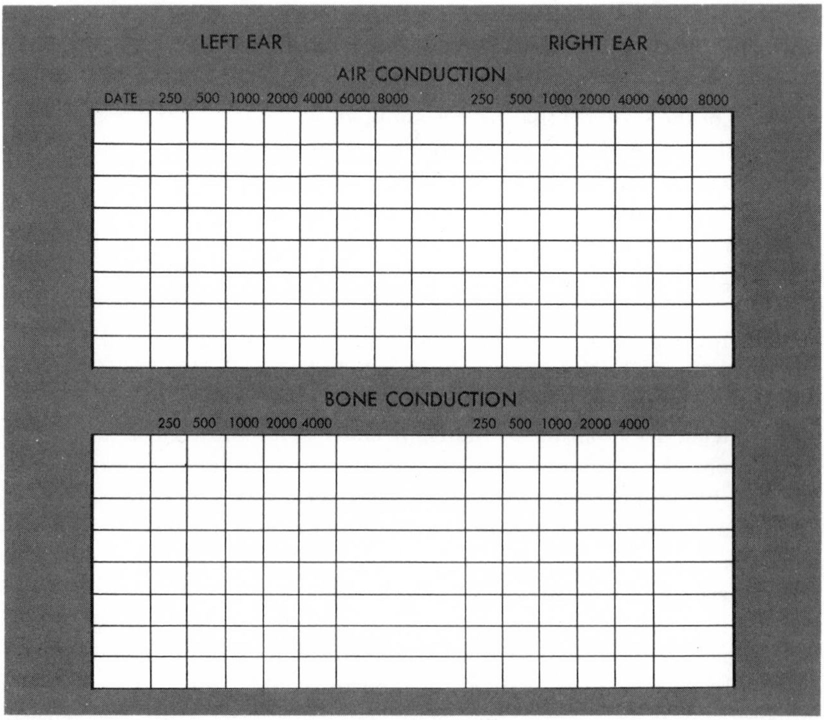

Figure 5-6.   Form for recording hearing levels in numbers.

INTERPRETING THE AUDIOGRAM

The purpose of hearing tests is twofold: first, to provide information which will assist the otologist in a diagnosis of the hearing impairment; and, second, to indicate what the patient's needs for aural rehabilitation might be. For both purposes, the audiogram requires expert interpretation.

As Aid to Diagnosis

To the otologist, the audiogram is useful for the information that it yields on the comparative sensitivity of the patient's air and bone conduction. Such information enables the otologist to diagnose the hearing impairment as being conductive, sensori-neural, or mixed in type. The course of treatment that the otologist prescribes will be based on his diagnosis. Naturally, his diagnosis depends not only on the hearing-test results but also on the results of the physical examination and the patient's medical history.

By definition, a "pure" conductive loss results from pathology or malfunctioning of the outer or middle ear with a normal inner ear. This means that a patient with a conductive loss should present an audiogram showing losses by air conduction but normal hearing by bone conduction. Figure 5-7 illustrates a typical audiogram of a patient with conductive loss.

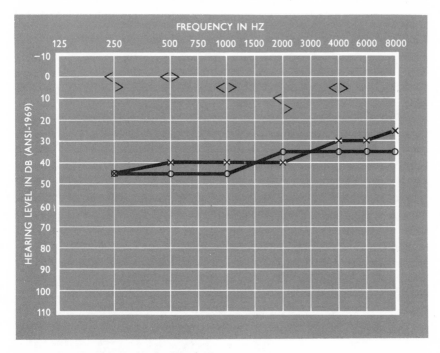

Figure 5-7. Typical conductive impairment.

Although a diagnosis of conductive impairment can be made only by comparing the air- and bone-conduction losses, it is possible to make some generalizations concerning the appearance of the air-conduction curve alone. Generally, in a conductive impairment, the air-conduction losses will be fairly equal at all frequencies, with perhaps slightly greater loss appearing for the lower frequencies. Reference to Figure 5-7 will demonstrate this observation. Yet, to reiterate, diagnosis cannot be made from the air-conduction curve alone since sensori-neural losses may also be fairly uniform at all frequencies. Also, there are instances of conductive loss that show poorer hearing for the high frequencies.

The cause of a particular conductive loss cannot be ascertained from an examination of the audiogram. There are some differences in the audiometric pictures of otitis media and otosclerosis, but these can be learned only through experience. No statements concerning etiology can be made, however, without the additional information derived from the physical examination and the medical history. Incidentally, it should be stated here that diagnosis of hearing impairment is not the responsibility of the audiologist. Because hearing loss is a medical disability, only a physician is legally qualified to make a diagnosis. The audiologist must be careful not to get into the position of "practicing medicine" or making medical pronouncements on the basis of his audiological work-ups.

Sensori-neural impairments are characterized usually but not always by greater losses at the higher frequencies on the audiogram. The audiogram

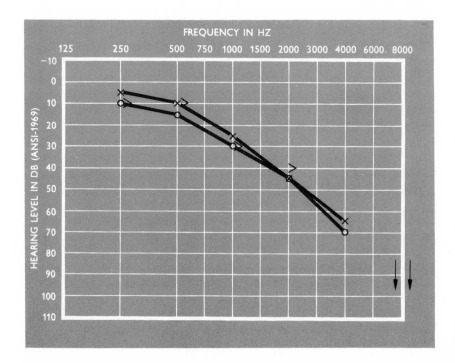

Figure 5-8. Typical sensori-neural impairment.

may show normal or close-to-normal hearing at the lower frequencies, with a rapid decrease in hearing sensitivity as the test proceeds through the higher frequencies. Figure 5-8 represents a more or less typical sensori-neural impairment. It will be noticed that the bone-conduction thresholds are approximately the same as the air-conduction thresholds, which, of course, is the important diagnostic indication of a sensori-neural loss. Since the bone-conduction thresholds of the right ear indicated that thresholds by bone were approximately equal to those by air, it was not necessary to test the bone conduction of the left ear. Because of the minimal interaural attenuation for bone conduction, it is obvious that the bone conduction of the left ear cannot differ significantly from that of the right. In this instance, the patient's loss at 8000 Hz exceeded the air-conduction limits of the audiometer. The arrows which point downward at the 90-dB level indicate that the patient did not respond at the maximum hearing level available at 8000 Hz. No bone-conduction threshold hearing levels are shown at 4000 Hz. The limit of intensity available by bone conduction in most audiometers is a hearing level of 65 or 70 dB. A notation should be made under "Remarks" on this audiogram that the patient did not respond to bone conduction at 4000 Hz at the maximum available hearing level.

The etiology of sensori-neural impairments cannot be determined from

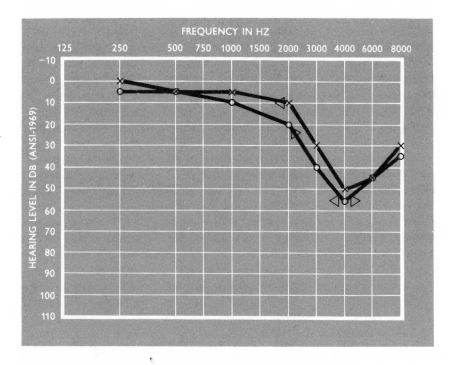

Figure 5-9.   Sensori-neural impairment resulting from noise exposure.

the audiogram alone, although certain causes do produce somewhat typical audiometric pictures. Noise-induced hearing loss—exposure to extreme noise for long enough periods to produce permanent hearing loss— usually is reflected in the audiogram by occurrence of the greatest amount of loss around 4000 Hz, with perhaps some recovery at higher frequencies. Figure 5-9 is an audiogram which is typical of sensori-neural loss caused by exposure to noise.

Sometimes a patient has extreme losses in one ear whereas the other ear is essentially normal. Where differences of 40 dB or more exist between the air-conduction curves, or between the air-conduction threshold hearing levels of the test ear and the bone-conduction threshold hearing levels of the nontest ear, masking should be applied in the better ear in order to obtain an accurate picture of the hearing in the poorer ear. Figure 5-10 is the audiogram of a girl in her twenties who had lost most of the hearing in one ear owing to a skull fracture. Both the masked and unmasked threshold hearing levels for the left ear are shown on the audiogram. It can be seen that, without masking, an entirely false picture of the hearing of the left ear would have been obtained. In this audiogram, the unmasked air-conduction threshold configuration of the left ear is an excellent example of a shadow curve. It

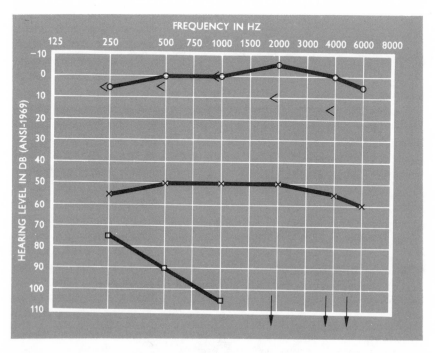

Figure 5-10.   Comparison of masked and unmasked threshold hearing levels in unilateral sensori-neural loss.

mirrors the curve of the right ear, because it is actually the right ear that is responding when the signal is being delivered to the left ear. When masking was used in bone-conduction testing, no responses within the intensity limitations of the bone-conduction circuit were obtained.

A mixed impairment will produce an audiogram which shows some loss by bone conduction but a more severe loss by air conduction. Or perhaps the mixed impairment will be manifested by conductive loss in the lower frequencies and sensori-neural loss in the higher frequencies. Figure 5-11 represents a mixed impairment.

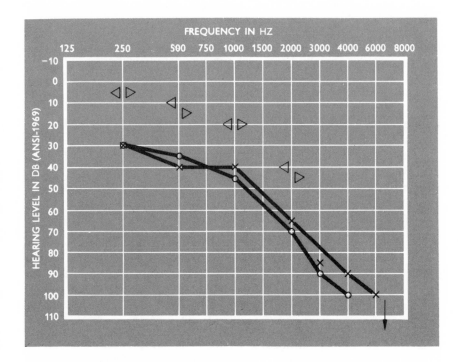

Figure 5-11.   A mixed impairment.

As Guide to Rehabilitation

The audiogram is useful in pointing to the need for rehabilitative measures, such as a hearing aid, for example, or instruction in speech reading. The audiogram can also serve to differentiate between children who are deaf and thus need full-time special education, and children who are hard-of-hearing and can fit into the framework of the regular classroom. Naturally, the audiogram is not the only criterion in making such determinations, but it is an important guide to rehabilitative needs.

The handicap of a hearing loss is in direct proportion to the effect that the loss has on the patient's communicative ability. Hence, it is important that the audiogram yield some information as to how hearing for speech has been impaired. If speech audiometric equipment is available, of course, this information can be obtained directly. Lacking speech-testing equipment, however, an estimate of the effect of the hearing loss on speech can be made from the pure-tone audiogram. In estimating the effect on speech of a particular hearing loss, two things are important: the amount of loss through the so-called speech frequencies and the configuration of the audiogram curve.

The speech frequencies are 500, 1000, and 2000 Hz. They are designated as speech frequencies because many studies have shown that there is a high correlation between the average hearing level at these three frequencies and the loss for speech as measured directly on a speech audiometer. The hearing level for speech in each ear can thus be predicted by adding the levels at each of these frequencies and dividing the sum by three. There is an important exception to this rule of averaging three frequencies to predict level for speech. If the shape of the audiogram curve is such that there is an abrupt increase in hearing level in proceeding from low to high frequencies, so that the difference in hearing level between 500 and 1000 Hz and between 1000 and 2000 Hz equals 20 dB or more, averaging the three frequencies will exaggerate the actual hearing level for speech. In such a situation, therefore, the rule is that the level for speech can be predicted by disregarding the frequency that shows the greatest loss and averaging the other two speech frequencies. This is called the *two-frequency* method of predicting hearing level for speech. Fletcher advocates that the two-frequency method be chosen for predicting the loss for speech regardless of the shape of the air-conduction curve on the audiogram.[35] At the present writing, audiological opinion is divided on this point.

Information concerning a patient's need for a hearing aid can be obtained by inspection of the hearing levels at the speech frequencies (500, 1000, and 2000 Hz), although it is no longer advisable to state the minimum hearing levels at which a hearing aid would be indicated. The oft-quoted rule that a hearing aid would not be considered unless the hearing loss for speech in the better ear is at least 30 dB no longer applies, since there are so many exceptions to the "rule." Today's hearing aids are easily put on and taken off. They operate quietly, and many patients with only minimal hearing loss for speech find hearing aids helpful to them, even though they may not be used at all times. A hearing aid is usually of little help to a person who has one normal ear, since in most situations he can hear speech adequately with his one good ear, but even this type of patient may find some benefit from a hearing aid in certain situations.

Losses for speech up to 80 dB can usually be "corrected" with the ampli-

[35] Harvey Fletcher, "A Method of Calculating Hearing Loss for Speech from an Audiogram," *Journal of the Acoustical Society of America*, Vol. 22 (January, 1950), pp. 1-5.

fication of a hearing aid. "Correction" does not mean restoration of the hearing function to normal—or zero hearing level on the audiometer. Rather, it refers to the restoration of the patient's hearing to a useful level. Losses for speech in excess of 80 dB *may* be "corrected" by means of amplification. Each patient must be considered individually, and frequently a decision cannot be made without a period of experimentation with amplification, which may extend over several weeks or months. It is doubtful that any patient whose loss for speech in the better ear is as great as 100 dB can be successfully rehabilitated by means of amplification alone. On the other hand, it cannot be said that such a patient would obtain no benefit from amplification. Here again experimentation is necessary. The subject of hearing aids and their selection will be discussed more fully in Chapter 10.

Before speech audiometry became common as a diagnostic tool, it was necessary to have some means of expressing the amount of handicap produced by a hearing loss, based on the pure-tone audiogram. In medicolegal cases, the amount of compensation for a hearing loss is based on the degree of handicap. The concept of *percentage of hearing loss* was introduced to meet this need. For a number of years percentage hearing loss was computed by what was termed the A.M.A. method, since it was published under the aegis of the American Medical Association. In the A.M.A. method, only four frequencies on the audiogram are given consideration: 500, 1000, 2000, and 4000 Hz. These frequencies are weighted in their importance to the total speech-hearing function, as follows: 500 Hz = 15 per cent; 1000 Hz = 30 per cent; 2000 Hz = 40 per cent; and 4000 Hz = 15 per cent. Losses in dB at each of these frequencies are assigned percentage values according to a chart which is used in conjunction with the pure-tone audiogram or sometimes is included as part of the audiogram. Losses for each ear are converted to percentages, and a formula is applied for computing the binaural percentage loss.

The disadvantage of the A.M.A. percentage method of expressing the handicap of a hearing loss is that it tells little about the patient's ability to communicate. Neither does it shed light on his ability to compensate for his loss by means of a hearing aid. Two patients with very different-appearing audiograms may actually have the same percentage of hearing loss when computed by the A.M.A. system, yet one patient may be considerably more handicapped in communication than is the other.

In 1959 a new method for computing percentage hearing impairment was published under the sponsorship of the American Academy of Ophthalmology and Otolaryngology, and hence it is referred to as the AAOO method.[36] The AAOO method has almost entirely replaced the

---

[36] "Guide for the Evaluation of Hearing Impairment," *Transactions American Academy of Ophthalmology and Otolaryngology* (March-April 1959) pp. 235-238.

The values in this article were based on ASA–1951 audiometric calibration standards. They have been corrected here to ANSI–1969 calibration standards.

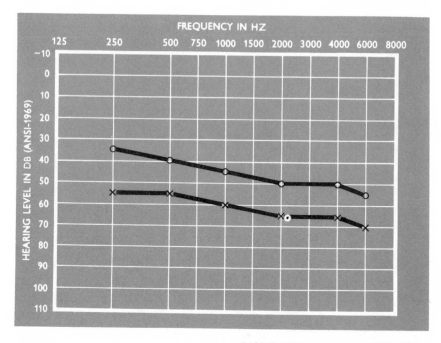

	RIGHT EAR	LEFT EAR
500	40	55
1000	45	60
2000	50	65
	3)135	3)180
average	45	60
	−26	−26
	(low fence)	(low fence)
net hearing level	19	34
	X 1½%	X 1½%
monaural %age impairment	29%	51%
	(rounded)	
	X 5	
	(weighting)	
	145	
impairment poor ear	+ 51	
	6)196	
binaural %age impairment	33%	
	(rounded)	

Figure 5-12.   Computation of percentage impairment by the AAOO method.

A.M.A. method for determining, on the basis of pure-tone audiometric information, the percentage of impairment. In the AAOO method, only the speech frequencies are assigned any percentage values. Percentage impairment is computed for each ear separately by averaging the air-conduction hearing levels at 500, 1000, and 2000 Hz, subtracting 26 dB from this average, and multiplying the remainder by 1½ per cent. The binaural percentage impairment is computed by multiplying the percentage impairment of the *better* ear by five, adding this product to the percentage impairment of the poorer ear, and dividing this sum by six. The computation of percentage hearing impairment by the AAOO method is illustrated in Figure 5-12.

The rationale of this method is that hearing is "impaired" only when the speech frequencies are affected, since the principal use to which our hearing is put is in listening to speech. Hearing impairment is confined between two "fences." The "low fence" is an average hearing level through the speech frequencies of 26 dB; until hearing level for speech exceeds 26 dB there is no impairment. In other words, the range of normal hearing is considered to extend to hearing levels of 26 dB. Thus before determining percentage of hearing impairment, 26 dB is subtracted from the average hearing level for the speech frequencies. The "high fence," or 100 per cent hearing impairment, is considered to be an average hearing level through the speech frequencies of 93 dB. Subtracting 26 dB (the low fence) from 93 dB (the high fence) leaves a remainder of 67 dB as the span of hearing loss from zero to 100 per cent. Thus each dB of this span is worth $1\frac{1}{2}$ per cent.

Since a unilateral hearing impairment is not nearly so handicapping as a bilateral impairment, the formula for combining the percentage impairments of the two ears into percentage binaural impairment weights the "better" ear five times the value of the "poorer" ear. The "inflated" percentage impairment of the better ear is then added to the percentage impairment of the poorer ear. Since this sum then contains six parts—five for the better ear and one for the poorer ear—the sum is divided by six. Naturally, because of the weighting, the resulting binaural percentage impairment is much closer to the value assigned to the better ear than it is to the percentage computed for the poorer ear.

While the AAOO method of computing percentage impairment represents an improvement over the A.M.A. method and is probably as good as any method based on the pure-tone audiogram alone could be, it is not as satisfactory a method of representing a communicative handicap as the results of clinical speech audiometry, as we shall see in the next chapter. The AAOO method is used extensively in medicolegal contexts as will be seen later in Chapter 9.

In this discussion of the value of the pure-tone audiogram in determining rehabilitative needs, so far we have considered only the extent of loss. The shape or configuration of the audiometric air-conduction curve and the type of hearing impairment are also important. The patient with a steeply sloping curve (greater losses for the higher frequencies) will usually present more difficult rehabilitation problems than the patient whose audiometric configuration is relatively "flat," that is, approximately equal at all frequencies. The flatness or slope of the curve is important primarily in the area of the speech frequencies—from 500 through 2000 Hz. If the losses at 1000 and 2000 Hz are markedly greater than at 500 Hz, the patient may confuse many consonants whose distinguishing characteristics are primarily in the higher frequencies. These consonants are generally the voiceless ones, such as *p, k, s, t, f, sh, ch,* and the voiceless *th.*

The patient who has a flat loss throughout the speech frequencies can usually make good use of amplification, because all speech sounds will be amplified equally. His handicap lies only in his inability to hear speech well. As speech is made louder through amplification, his handicap is diminished for he can understand what he hears.

A flat audiogram curve does not guarantee good performance with a hearing aid, however. Some patients with flat sensori-neural losses show very poor understanding of speech with amplification. On the other hand, the patient whose curve slopes steeply through the speech frequencies will not receive as much benefit from amplification because even with amplification his response to different frequencies will be unequal. In theory, the principle of selective amplification, that is, amplifying only the frequencies for which sensitivity is diminished and by an amount equal to the extent of the loss at those frequencies, should operate to provide usable amplified speech. Unfortunately, in practice, selective amplification has not been found to be generally useful. Modifications of the earpiece that connects the receiver of the aid with the ear may be helpful in reducing the distortion of amplified speech for patients with sloping audiograms, however, as we shall see in Chapter 10.

Although the audiogram yields important information concerning the rehabilitative needs of patients, it is most valuable when the information it conveys is combined with the results of clinical speech audiometric tests, which measure directly a patient's ability to hear and understand speech. After all, the measure of the handicap of a hearing loss is how one's communicative ability is affected. Whereas predictions of how communication is affected can be made from the pure-tone audiogram with some confidence, actual measures of the communicative ability can be derived through speech audiometry.

CAUTIONS FOR THE EXAMINER

Before moving into the subject of speech audiometry, we should mention two items of caution for the examiner—one concerning possible misinterpretation of test results, and the other concerning earphone hygiene.

Collapsed Canal

Some patients have very small or slitlike external canals that will seal shut with the relatively slight pressure exerted by the earphones. Since the blocked canals prevent the effective transmission of the air-borne sound wave to the eardrum, the patient will present the diagnostic indication of a conductive or mixed loss—an air-bone gap—when in fact no gap exists, or the hearing may even be normal. Whenever the test results reveal an air-bone gap, the examiner should inspect the patient's ears and check to see if the canals seal shut when pressure is applied to the pinnas. If so, a short length of hollow tubing should be inserted in the canal while the air-conduction test is repeated. The tubing prevents the canal from collapsing under the pressure of the earphone. Air-conduction threshold improvements of from 15 to 30 dB have been reported when this retest procedure was followed.[37]

Earphone Contamination

Talbott has directed attention to the danger of spreading infection from earphone cushions.[38] He found that the MX-41/AR cushions used in routine testing in a hospital audiology clinic contained numerous colonies of bacteria of the type associated with otitis media and otitis externa. While he presented no evidence of patients incurring infections from the cushions, he concluded that the potential for infection was present. He reported that irradiation of the cushions with ultraviolet light for a period of five minutes eliminated 90 per cent of the bacteria.

The most common way of disinfecting earphone cushions is to wipe them off with an ethanol sponge. There is no information available as to the relative effectiveness of this method of disinfecting the cushions and ultraviolet irradiation. The use of any disinfecting liquid, however, can be potentially harmful to the cushions—or to the earphone itself if the liquid reaches the diaphragm of the phone. Alcohol or other disinfecting agents are probably more readily available to the average audiology clinic, however, than the proper kind of ultraviolet irradiation.

It is probably true that most clinics make no attempt to disinfect earphone cushions after each patient's use, and it is also probably true that in most cases no harm results. If a patient is referred with an active otitis media, or with an external otitis, however, the audiologist should take every possible precaution to protect following patients from infection by cleansing the cushions with whatever antibacterial agents are available. An added precaution in testing patients with known infections is to cover the patient's pinnas with sterile gauze pads before putting the earphones in place. Of course the best procedure would be to disinfect the cushions after every patient. Incidentally, while the chances are remote that patients will be harmed in any way through audiological procedures, audiologists should protect themselves by carrying malpractice insurance—or making sure that they are covered under blanket policies issued to institutions where they work.

[37] Ira Ventry, Joseph B. Chaiklin, and William F. Boyle, "Collapse of the Ear Canal During Audiometry," *A.M.A. Archives of Otolaryngology*, Vol. 73 (1961), pp. 727-731.

Victor H. Hildyard and Milton A. Valentine, "Collapse of the Ear Canal During Audiometry," *A.M.A. Archives of Otolaryngology*, Vol. 75 (1962), pp. 422-423.

Mark Ross and C. A. Tucker, "A Case Study of Collapse of the Ear Canal During Audiometry," *Laryngoscope*, Vol. 75 (1965), pp. 65-67.

Earl W. Stark, "Collapse of the Ear Canal During Audiometry: A Case Report," *Journal of Speech and Hearing Disorders*, Vol. 31 (November, 1966), pp. 374-376.

[38] Richard E. Talbott, "Bacteriology of Earphone Contamination," *Journal of Speech and Hearing Research*, Vol. 12 (June, 1969), pp. 326-329.

6

TESTING THE HEARING FUNCTION: SPEECH AUDIOMETRY

EQUIPMENT REQUIRED

Speech audiometers have been produced commercially only since the early 1950s. Prior to that time it was necessary to have speech audiometers custom designed and built. Several companies build speech-testing equipment today, usually as part of a console that incorporates pure-tone circuitry as well. Since most of these "clinical hearing evaluators" provide two channels and a variety of inputs and outputs, they constitute extremely flexible (and expensive) instruments with which the most sophisticated pure-tone and speech tests may be performed. Thus, since the first standards for speech audiometers were published in 1953, speech-testing equipment has advanced from a simple turntable connected to a headset of two air-conduction earphones through an amplifier and attenuator to the complex circuitry of a modern console. The standards for speech audiometers are now incorporated with the standards for pure-tone diagnostic and screening audiometers.[1]

Speech audiometry requires a two-room suite. The test room ideally should be at least eight feet square (inside dimensions), constructed so that it is isolated acoustically from surrounding space. The test room should be joined with the control room by a triple-paned window (for acoustic insulation purposes) through which the tester may observe the patient. Access to the test room should be through a specially designed acoustic door. The dimensions of the control room are unimportant, so long as there is sufficient

[1] "American National Standard Specifications for Audiometers" (ANSI S3.6–1969, New York, American National Standards Institute, 1970).

room for the equipment and the examiner. It is not necessary to have the control room acoustically isolated unless the adjacent spaces are particularly noisy, or unless the noises emanating from the control room might disturb others working nearby. It is usually more satisfactory to make use of pre-fabricated sound-isolated rooms than to attempt to build one's own test suite. Single- or double-walled prefabricated panels, depending on the amount of attenuation required, can be combined to provide any size room desired.

Assuming the desirability of combining pure-tone and speech audiometric equipment, the audiometer used in a two-room suite should provide the following:

1. Inputs
   a. microphone
   b. turntable
   c. masking noise generator(s)
   d. stereo tape recorder with delayed auditory feedback equipment
   e. two pure-tone generators
2. Two input channels
3. Two volume controls and VU meters
4. Two selector switches for choosing inputs—one for each channel
5. Amplifiers
6. Attenuators
7. Outputs
   a. air-conduction earphones
   b. bone-conduction vibrator
   c. one or two loudspeakers
8. An output selector switch permitting selection of either or both input channels for any of the outputs
9. Monitoring and patient talk-back system, including microphone for patient, amplifier, and earphones and/or loudspeaker for examiner
10. Patient signaling device

With such equipment, all the standard and special speech tests, including those for functional or nonorganic hearing problems, can be administered. Figure 6-1 is a photograph of the console of a two-channel combined speech and pure-tone audiometer. Figure 6-2 shows this audiometer mounted on a table next to a cabinet containing, from top to bottom, a turntable, an X-Y recorder (for use in Békésy audiometry, to be described in Chapter 7), and a tape deck.

Volume indicator meters (VI meters or more often VU for "volume units") are needed to enable the examiner to monitor the inputs to the amplifiers. The output of the amplifiers must be calibrated in terms of a specific level of input signal. Once the calibration is established, whatever input is selected must be adjusted to the particular input level that was used in

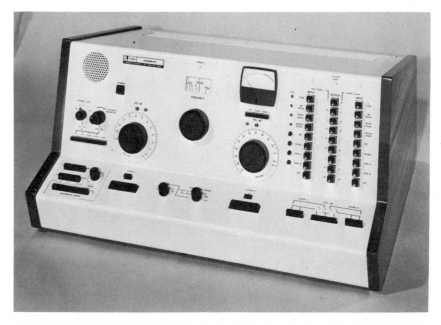

Figure 6-1.   Console of the Grason-Stadler 1701 audiometer. (Reproduced by permission of Grason-Stadler, a GR Company, Concord, Mass.)

calibration; otherwise the output level will fluctuate with changes in input level. It is customary to monitor all inputs to an average peak reading of zero dB on the VU meter. The input level is controlled by a potentiometer (volume control). The examiner compensates for differences in levels of recording or for differences in vocal intensity in live-voice testing by turning the input volume control until the needle on the VU meter is peaking on the average at zero dB.

The American National Standard calls for the output of speech audiometers to cover a range of at least 100 dB, from 0 to +100 dB in relation to the normal speech hearing threshold level in steps of 2.5 dB or less.[2] Actually, most speech audiometers will provide a range of 110 dB or more, with attenuator steps of 1 or 2 dB.

Speech-testing materials may be introduced either through the microphone, which is referred to as monitored live-voice testing, or by means of disc or tape recordings. Both methods have advantages. Live-voice testing is, of course, more flexible, in that the examiner can adapt his manner of testing to suit the particular patient with whom he is working. Thus, with an elderly patient, the examiner can slow down his presentation of test words to a rate that is suitable. The recorded tests, on the other hand, provide a greater

[2] *Ibid.*, p. 16.

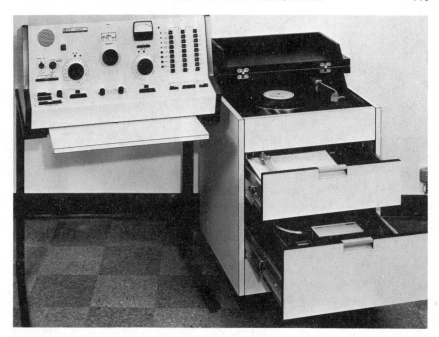

Figure 6-2. The 1701 audiometer with associated equipment. (Reproduced by permission of Grason-Stadler, a GR Company, Concord, Mass.)

standardization for speech tests, since they can be presented in the same way time and again. Recorded tests are essential in order to achieve equivalence of test results from one clinic or center to another, as, for example, in auditory tests given to veterans for purposes of rating disability. With monitored live-voice tests the examiner himself constitutes one source of variability. It is impossible for an examiner, no matter how skillful he may be, to present a list of words two or more times in precisely the same way. For accurate and reliable testing, therefore, recorded speech tests are preferable. There will be times, however, when, because of a patient's inability to respond to the standard test materials in recorded form, it will be necessary to adopt the live-voice technique and perhaps to improvise materials and procedures. At such times the examiner must realize that he is departing from the standard procedures. and his test results must be interpreted accordingly. The beauty of speech audiometric testing is that it is possible to be flexible in approach and thus to obtain some measure of hearing level for speech for almost any patient who understands spoken language. Special techniques for testing very young children with the speech audiometer will be discussed in the next chapter. The remainder of this chapter will deal with the standard techniques of speech audiometry as applied with adults and with older children.

MEASURES SOUGHT

Speech-Reception Threshold

Just as in pure-tone testing we seek to obtain the patient's threshold for individual frequencies, so in speech audiometry a measure that we are after is the patient's threshold hearing level for speech. We want to know how intense simple speech must be before the patient can just understand it. We are not interested at this point in the level at which the patient can barely detect the presence of speech (threshold of speech detectability), but rather in the level at which the patient can repeat simple words or can understand simple running (connected) speech. This level we refer to as the patient's *speech-reception threshold,* abbreviated SRT. The SRT is measured in dB from the level at which the average normal ear's SRT has been established. The sound pressure level of zero-dB SRT will vary according to the specific test materials employed, the particular methodology used in arriving at threshold, and the "test sophistication" of the listeners. The American National Standard specifies that zero-dB hearing level for speech is a sound pressure level of 19 dB when normal threshold is based on 50 per cent intelligibility of spondee words.[3] When the test earphone is a Telephonics TDH-39 instead of the Western Electric 705-A employed in the ANSI standard, the sound pressure level for speech audiometric zero becomes 20 dB instead of 19 dB.[4] The calibration of the speech audiometer is checked by measuring the rms (root-mean-square) level in a 6 cc coupler of a 1000 Hz tone in an earphone that produces a VU meter reading that agrees with the average peaks of the VU meter for the speech signal.[5] The allowable limits for calibration are ± 3 dB, or, in other words, between 17 and 23 dB for the TDH-39 earphone.[6] In the past, various investigators have reported sound pressure levels for zero-dB SRT within these allowable limits.[7]

In the 1953 American standard for speech audiometers, zero-dB SRT was defined as a sound pressure level of 22 dB when the speech threshold was determined as the 50 per cent intelligibility level of spondee words. Speech audiometric zero was established at 22 dB SPL at that time for two reasons: (1) this was the average of levels reported from laboratory studies of normal-

---

[3] *Ibid.,* p. 12.

[4] *Ibid.,* p. 21.

[5] *Ibid.,* p. 15.

[6] *Ibid.,* p. 16.

[7] Ira J. Hirsh, Hallowell Davis, S. Richard Silverman, Elizabeth G. Reynolds, Elizabeth Eldert, and Robert W. Benson, "Development of Materials for Speech Audiometry," *Journal of Speech and Hearing Disorders,* Vol. 17 (September, 1952), p. 328.

James F. Jerger, Raymond Carhart, Tom W. Tillman, and John L. Peterson, "Some Relations Between Normal Hearing for Pure Tones and for Speech," *Journal of Speech and Hearing Research,* Vol. 2 (June, 1959), pp. 126-140.

Joseph B. Chaiklin, "The Relation Among Three Selected Auditory Speech Thresholds," *Journal of Speech and Hearing Research,* Vol. 2 (September, 1959), pp. 237-243.

hearing subjects available then, and (2) the assumption was made that the threshold of intelligibility for spondee words should be about 6 dB higher than the normal threshold hearing level for 1000 Hz, which by the ASA-1951 standard was defined as 16.5 dB SPL. It was assumed that establishing zero-dB SRT at 22 dB SPL would result in good agreement between a normal-hearing subject's SRT and the arithmetic average of his threshold hearing levels for the "speech frequencies"—500, 1000, and 2000 Hz. Actually, research demonstrated that for normal-hearing subjects the threshold of intelligibility for spondee words was on the average 13 dB higher in sound pressure level than the threshold hearing level at 1000 Hz.[8] So, in order to secure good agreement between the average threshold hearing level for the speech frequencies and the SRT, it was necessary to peg zero-dB SRT at a sound pressure level of 29 dB (about 13 dB higher than the ASA-1951 standard of 16.5 dB SPL for 1000 Hz).

Until the ISO-1964 standard for calibration of pure-tone audiometers was generally adopted, there was confusion regarding the sound pressure level of zero-dB SRT. Some audiometer manufacturers followed the reasoning of Jerger et al. and set zero-dB SRT at 29 dB SPL, while others continued to adhere to the 1953 standard of 22 dB SPL. The ISO-1964 standard defined audiometric zero for 1000 Hz as 6.5 dB SPL. Now adding 13 dB to the normal threshold hearing level for 1000 Hz resulted in a sound pressure level of 19.5 dB (rounded to 20 dB) for the theoretically valid zero-dB SRT. This is exactly the value specified (for the Telephonics TDH-39 earphone) in the ANSI-1969 standard.

Although a variety of speech materials are suitable for arriving at the SRT, one test is much more common than the others. This consists of lists of two-syllable words, referred to as *spondees,* although most of these words would normally not be pronounced with equal stress on both syllables. They are words such as *doorway, footstool, airplane,* and *armchair.* Two recorded forms of the spondee test are available. They are called Auditory Tests W-1 and W-2: spondaic word lists.[9] Test W-1 consists of lists of thirty-six spondaic words which have been recorded at a constant level. The audiometrist introduces as much attenuation as he needs in the course of the test to arrive at the patient's SRT. Test W-2 consists of the same lists of words but with attenuation at an average of 1 dB per word built into the record. For most speech audiometric installations, Test W-1 would be preferable.

The SRT by spondees is defined as the hearing level at which the patient can repeat 50 per cent of the words correctly. It is not always practical to follow this definition literally. The tester must sometimes estimate the point at which the patient is right approximately half the time.

[8] Jerger et al., op. cit., p. 138.

[9] These tests were adapted by Central Institute for the Deaf from Auditory Test No. 9, originated by the Psycho-Acoustic Laboratory, Harvard University. The records are manu-factured and distributed by Technisonic Studios, 1201 South Brentwood Blvd., Richmond Heights, Missouri 63117.

The test is administered monaurally (to each ear separately) through ear-phones and then again, if the occasion requires it, through the loudspeaker. Loudspeaker testing is referred to as "sound-field" testing, because the sound is not confined, as it is in an earphone, but circulates in a field about the head of the patient. Unless we are talking over the telephone, or for some reason listening through earphones, all our listening throughout the day is of the sound-field type. It is to judge how the patient hears in a typical, sound-field listening situation that we give speech tests through a loudspeaker.

The method of administering the test is to start the record (or the delivery of the words by live voice) at a level above the patient's presumed threshold. As the patient repeats two or three words successfully, decrease the intensity by a few dB. After two or three more words have been repeated correctly at this new level, decrease the intensity further. Continue in this way until the patient misses some words. Then by following the procedure described later in this chapter, determine the level at which the patient is correct in his responses about half the time. This is his SRT by spondees. The W-1 spondee word lists appear in the Appendix to this book.

A second test which is not so frequently used for establishing the SRT as it is for other speech audiometric measures is the so-called "cold running-speech" test. "Running speech" means simply *connected speech*. "Cold" refers to the fact that the speech is informative in content and delivery, rather than emotional. Again, this test may be administered by either the live-voice or the recorded technique. If records are to be played, they should be chosen carefully to represent good, average American speech. For many years, it was the practice in clinics and centers to select recordings of news commentaries by Fulton Lewis, Jr. for running speech tests. Actually, any recording of informative running speech is satisfactory, provided that the speaker's rate is right for easy listening and the average intensity level of his voice remains fairly constant, making the recording easy to monitor.

The test for establishing threshold for running speech is administered by having the patient say "yes" every few seconds as long as he can understand the connected discourse. The record is started at a level above the patient's presumed threshold. The intensity is then decreased in small steps until the patient responds "no," meaning that he can no longer follow the train of thought. The point at which he is just barely able to understand the speaker is termed his SRT by running speech or connected discourse. This test may also be administered monaurally and by sound-field, and the results should show close agreement with the SRT for spondee words.

Most Comfortable Loudness

The second measure sought in speech audiometry is the hearing level at which speech is most comfortable for the patient. This measure and the next one to be described have significance in determining the limits of amplification that are suitable for the patient who is a candidate for a hearing aid. The patient's most comfortable loudness, abbreviated MCL, is measured by means of running speech. The patient is instructed to signal when the speech is most comfortably loud for him as the examiner varies the intensity at supra-threshold levels. The MCL is measured in dB above zero SRT monaurally and if desired by sound-field.

Tolerance Level

The tolerance level, sometimes called the threshold of discomfort (TD), or the uncomfortable level (UCL), is the hearing level at which speech becomes uncomfortably loud. The purpose of this measure is to find the upper limit of the patient's range of hearing for speech, so that the tests which follow can be given within that range, Also, the tolerance level represents the maximum amplification that the patient can accept in a training situation or in a hearing aid. Tolerance level is expressed in dB above zero SRT. The normal ear should be able to tolerate speech at hearing levels of 90 to 100 dB without experiencing discomfort. It should be remembered that, according to the American National Standard, zero SRT is 20 dB (for the TDH-39 earphone) above the standard reference pressure of 0.0002 dyne/cm^2, so that a hearing level of 100 dB would be a sound-pressure level of 120 dB. It will be recalled from the discussion in Chapter 2 that the average threshold of discomfort is at a sound-pressure level of 120 dB.

The same running speech for measuring MCL can be used to determine the tolerance level. The intensity of the running speech is increased gradually above the MCL until the patient signals that it is uncomfortably loud. This hearing level is then recorded as the patient's tolerance level. The test is performed monaurally and also may be presented by sound-field. The patient should be instructed not to signal until the speech becomes so loud that it actually causes him to feel physiological discomfort in the ear, as if a further increase would produce pain.

Dynamic Range

The patient's dynamic range is computed by subtracting the SRT from the tolerance level. The dynamic range represents the limits of useful hearing that the patient has in each ear, and by sound-field. This is important in diagnosis and in planning for the patient's rehabilitation, as will be brought out later in this chapter.

Discrimination

In addition to the measures of sensitivity for speech, an indication of the patient's speech-discrimination ability is desirable. The handicap of a hearing loss may consist not only of a decrease in sensitivity to sound but also of an impairment in understanding what is heard. With many patients, the primary difficulty is one of interference with the intelligibility of speech. As we have seen in the previous chapter, speech intelligibility is probably related to the audiometric configuration, the type of pathology, the degree of impairment, and perhaps other factors. The term *articulation* is used audiologically for the function of speech discrimination. In this context, an articulation test is one which examines a patient's ability to discriminate among similar sounds or among words that contain similar sounds. It is unfortunate that the word *articulation* has other connotations for individuals whose orientation is in the field of speech. In this chapter we shall apply the terms *articulation* and *speech discrimination* interchangeably.

The articulation or discrimination function is usually measured clinically by administering so-called *phonetically balanced* (PB) word lists at levels well above the patient's SRT. Each list contains fifty monosyllabic words, chosen systematically in order that each list will contain samples of speech sounds in approximately the same proportion in which they occur in English running speech. Actually, as Lehiste and Peterson have pointed out, the lists should more properly be designated as "phonemically balanced" lists,[10] since they were designed to include the various phonemes of the language in correct proportion rather than balancing all the physiological and acoustical properties of speech implied by the term "phonetics."

The original PB lists were created at the Harvard Psycho-Acoustic Laboratory.[11] The twenty lists, consisting of 1000 words in all, were recorded by Rush Hughes, a radio announcer in St. Louis. These are referred to as the PB-50 lists to differentiate them from the PB word lists developed at Central Institute for the Deaf by Hirsh and his associates.[12] Hirsh *et al.* developed a list of 200 PB words, of which 180 were taken from the 1000 words in the Psycho-Acoustic Laboratory (PAL) lists. Hirsh recorded on magnetic tape the 200 words in four lists of fifty words each. Each list was then "scrambled" six times to give different word orders, so that there are twenty-four lists in all. These PB word lists are available in disc-recorded form as Auditory Test W-22.[13] They may, of course, be delivered by live voice as well. If they are given by live voice, the examiner must avoid the temptation to monitor each word to the same point on the VU meter. Since there is a wide difference in the phonetic power of various speech sounds, monitoring the words to the same level on the VU meter can result in inaccurate discrimination scores. The words should be spoken with equal effort rather than with equal intensity as measured on the meter. Not only are the lists phonemically balanced with English speech, they are also

---

10 Ilse Lehiste and Gordon E. Peterson, "Linguistic Considerations in the Study of Speech Intelligibility," *Journal of the Acoustical Society of America,* Vol. 31 (March, 1959), p. 281.

11 J P Egan, "Articulation Testing Methods," *Laryngoscope,* Vol. 58 (1948), pp. 955-991.

12 Hirsh *et al., op. cit.*

13 The records are manufactured and distributed by Technisonic Studios, 1201 South Brentwood Blvd., Richmond Heights, Missouri 63117.

balanced with each other. There should be very little variation in a patient's score from list to list, therefore. While it is possible to obtain a rough estimate of a patient's discrimination ability by using just twenty-five words of a list, it is advisable to use an entire list of fifty words for each discrimination test, since the first half of a list has not been balanced with the second half. The twenty-four W-22 lists are reproduced in the Appendix to this book.

A great deal of research has been done with both the Harvard PB-50 lists and with the W-22 PB lists in defining what has been termed the articulation function. The research has been with normal ears, as well as with impaired ears of all types. "Articulation curves" have been constructed, showing how the scores on PB tests for normal and impaired ears are affected by the intensity at which the word lists are presented. As the intensity is increased above the individual's threshold for speech, scores on the tests increase rapidly until the intensity at which the PB words are presented reaches a level of 35 to 40 dB greater than the individual's SRT. At this point the articulation curve flattens out. With increasing intensity above this point there is a negligible increase in discrimination score. It is important, in administering the PB tests clinically, that they be presented at a level which will result in obtaining the patient's maximum discrimination score—referred to as "PB-Max." Usually, but not always, the patient's PB-Max will be found at a sensation level of 40 dB.

The best method of administering the PB tests is to have the patient write his responses on a paper with fifty numbered blank spaces. In this way there can be little doubt as to whether or not the patient has heard the words correctly, and there is the added advantage that a permanent record of the patient's responses is available for analysis of his discrimination errors. If you have the patient repeat the words to you while you listen over the talkback earphones or loudspeaker, you are testing your own discrimination for the patient's speech. Of course, sometimes there will be no alternative but to have the patient repeat the words, since writing is impossible or difficult for some patients. In this situation, if it is feasible to do so, it is a good idea to have the patient spell each word as he hears it, rather than repeat it, in order to reduce the chances of error in scoring the test.

The discrimination tests are scored in terms of the percentage of words heard correctly. Since there are fifty words to a list, the percentage correct can easily be computed by counting the number of correct responses and multiplying by two. The percentage of correct responses is the patient's discrimination score. Subtracting this number from 100 yields the patient's *discrimination loss*, one of the dimensions used in determining the patient's social adequacy index, the next measure to be described. As is true of the previously described measures, the discrimination tests may be administered both monaurally and by sound-field.

Since the appearance of the W-22 test and its incorporation into standard clinical procedures in place of the older Rush Hughes recordings of the PB-50 lists, there have been many attempts to develop improved tests of discrimination or speech intelligibility. Fairbanks[14] devised the Rhyme Test, which is a completion type of test requiring the subject to supply the initial consonant to a "stem." The subject has a list of fifty stems. He writes in the missing letter as he hears the word pronounced by the speaker. The words in the test were selected so that there are at least five rhyming choices the subject can make for each word. Thus for the stem "–ame," some choices would be "tame, same, lame, came, name, dame." With this test it is easy to categorize the constant errors the subject makes.

House *et al.*[15] developed a "closed-response set" discrimination test that has come to be known as the Modified Rhyme Test (MRT). Instead of allowing the subject to select a letter to add to a stem as was done in the Rhyme Test, the authors supply the subject with six rhyming words for each of fifty stimulus items. The subject must then draw a line through the word he thought he heard. The MRT consists of twenty-five items that differ only in the initial consonant (e.g., "sip, rip, tip, dip, hip, lip") and twenty-five items that are differentiated by the final consonant (e.g., "map mat, math, man, mass, mad"). To make the listening task sufficiently difficult, both the Rhyme Test and MRT are administered in the presence of a broad-band noise.

The MRT was developed originally as a test to differentiate communication systems, although its authors recognized its possibilities as a clinical tool. Kreul *et al.*[16] refined the MRT by changing some items and prepared tape recordings of the test to be used in the clinical assessment of discrimination ability. The recordings are furnished with both male and female speakers and with three signal-to-noise ratios (S/N).

Because they were dissatisfied with the PB words as a discrimination test to be used as a research tool, Lehiste and Peterson[17] constructed ten lists of fifty monosyllabic words each (500 different words) which are more rigorously phonemically balanced and more carefully selected on the basis of frequency of occurrence in American English than were the Harvard PB-50 lists and the W-22 lists of PB words. They referred to their lists as CNC lists (consonant-nucleus-consonant). Later the authors revised the lists by eliminating some rare and literary words and suggested that the revised

14 Grant Fairbanks, "Test of Phonemic Differentiation: the Rhyme Test," *Journal of the Acoustical Society of America*, Vol. 30 (July, 1958), pp. 596-600.

15 Arthur S. House, Carl E. Williams, Michael H. L. Hecker, and K. D. Kryter, "Articulation Testing Methods: Consonantal Differentiation with a Closed-Response Set," *Journal of the Acoustical Society of America*, Vol. 37 (January, 1965), pp. 158-166.

16 E. James Kreul, James C. Nixon, Karl D. Kryter, Donald W. Bell, Janna S. Lang, and Earl D. Schubert, "A Proposed Clinical Test of Speech Discrimination," *Journal of Speech and Hearing Research*, Vol. 11 (September, 1968), pp. 536-552.

17 Lehiste and Peterson, *op. cit.*, pp. 280-286.

CNC lists would be useful both in auditory research and in clinical testing of discrimination.[18]

Attempts have been made also to develop discrimination tests based on sentences rather than single words, on the theory that a sentence test is more analogous to everyday listening situations than isolated words and thus a more valid test of an individual's discrimination abilities. Davis[19] discusses sentence tests and reproduces some of them, including a new list devised at Central Institute for the Deaf to represent "everyday American speech." Speaks and Jerger[20] constructed a test consisting of closed-message sets of "synthetic" or artificial sentences. These sentences do not bear much resemblance to real sentences, since they consist of words strung together without regard for syntax or meaning. The listener's task is to select which "sentence" of a set was spoken by the talker. The synthetic sentence test was designed primarily for experimental use when the speech signal is filtered, distorted, or masked in various ways.

While the various "improvements" on the PB lists have their adherents and no doubt will be used in audiology clinics for clinical as well as research purposes, the CID W-22 recordings continue to be the standard tool for the clinical assessment of speech discrimination. Perhaps the most compelling reason for continuing with the W-22 recordings is that the Veterans Administration has based compensation for service-connected hearing impairment on speech audiometric results obtained with the W-22 recordings. Obviously a change in the test for measuring discrimination might necessitate a change in the rating schedule and a re-evaluation of all those veterans whose compensation was based on the W-22 test. The economic implications of such a move are enormous.

Social Adequacy Index

In pure-tone audiometry, the only way of expressing the patient's hearing handicap in meaningful form is to compute the percentage of hearing loss monaurally and binaurally. In the last chapter, the limitations of this method of expressing the degree of handicap were discussed. The principal limitation is that percentage of pure-tone loss does not tell us anything directly about the patient's communicative ability. What is needed is some measure based on the results of speech audiometry which will represent the degree of handicap so far as hearing and understanding speech are concerned. One such measure is the social adequacy index (SAI), conceived and devel-

18 Gordon E. Peterson and Ilse Lehiste, "Revised CNC Lists for Auditory Tests," *Journal of Speech and Hearing Disorders,* Vol. 27 (February, 1962), pp. 62-70.

19 Hallowell Davis, "Audiometry: Pure Tone and Simple Speech Tests," in Hallowell Davis and S. Richard Silverman, eds. *Hearing and Deafness* (New York, Holt, Rinehart and Winston, 1970), pp. 213-214, 489-495.

20 Charles Speaks and James Jerger, "Method for Measurement of Speech Identification," *Journal of Speech and Hearing Research,* Vol. 8 (June, 1965), pp. 185-194.

oped at Central Institute for the Deaf.[21] The SAI is a measure that is computed from the results of the speech-reception threshold and articulation tests. It can be found by means of a table in which the two dimensions are SRT and discrimination loss. The table for computing the SAI is reproduced in Figure 6-3.

SAI scores have been correlated with patients' reports of their degree of handicap in various business and social situations, so that values of handicap could be assigned to certain points along the SAI scale from 0 to 100. The limits of SAI for the normal ear are from 94 to 100. At an SAI of 67, the patient begins to notice difficulty with his hearing in some situations. The "threshold of social adequacy" is an SAI of 33. In other words, with an SAI of 33, a patient can "get by" in business and social situations only with great difficulty. With an SAI as low as 10 to 15, it is impossible for a patient to function communicatively without amplification.

Although the SAI is scaled from 0 to 100, it is not to be regarded as a percentage scale of speech hearing, comparable to the percentage loss for pure tones. What the SAI really represents is a patient's ability to understand PB words at three standard levels of intensity. In the original research on the SAI, each patient was given three PB tests: one at a level of 33 dB, one at 48 dB, and one at 63 dB, all levels in relation to zero SRT, defined at that time as an SPL of 22 dB. These three hearing levels had been empirically defined as the average levels of faint, average, and loud conversational speech, respectively. The scores made by the patient on these three tests were averaged, and the result was called the social adequacy index. Thus the SAI is actually the average percentage of correct responses a patient makes (or could, theoretically, make) on PB tests at three standard levels of intensity. The table for computing the SAI was evolved as a short-cut method, since the administration of three PB tests in each ear and again binaurally is time-consuming and tiring. With the table, the patient's SRT and his score on a single PB test given at a minimum sensation level of 40 dB can serve as the basis for predicting what his performance would be if the lengthier procedure of administering several PB tests were to be followed.

It should be mentioned at this point that the original articulation curve and SAI table were derived with recordings of the Harvard PB words, and not with the later recordings of the modified Harvard list, known as Auditory Test W-22. There is evidence that most people will make higher scores on the W-22 test than they could on the older recordings of the Harvard PB words. If this is so, their SAI would be somewhat higher when computed with the W-22 scores. Thus, the interpretation of the degree of handicap represented by a particular SAI based on W-22 scores should be made with caution. Also, the data on which the degrees of handicap were based came from a very limited sampling of hearing-impaired patients—only those with

[21] Hallowell Davis, "The Articulation Area and the Social Adequacy Index for Hearing," *Laryngoscope*, Vol. 58 (1948), pp. 761-768.

Social Adequacy Index

Discrimination Loss (% PB words missed at high intensity)	\ Hearing Loss for Speech in Decibels →	0	2	4	6	8	10	12	14	16	18	20	22	24	26	28	30	32	34	36	38	40	42	44	46	48	50	52	54	56	58	60	62	64	66	68	70	72	74
0		99	98	97	96	94	93	92	90	88	85	82	79	75	69	64	61	57	52	48	44	41	37	33	28	24	20	17	15	12	10	7	4	2	1	0	0	0	0
5		94	93	92	91	90	89	88	87	85	82	79	76	72	67	63	59	55	51	47	43	40	37	32	28	24	20	17	15	12	9	7	4	2	1	0	0	0	0
10		89	89	88	86	85	85	84	83	81	78	76	73	70	65	61	57	53	49	46	42	40	37	31	27	23	19	16	14	11	9	7	4	2	1	0	0	0	0
15		84	84	83	83	82	81	80	79	77	75	72	70	67	63	59	55	53	47	44	41	39	36	30	26	23	19	16	14	11	9	7	4	2	1	0	0	0	0
20		79	79	78	78	78	77	76	75	73	71	69	67	64	61	57	53	50	46	43	40	37	34	29	26	22	19	16	13	11	9	6	4	2	1	0	0	0	0
25		75	75	74	74	73	72	71	70	69	67	65	63	61	58	55	51	47	44	40	38	36	33	28	25	21	18	15	13	10	8	6	4	2	1	0	0	0	0
30		70	70	69	69	68	67	66	66	65	63	62	60	58	55	52	48	44	41	38	36	34	31	27	24	21	18	15	12	10	8	6	4	2	1	0	0	0	0
35		65	65	64	64	63	63	62	61	60	59	58	56	54	52	48	45	42	39	36	34	32	29	26	23	20	17	15	12	10	8	6	4	2	1	0	0	0	0
40		60	60	59	59	59	58	58	57	56	55	54	53	51	48	46	43	40	37	34	32	30	28	25	22	19	16	14	12	10	8	6	4	2	1	0	0	0	0
45		55	55	55	54	54	54	53	53	52	51	50	49	47	45	41	40	37	34	32	30	28	26	24	21	18	16	13	11	9	7	5	4	2	1	0	0	0	0
50		50	50	50	50	50	49	49	49	48	46	45	44	43	41	39	37	34	32	29	27	26	24	22	20	17	14	12	10	9	6	5	3	2	1	0	0	0	0
55		45	45	45	45	45	45	44	44	43	42	41	40	39	38	36	34	31	29	27	25	24	22	19	16	14	11	9	8	7	5	4	3	2	1	0	0	0	0
60		40	40	40	40	40	40	39	39	38	37	36	35	34	32	30	28	26	24	21	19	17	16	13	11	9	8	7	6	6	4	3	3	2	1	0	0	0	0
65		35	35	35	35	35	35	34	34	33	33	33	32	31	30	29	27	25	23	20	18	16	15	13	11	8	7	6	5	4	3	2							
70		30	30	30	30	30	30	25	29	29	29	24	28	27	26	25	23	22	21	20	15	15	14	13	11	9	8	6											
75		25	25	25	25	25	25	25	24	24	24	24	23	23	22	20	19	17	16	15	13	11	10	9															
80		20	20	20	20	20	20	20	20	20	19	19	19	19	18	18	17	16	14	12	11	10	9																
85		15	15	15	15	15	15	15	15	15	15	15	14	14	14	13	13	12	11	9	8	7																	
90		10	10	10	10	10	10	10	10	10	10	10	10	10	10	9	9	8	8	7																			
95		10	10	10	10	10	10	10	10	10	10	10	10																										
100		0	0	0	0	0	0	0	0	0	0	0	0	0	0	0	0	0	0	0	0	0	0	0	0	0	0	0	0	0	0	0	0	0	0	0	0	0	0

When the discrimination loss is greater than about 90% ordinary speech is not understood at any intensity, and it becomes difficult or impossible to measure the hearing loss for speech.

Hearing Loss for Speech in Decibels

Figure 6-3. Table for finding the social adequacy index.

129

a diagnosis of clinical otosclerosis who were candidates for fenestration surgery. It is likely that a broader spectrum of patients, that is, patients with a variety of conductive and sensori-neural pathologies, would yield quite different findings as to the levels of SAI associated with degrees of handicap. The SAI concept is presented here not as a calibrated clinical tool but as one possible approach to the problem of expressing a patient's communicative handicap based on speech audiometry instead of pure-tone results as in the AAOO method of computing percentage hearing loss. A valid procedure for translating audiometric results into degree of communicative handicap should be most useful in medicolegal contexts.

STEP-BY-STEP PROCEDURE IN SPEECH AUDIOMETRY

The procedure described below is designed for adults or older children and for a typical two-room testing situation. The assumption is made that recorded tests will be used and that the patient is capable of writing responses where necessary. Instructions to the patient will be covered in the procedure. Many audiologists have the patient read over a list of the words that appear in the spondee test so that he is familiar with the vocabulary. Of course when presented in test form the words would be in a different order.

1. Inform the patient that the first test will be through earphones, one ear at a time, and will consist of two-syllable words, such as *doorway* and *footstool*. The words will start out fairly loud, and decrease in loudness gradually. The patient is to repeat each word as he hears it, guessing at the word if necessary. You should tell him that the object of the test is to find the point at which he misses about half of the words, and therefore he is not to become upset or angry with himself if he finds that he is missing some words.

2. Place the earphones on the patient's head, making sure that they fit snugly and comfortably over each ear. From the pure-tone test which you have already administered, you will know whether masking will be necessary in either ear for the speech tests (if it is necessary, explain to the patient what you are doing and why). Switch the input selector to "turntable." Switch the output selector to "earphone," either left or right. Then put on one of the W-1 records. Follow the instructions that accompany the records for determining the proper setting of the input volume control. This involves adjusting the control until the VU meter registers the correct value for a 1000 Hz calibrating tone which is cut in the record. Having set the input control properly, adjust the attenuator to produce an output level that you estimate will be about 15 to 20 dB above the patient's threshold in that ear. After the patient has repeated three or four consecutive words correctly, decrease the output level by 5 dB. Repeat this procedure until you reach a point at which the patient is missing some words. Then increase the level by 5 or 6 dB to reach an even step on the attenuator. At this level present three spondee

words. If the patient repeats them correctly, decrease the level by 2 dB and present more spondee words. If the patient misses one or more of the three words presented, continue with spondee words at the same level until a maximum of six words have been presented. If the patient misses four of the six words, increase the level by 2 dB and present up to six additional words. As soon as the patient gets three words of a series correctly, decrease the level by 2 dB and start another series. Thus at each even step on the hearing-level dial, at least three and up to six words will be presented, depending on the patient's responses. You are seeking the minimum hearing level (in even numbers of decibels) at which the patient can repeat three spondee words correctly. Continue decreasing the hearing level in 2 dB steps until the patient misses at least four out of six words at three consecutive decrements of intensity. This step is a precaution against premature acceptance of too high an SRT. The threshold criterion to be applied is a 50 per cent level of correct response, that is, at least three out of six words repeated correctly. Record the lowest hearing level at which the patient achieved this 50 per cent criterion as his SRT by spondees for the ear being tested.[22] While the method just described will yield the patient's SRT to the nearest 2-dB step on the hearing-level control, it is faster and—according to Chaiklin and Ventry—just as valid to use 5-dB steps in arriving at SRT and to express the patient's SRT to the nearest 5-dB step on the hearing-level control.[23] In testing veterans for compensation purposes, however, it is necessary to find the SRT to the nearest 2-dB step.

With the W-1 records, on which the calibrating tone and carrier phrase "You will say . . ." have been recorded at a level of 10 dB greater intensity than the test words, you must be careful to record the correct hearing level as the patient's SRT. Speech audiometers are calibrated to zero dB as the average, normal speech-reception threshold for *test words*, not the carrier phrase. In other words, assuming that audiometric zero equals a sound pressure level re 0.0002 dyne/cm^2 of 20 dB, the output of the amplifier is set so that, when the attenuator dial reads 0, the average normal ear can just understand approximately 50 per cent of the spondee words when the *words* are monitored to 0 on the VU meter. When the W-1 records are used, the VU meter is set to 0 for the calibrating tone and carrier phrase, and the spondee words themselves will peak an average 10 dB below 0 on the meter. This means that the output level of the spondee words will be 10 dB less than the indicated hearing level on the attenuator dial. It will be necessary for you, when using the W-1 records, to subtract 10 dB from the obtained SRT in order to arrive at the actual SRT. It is awkward to have to make this correction every time a recorded spondee test is administered. With the situ-

[22] The technique for arriving at SRT by spondees described here is adapted from the method described by Chaiklin, *op. cit.,* p. 240.

[23] Joseph B Chaiklin and Ira M Ventry, "Spondee Threshold Measurement: A Comparison of 2- and 5-dB Methods," *Journal of Speech and Hearing Disorders,* Vol. 29 (February, 1964), pp. 47-59.

ation that pertains currently, it is much simpler to secure the SRT for spondees by means of live voice, monitoring the level of the spondees with the input volume control and the VU meter. As mentioned before, however, recorded tests should be given for the purpose of obtaining greater standardization of results from clinic to clinic. Some audiologists prefer to make their own recordings of spondee words on magnetic tape. If you make your own recordings, the carrer phrase and test words can be recorded at the same level, thus obviating the need for any correction for difference in level between them.

3. Now switch the ouput selector to the opposite ear, turn up the level until the spondees are being delivered at about 15 to 20 dB above the patient's supposed threshold in that ear, and proceed to determine the SRT by spondees in the same manner as in step 2. Record this result.

4. If it is desirable for any reason to obtain the patient's threshold of intelligibility for running speech, next explain to the patient (switching the input selector to "microphone" and increasing the amplification until he can hear your explanation easily) that you are going to put on a record of running speech. Tell him that he will hear the running speech in one ear at a time, that at the beginning he will hear the speech well, but that you are going to make it progressively softer until finally he will not be able to understand what the speaker is saying. Instruct him to say "yes" every few seconds as long as he can understand the speaker, "no" when he can no longer understand him. Tell the patient that he may miss some individual words and yet be able to follow the thought being expressed, and as long as he can follow the train of thought he should say "yes."

5. Switch the input selector back to "turntable," and put on the running-speech record. Adjust the input volume control until the needle on the VU meter is peaking zero dB on the average. Again, start the record at an output level that you know will be well above the patient's threshold. After the patient has responded "yes" two or three times, decrease the output level by a few dB, allow him to respond "yes" two or three times, and decrease the output level again. Follow this procedure until you reach the point at which the patient says "no." The hearing level at which the patient last responded "yes" should be noted as the patient's SRT by running speech. If you have reason to question the validity of the patient's "yes" responses, you should ask him some simple questions concerning the material he has heard.

6. Switch the output selector to the other ear, and go through the same process in establishing the SRT by running speech for that ear. Record the result.

7. You now have SRT's for each ear both by spondees and by running speech. Average the thresholds obtained by the two methods for each ear, and record the results as the patient's monaural SRT's. Many audiologists do not bother to obtain SRT's by running speech, and you may well decide to skip steps 4 through 7 of these procedures.

8. Switching back to "microphone," explain to the patient that now you are going to make the running speech louder. Tell him that you want him to signal when the speech is at a level which is "most comfortable" for him to listen to. Tell him that you want him to be sure that the level he picks is the most comfortable, that he should therefore direct you to make the speech louder and softer two or three times until he is certain of his decision.

9. Switch back to "turntable," and put on the running-speech record again. Then gradually increase the intensity of the speech until the patient signals that it is most comfortably loud. Make him repeat this judgment until you and he are sure that the most comfortable level has been found. Record this hearing level as the patient's MCL. Switch to the other ear, and repeat the procedure to establish the MCL in that ear.

10. Switching back to "microphone," explain to the patient that now you are going to make the running speech louder still. Tell him that you want to find out whether the speech gets so loud that it causes him to feel a sensation of discomfort in the ear. Inform him that the speech will be louder than he would care to listen to, but that you want to find out if it gets so loud that it causes him physiological discomfort, such as a tickling sensation, in the ear. If it should get that loud he is to push the button, which will illuminate a light on your control panel, and tell him that when you see the light you will immediately turn off the loud speech.

11. Switch back to "turntable," and put on the running-speech record again. Gradually increase the intensity of the speech, watching the patient through the window. It is a good idea to keep your hand on the input volume control while you are increasing the output. As soon as the patient signals that the speech is uncomfortably loud, immediately turn the input volume control counter-clockwise all the way, thus cutting the signal off without disturbing the setting of the output attenuator. Note what the hearing-level reading is, and record this figure as the patient's tolerance level for that ear. Switch the output selector to the other ear, and repeat the procedure to obtain the tolerance level for that ear.

12. Subtract the patient's average SRT from his tolerance level in each ear and record the difference as his dynamic range.

13. Switching back to "microphone," explain to the patient that now you are going to put on a recording of a man speaking one-syllable words, that there will be no difficulty in hearing the words because you will make them loud enough to be heard easily. Tell him that though each word will be preceded by the phrase "You will say . . ." he is to write the word that he hears on the blank you have given him, rather than repeat it. Tell him that he is to write down what he thinks the word is each time, but, if he has no idea what the word is, he is to leave that space blank. Explain that there will be fifty words in the list and that, when one list has been completed, you will switch to the other ear and present another list. In order to reduce the effect of learning on the test scores, many audiologists present a practice

list of 25 or 50 PB words to the patient before beginning the actual test. The practice list should not be the same one used in the test.

14. Switch the input selector to "turntable," and put on one of the W-22 records. Adjust the input volume control so that the calibrating tone on the record will peak the needle on the VU meter at zero dB. On the W-22 records, the calibrating tone and the carrier phrase are recorded at the same level as the test words. When the input volume control is properly set for the calibrating tone, the carrier phrase will peak consistently at the same place on the VU meter. The PB words will not all peak the same, however, as the words differ in their phonetic power. Once the proper level for the calibrating tone and carrier phrase has been established, the input volume control should not be touched. Adjust the output attenuator so that the output is 40 dB greater than the SRT for the ear being tested, unless adding 40 dB to the SRT will result in an output that equals or exceeds the tolerance level for that ear. In that event, it will be necessary for you to present the PB list at a level less than 40 dB above the SRT, for you cannot present the words at a level that will cause discomfort to the patient. Then start the discrimination test.

15. Switch the output selector to the opposite ear, adjust the attenuator to a level of 40 dB above the SRT in that ear, if that is possible, and put on another W-22 record.

16. You have now completed the monaural tests. Score the PB test papers, and enter the percentage correct for each ear on the speech audiogram after "Discrimination."

17. Remove the earphones from the patient's head. If it is desirable to obtain information about the patient's hearing for speech in a sound field (as it would be in the case of a hearing-aid consultation, for example), explain to him that now you are going to repeat the same series of tests while he listens to a loudspeaker; that first there will be the two-syllable words, then the running speech which will be first soft, then comfortably loud, and finally very loud; and that to complete the test there will be an additional list of 50 monosyllabic words to write out.

18. Switch the output selector to "speaker." Then repeat the test procedures detailed above. You will now have sound-field measurements of SRT (by spondees, and by running speech, if desired), MCL, dynamic range, tolerance level, and discrimination.

19. With the aid of the SAI table, you may compute the social adequacy index for each ear separately, and again for sound-field, and record the results on the speech audiogram blank. Since many audiologists do not make use of the SAI computation, this step is optional.

INTERPRETING RESULTS

The results of speech audiometry are recorded on a speech audiogram, a sample of which is shown in Figure 6-4, or they may be recorded on such

SPEECH AUDIOMETRIC EXAMINATION

Patient_____ Examiner_____ Date_____

	MONAURAL		SOUND FIELD
	Right	Left	
SPEECH RECEPTION THRESHOLD (dB hearing level)	_____	_____	_____
MOST COMFORTABLE LOUDNESS (dB hearing level)	_____	_____	_____
TOLERANCE LEVEL (dB hearing level)	_____	_____	_____
DYNAMIC RANGE (difference in dB between SRT and tolerance level)	_____	_____	_____
DISCRIMINATION (PB-MAX) (percentage correct at sensation level of 40 dB)	_____	_____	_____
SOCIAL ADEQUACY INDEX (average discrimination score for faint, average, and loud speech--obtained from table using SRT and discrimination)	_____	_____	_____

COMMENT ON EXAMINATION; RECOMMENDATIONS

Figure 6-4.   A sample speech audiogram form.

a form as that shown in Figure 5-5, in the preceding chapter, in combination with a pure-tone audiogram.

As Aid to Diagnosis

While the speech audiometric results alone have limited diagnostic value, in combination with the pure-tone audiogram they provide information that assists the otologist in arriving at a diagnosis as to whether an impairment is conductive or sensori-neural in type, and if the latter, whether or not it is cochlear in origin. More will be said concerning the use of speech audiometry in differentiating between cochlear and retrocochlear sensori-neural lesions in the next chapter. Also in the next chapter the contribution of speech audiometry to the diagnosis of functional or nonorganic hearing problems will be discussed.

If the dynamic range is restricted because of a lowered tolerance level, which might be an indication of the presence of recruitment, especially if in addition there are relatively low discrimination scores, the probability is high that the patient has a sensori-neural impairment. On the other hand, if there is no lowering of the tolerance level and the discrimination scores are high, there is no assurance that the patient does not have sensori-neural impairment. Ordinarily normal tolerance and high discrimination scores would be representative of conductive impairment, but there are some patients with sensori-neural involvement whose speech audiometric scores would be indistinguishable from those of conductively impaired patients. Thus it is as risky to attempt a diagnosis from speech audiometric results alone as it would be to attempt to delineate the type of impairment from a patient's pure-tone air-conduction curve alone.

Keeping the diagnostic limitations of speech audiometry in mind, let us examine the speech audiograms that accompany some of the pure-tone audiograms depicted in Chapter 5. Figure 6-5 is the speech audiogram obtained for the patient whose pure-tone audiogram is shown in Figure 5-7. It can be seen from a comparison of Figures 5-7 and 6-5 that the obtained SRT's agree well with the predicted loss for speech secured by averaging the losses at 500, 1000, and 2000 Hz in each ear. As would be expected because of the flatness of the audiogram curve through the speech frequencies in Figure 5-7, speech tests reveal high discrimination scores, as shown in Figure 6-5. Since a conductive impairment is not characterized by recruitment, we would expect that the tolerance level and dynamic range would be normal, which is borne out in Figure 6-5.

Figure 6-6 is the speech audiogram for the patient whose pure-tone audiogram is shown in Figure 5-8. Because this patient has a gradually sloping audiogram curve, rather than an abruptly sloping one, the predicted speech loss is better computed by the three-frequency method than the two-frequency one, and we find that the SRT's obtained in speech audiometry

SPEECH AUDIOMETRIC EXAMINATION

Patient_____ Examiner_____ Date_____

	MONAURAL		SOUND FIELD
	Right	Left	
SPEECH RECEPTION THRESHOLD (dB hearing level)	42	42	40
MOST COMFORTABLE LOUDNESS (dB hearing level)	82	80	76
TOLERANCE LEVEL (dB hearing level)	108	104	102
DYNAMIC RANGE (difference in dB between SRT and tolerance level)	66	62	62
DISCRIMINATION (PB-MAX) (percentage correct at sensation level of 40 dB)	90%	94%	96%
SOCIAL ADEQUACY INDEX (average discrimination score for faint, average, and loud speech--obtained from table using SRT and discrimination)	37	37	40

COMMENT ON EXAMINATION; RECOMMENDATIONS

Figure 6-5.   Speech audiogram obtained for the patient whose pure-tone audiogram is shown in Fig. 5-7.

SPEECH AUDIOMETRIC EXAMINATION

Patient_____ Examiner_____ Date_____

| | MONAURAL | | SOUND FIELD |
	Right	Left	
SPEECH RECEPTION THRESHOLD (dB hearing level)	28	22	24
MOST COMFORTABLE LOUDNESS (dB hearing level)	44	40	40
TOLERANCE LEVEL (dB hearing level)	88	85	82
DYNAMIC RANGE (difference in dB between SRT and tolerance level)	60	63	58
DISCRIMINATION (PB-MAX) (percentage correct at sensation level of 40 dB)	70%	74%	72%
SOCIAL ADEQUACY INDEX (average discrimination score for faint, average, and loud speech--obtained from table using SRT and discrimination)	52	62	59

COMMENT ON EXAMINATION; RECOMMENDATIONS

Figure 6-6.   Speech audiogram obtained for the patient whose pure-tone audiogram is shown in Fig. 5-8.

show a fairly close agreement with those predicted. Since the patient has a sensori-neural impairment, there is the possibility that recruitment of loudness might occur. The lowered tolerance level reported in Figure 6-6 suggests the presence of recruitment. Incidentally, it should be noted that the dynamic range alone cannot be used as an indicator of the presence of recruitment, since the patient whose scores are reported in Figure 6-6 has dynamic ranges about on a par with those of the patient with conductive impairment whose scores are shown in Figure 6-5. The reason for the similarity of their dynamic range is that the patient whose scores are depicted in Figure 6-5 has higher SRT's than the patient whose scores are given in Figure 6-6. It will be noted that the discrimination scores reported in Figure 6-6 are relatively low. The shape of this patient's pure-tone air-conduction curve (see Figure 5-8) undoubtedly contributes to his discrimination loss.

A mixed impairment is represented by the pure-tone audiogram in Figure 5-11. Figure 6-7 shows the speech audiogram for this patient. The obtained SRT's are somewhat better than would be predicted from the audiogram by the three-frequency method. The patient's tolerance levels are slightly reduced and there is some discrimination loss in each ear which is probably related to the sensori-neural component and the configuration of the air-conduction curve.

Before we leave the subject of the diagnostic significance of speech audio-metry, an additional word should be said concerning the need for masking when there is a difference between the ears. As is true in pure-tone air-conduction audiometry, a speech signal can be heard in the ear not under test when the difference in sensitivity between the ears is on the order of from 40 to 60 dB. To prevent the contralateral ear from participating it is necessary in such instances to apply a masking noise. The preferred masking noise for speech audiometry is either white noise, or a noise "shaped" to resemble the speech spectrum. In speech testing, as in pure-tone air-conduction testing, there is little if any danger that too high a level of masking will be used, that is, so intense a masking noise that the threshold of the ear under test would be affected. Instead there is danger that the level of the masking signal may not be sufficiently high to rule out the participation of the better ear. It is best, therefore, to set the level of the masking noise as high as the patient will tolerate it without complaining.

While the indications for the use of masking during theshold determination are fairly clear, it may not always be apparent that masking should be employed while testing the patient's discrimination. If there is sufficient difference in sensitivity between the ears to justify the use of masking while obtaining the SRT, then of course masking should be utilized also in the discrimination test of the poorer ear. There are occasions, however, when threshold differences between the ears are not sufficient to require masking while measuring SRT, and yet masking is required to prevent the participation of the better ear in discrimination testing. Such an instance is illustrated in

SPEECH AUDIOMETRIC EXAMINATION

Patient_____ Examiner_____ Date_____

	MONAURAL		SOUND FIELD
	Right	Left	
SPEECH RECEPTION THRESHOLD (dB hearing level)	44	42	42
MOST COMFORTABLE LOUDNESS (dB hearing level)	60	60	59
TOLERANCE LEVEL (dB hearing level)	88	90	86
DYNAMIC RANGE (difference in dB between SRT and tolerance level)	44	48	44
DISCRIMINATION (PB-MAX) (percentage correct at sensation level of 40 dB)	80%	82%	84%
SOCIAL ADEQUACY INDEX (average discrimination score for faint, average, and loud speech--obtained from table using SRT and discrimination)	29	35	36

COMMENT ON EXAMINATION; RECOMMENDATIONS

Figure 6-7. Speech audiogram obtained for the patient whose pure-tone audiogram is shown in Fig. 5-11.

AUDIOMETRIC EXAMINATION
(INTERNATIONAL THRESHOLD NORMS HAVE BEEN USED AS REFERENCE)

REASON FOR REFERRAL	NAME OF REFERRING STATION
Compensation Exam	Regional Office

AIR CONDUCTION

EXAMINER'S INITIALS	RIGHT							LEFT						
	125	250	500	1000	2000	4000	8000	125	250	500	1000	2000	4000	8000
		5	5	0	5	25	15	UM	5	10	30	50	80	70
								M			30	65	80	NR
MASKING LEVEL IN OPPOSITE EAR										70 dB white noise--				

BONE CONDUCTION

EXAMINER'S INITIALS	RIGHT						LEFT					
		250	500	1000	2000	4000		250	500	1000	2000	4000
			5	0	0	25			10	30	NR	NR
MASKING LEVEL IN OPPOSITE EAR									70 dB white noise			

ELECTRODERMAL RESPONSE

EXAMINER'S INITIALS	RIGHT						LEFT				
		250	500	1000	2000	4000		250	500	1000	2000	4000
										35		
MASKING LEVEL IN OPPOSITE EAR												

SPEECH AUDIOMETRY

EXAMINER'S INITIALS	SPEECH RECEPTION THRESHOLD				ITEM	DISCRIMINATION SCORE (PB MAX)				PURE TONE AVERAGES		
	1	2	3	4		1	2	3	4			
RIGHT EAR	4				RIGHT EAR	98%				EAR	TWO FREQ.	THREE FREQ.
					LIST 1A MASKING LEVEL							
LEFT EAR	26				LEFT EAR	88%	70%			RIGHT	3	3
MASKING LEVEL					LIST 2A MASKING LEVEL	3A 70				LEFT	20	35

INTER-TEST CONSISTENCY (RE)	WEBER TEST	INTER-TEST CONSISTENCY (LE)
Good	.	Good

REMARKS
Note deterioration of discrimination score in left ear when right ear is masked.

LAST NAME - FIRST NAME - MIDDLE INITIAL OF PATIENT	AGE	CLAIM NO.	SOCIAL SECURITY NO.
WRB	58	C-	

NAME OF EXAMINING STATION OR CLINIC	SIGNATURE OF EXAMINING AUDIOLOGIST OR PHYSICIAN	DATE OF EXAMINATION
VA Hospital	HDR	3/15/67

VA FORM MAY 1966 **10-2364**   SUPERSEDES VA FORM 10-2364, DEC 1962, WHICH WILL NOT BE USED.

Figure 6-8. Illustration of need for masking in testing speech discrimination.

Figure 6-8, which shows pure-tone and speech test results recorded on a special audiogram form used by the Veterans Administration. This patient has normal hearing in the right ear and a sharply sloping sensori-neural impairment in the left ear. The first air-conduction results recorded show unmasked (UM) hearing levels. The second set of air-conduction results was obtained with masking of the contralateral ear for the frequencies of 1000 Hz and above. With masking (M), it is seen that the threshold at 2000 Hz shifts 15 dB, which indicates that the slope of the air-conduction curve through the speech frequencies is even steeper than it appeared without masking. Now note the speech test results. Since there is only 22 dB difference between the ears in SRT, there is no indication that masking should be employed while obtaining the threshold measurement of the left ear. This is an insufficient difference in hearing level for the signal to be referred to the contralateral ear. The unmasked discrimination score for the left ear is 88 per cent—a relatively high discrimination score, considering the pure-tone configuration in the left ear, but still possible. But when a masking noise is applied to the right ear and the discrimination test is repeated on the left ear, we see that the discrimination score in that ear drops 18 per cent.

Why masking is needed in the case presented in Figure 6-8 becomes clear when we consider that a discrimination test is administered usually at a level that is 40 dB above the SRT. If we present a PB list to the left ear at a hearing level of 66 dB, then it is possible that there could be some participation of the right ear in the test, since the speech signal is now 62 dB above the SRT of the right ear and air-conducted signals can be referred to the opposite ear when this great a difference between the ears exists. The difference in PB scores in the left ear obtained when the right ear was masked suggests that this is indeed what happened. The unmasked discrimination score of 88 per cent for the left ear represents the discrimination ability of the left ear for a signal of 40-dB sensation level assisted by the discrimination ability of the right ear for a relatively weak signal.

Incidentally, the case shown in Figure 6-8 illustrates very well the type of air-conduction configuration with which the two-frequency method of predicting SRT should be used. Because of the steep slope of the air-conduction curve, a prediction of speech threshold based on a three-frequency average overestimates the SRT actually obtained by 9 dB. The two-frequency prediction underestimates the obtained SRT, but it is in error by only 6 dB.

As Guide to Rehabilitation

As a guide to a patient's rehabilitative needs, the speech audiogram is invaluable. It tells us directly how the patient is handicapped in communication by giving information on the degree of loss (the SRT) and the amount of difficulty in understanding what is heard (discrimination or articulation score). The SAI is a means of expressing the degree of handicap based on these two measures. In the preceding chapter, suggestions were made as to how information from the pure-tone audiogram could be applied in determining what the patient needs in the way of rehabilitation. The speech audiogram can be used in the same manner but with more assurance since with the pure-tone audiogram only speculation is possible as to the effect of the loss on speech-hearing, whereas the speech audiogram shows us this effect.

The comments made in the last chapter concerning the utilization of information from the pure-tone audiogram in determining whether or not a patient can benefit from amplification apply here too. The hearing aid should provide enough amplification to reach above the patient's threshold for speech, but at the same time it must not exceed the patient's threshold of discomfort. The dynamic range gives us the limits within which the hearing aid must operate. The MCL tells us at what level of amplification the patient will hear most comfortably.

The speech audiogram yields information as to how much difficulty the patient may be expected to experience in learning to use the hearing aid effectively. As a rule, a patient who has a poor discrimination score will have much more difficulty with the aid than someone who has a high score. All that the hearing aid can do is to make speech louder; as a general rule it cannot make it any clearer. If a patient's primary difficulty is one of not being able to understand what is said because of poor speech discrimination, he will no doubt be disappointed in a hearing aid. He will hear speech more loudly with the aid, but he will not be able to understand well what he hears. Such a patient needs training in making his hearing serve him most effectively (auditory training), and he may also need training in speechreading (lip-reading). If he can learn to take advantage of the minimal sound clues that he receives and can learn to distinguish among dissimilar sounds through their appearance on the speaker's mouth, he can communicate effectively.

The patient's SAI tells us generally the degree of communicative handicap he has by placing him somewhere on a scale from zero to one hundred. For reasons stated earlier in this chapter, the clinical significance of a particular SAI needs to be established with patients presenting a wide range of auditory impairments and aural pathologies. Nevertheless, the SAI is useful in giving a rough indication of how much discrimination ability the patient has over the usual range of conversational speech. The Veterans Administration employs a method for determining hearing disability for compensation purposes that takes into account both loss of sensitivity for speech (SRT) and discrimination score (PB-Max). Perhaps in the future courts of law and compensation boards generally will demand direct evidence of the degree of difficulty in communication a claimant is experiencing, instead of depending on the percentage of pure-tone loss as the sole yardstick for judging disability.

In the next chapter, speech audiometry serving special purposes will be discussed, including techniques in assessing the hearing sensitivity of very young children. The development of speech audiometry has added substantially to the audiologist's armamentarium.

7

SPECIAL PROBLEMS IN
HEARING TESTING

In the previous two chapters, the emphasis has been on the techniques and procedures of standard pure-tone and speech audiometry. In this chapter, attention will be paid to special problems in clinical audiometry and special tests for particular purposes.

PRE- AND POSTOPERATIVE AUDIOMETRY

In all aspects of audiology, the otologist and the audiologist work closely together for the benefit of the hard-of-hearing patient. One of the best examples of the closeness of their teamwork is in the selection of candidates for operative procedures and in the evaluation of the success of an operation in restoring hearing. As was mentioned in Chapter 3, there are a number of operations designed to improve the hearing in patients who manifest a primarily conductive impairment. Perhaps the most common operation is the tonsillectomy and adenoidectomy, usually referred to as a "T and A." The purpose of this operation, when it is performed for reasons of improving the hearing, is to restore the patency of the Eustachian tube and thus to correct a condition of retraction of the eardrum. The selection of a candidate for the T and A is frequently dependent on a recognition that the hearing is defective in the first place. The otologist turns to the audiologist for information concerning the patient's hearing. The comparison of the air-conduction and bone-conduction hearing reveals the amount of conductive impairment. Since usually a T and A is performed on a child, the measurement of the amount of conductive loss before the operation and the evaluation of the postoperative hearing may be difficult tasks. The last section of this chapter will be devoted to the special problems of assessing the hearing of young children.

The modified radical mastoidectomy has a dual purpose—the elimination of infection in the middle ear and mastoid process, and the improvement of the hearing. A tympanoplasty is designed to improve the hearing by reconstructive surgery on the eardrum or the middle ear. In both these operations, it is important for the otologist to know the extent of the preoperative hearing loss both by air conduction and by bone conduction. Postoperative testing, of course, reveals the amount of improvement in hearing that has occurred and thus measures how successfully the otologist has achieved one of the goals of the operation.

Important as the audiologist is in assisting the otologist in a selection of patients for the operations mentioned above, and in evaluating the success of these operative procedures, it is in the field of surgery for otosclerosis that the audiologist can make his greatest contribution in pre- and postoperative audiometry. For many years the fenestration operation was the only procedure which could effect an improvement in hearing in a case of otosclerosis. Since the fenestration is a major operation performed under a general anesthetic, and since in the course of the operation unalterable changes are made in the anatomy of the ear, the proper selection of candidates for this operation assumes tremendous importance. Otologists and audiologists worked together to develop audiometric procedures for the purpose of predicting the results of a fenestration in a specific patient. With careful methods of selection, the "batting average" of the surgeon in fenestration operations rose to the point where eight out of ten suitable candidates for the operation could anticipate the achievement of "functional" hearing in the operated ear.

The advent of the stapes mobilization procedure brought a decline in the popularity of the fenestration operation. Then when stapedectomy was introduced the stapes mobilization procedure became almost extinct. Because of its simplicity (for the patient) and the potential improvement in hearing to the level of preoperative bone conduction, the stapedectomy is the operation of choice for otosclerosis in almost every case. Occasionally the fenestration will still be performed when a stapedectomy has been unsuccessful or when in the judgment of the otologist there are contraindications for a stapedectomy.

As the operations for otosclerosis have improved over the years, there has been a decreasing emphasis on audiological contributions to the success of operative procedures. In the late 1940's and early 1950's during the period of popularity of the fenestration, great importance was attached to the proper selection of candidates for the operation. Fenestration was major surgery, and since at best it could result in a residual hearing loss of from 20 to 30 dB owing to the destruction of the ossicular chain, it was necessary to exercise great care in selecting candidates who reasonably could be expected to benefit from this operation. In the selection of patients, the otologist was dependent on information furnished by the audiologist.

In two outstanding instances, otologists and audiologists combined their talents to devise methods for predicting postoperative hearing levels on the basis of what were termed "fenestration surveys" performed in the audiology clinic. Davis and Walsh[1] described a method based on a combination of pure-tone and speech audiometric data for predicting the patient's post-operative SRT. Shambaugh and Carhart[2] predicted a patient's postoperative pure-tone air-conduction thresholds on the basis of a comparison of his pre-operative air-conduction and bone-conduction hearing levels at four frequencies. It was Carhart who reported that preoperative bone-conduction hearing levels could not be measured accurately in otosclerotics because the fixated stapes, interfering with the movement of cochlear fluids, was responsi-ble for producing an "inner ear conductive block." This conductive block resulted in an apparent depression of bone-conduction acuity that amounted on the average to 5 dB at 500 and 4000 Hz, 10 dB at 1000 Hz, and 15 dB at 2000 Hz. Thus a patient whose cochlear function was actually unimpaired would demonstrate preoperatively a depression of his bone-conduction curve that has come to be called the "Carhart notch." In order to obtain a more accurate assessment of an otosclerotic's cochlear function, it was necessary to correct his preoperative bone-conduction hearing levels for the Carhart notch.[3]

In stapes mobilization surgery, operating-room audiometry came into existence. Many otologists found it helpful to have an audiologist in the operating room, so that the progression of the patient's hearing improvement could be monitored audiometrically at various stages in the procedure. Goodhill[4] described the test sequence in operating-room audiometry, and Goodhill and Holcomb devised a graphical means of recording the audio-metric results obtained at stages in the operation as a guide to the surgeon on the success of his mobilization attempts.[5]

Since both the fenestration and the stapes mobilization operations are largely of only historical interest at the present time, no description will be given of the techniques devised for predicting the outcome of the fenestration operation or monitoring the progression of the stapes mobilization procedure. The student who is interested in reading about these audiological innovations will find a full discussion of them in the first edition of this book (1958).

[1] Hallowell Davis and Theodore Walsh, "The Limits of Improvement of Hearing Following the Fenestration Operation," *Laryngoscope*, Vol. 60 (April, 1950), pp. 273-295.

[2] George E. Shambaugh and Raymond Carhart, "Contributions of Audiology to Fenestra-tion Surgery, Including a Formula for the Precise Prediction of the Hearing Result," *A.M.A. Archives of Otolaryngology*, Vol. 54 (December, 1951), pp. 699-712.

[3] Raymond Carhart, "Bone-conduction Advances Following Fenestration Surgery," *Transactions American Academy Ophthalmology and Otolaryngology*, Vol. 56 (July-August, 1952), pp. 621-629.

[4] Victor Goodhill, "Surgical Audiometry in Stapedolysis (Stapes Mobilization)," *A.M.A. Archives of Otolaryngology*, Vol. 62 (November, 1955), pp. 504-508.

[5] Victor Goodhill and Arthur L. Holcomb, "The Surgical Audiometric Nomograph in Stapedolysis (Stapes Mobilization)," *A.M.A. Archives of Otolaryngology*, Vol. 63 (April, 1956), pp. 399-410.

The selection of candidates for the stapedectomy operation is a matter of making a careful assessment of bone conduction. The success of any middle ear surgery is dependent on the state of the cochlear function, since the best result that can be achieved in such surgery is the complete elimination of the air-bone gap on the audiogram. The patient who has preoperative bone-conduction hearing levels of from 40 to 50 dB through the speech frequencies cannot expect to achieve functional hearing through a stapedectomy operation. On the other hand, such a patient may consider the operation well worthwhile if his preoperative air-conduction hearing levels were at the limits of the audiometer, since if his air-bone gap were completely eliminated he could utilize a hearing aid more effectively following the operation. In assessing a patient's preoperative bone conduction, cognizance should be taken of the Carhart notch, referred to earlier in this chapter. Since it is most difficult to rule out the participation of the contralateral ear in measuring bone-conduction hearing levels in cases of extreme conductive impairment, care must be taken to employ proper masking procedures. The Rainville type of bone-conduction testing, as discussed in Chapter 5, will be found to be useful as an adjunct to or perhaps in place of standard bone-conduction methodology.

Holcomb and Goodhill[6] suggested a method for determining the degree of success of an operative procedure on the middle ear that is as useful in stapedectomy as it was in stapes mobilization. The method consists of computing the preoperative air-bone gap by subtracting the "equivalent SRT" by bone conduction from the "equivalent SRT" by air conduction in order to determine the maximum gain that can be achieved by the operation. "Equivalent SRT" is a term coined by Goodhill and Holcomb.[7] It is computed by averaging the two out of the three speech frequencies (500, 1000, and 2000 Hz) that show the lesser amount of loss. This is the Fletcher system for predicting speech loss from the pure-tone audiogram.[8] Following the operation, the air-bone gap in terms of equivalent SRT is computed again. The reduction in air-bone gap achieved by the operation is computed by subtracting the postoperative air-bone gap in terms of equivalent SRT from the preoperative air-bone gap. The percentage of success of the operation is then determined by dividing the preoperative air-bone gap into the reduction in air-bone gap, or what Holcomb and Goodhill refer to as the "air-conduction gain." Thus if the operation eliminates the air-bone gap completely it has been 100 per cent successful. If half the air-bone gap has been eliminated the operation is 50 per cent successful.

6 Arthur Holcomb and Victor Goodhill, "Evaluation of Surgery in Conductive Deafness by 'Per Cent Improvement,'" *A.M.A. Archives of Otolaryngology*, Vol 69 (February, 1959), pp. 163-169.

7 Goodhill and Holcomb, *op. cit.*

8 Harvey Fletcher, "A Method of Calculating Hearing Loss for Speech from an Audiogram," *Journal of the Acoustical Society of America*, Vol. 22 (January, 1950), pp. 1-5.

To illustrate the Holcomb and Goodhill method let us assume the following preoperative and postoperative audiometric data expressed for the speech frequencies only in the operated ear.

	PREOPERATIVE Hearing Levels in dB		POSTOPERATIVE Hearing Levels in dB	
	AC	BC	AC	BC
500	80	20	40	20
1000	85	25	50	20
2000	90	40	55	25
Equivalent SRT	83	23	45	20
Air-bone Gap	60		25	

The reduction in the air-bone gap in this illustration turns out to be 35 dB (60-25). The operation is seen to have been almost 60 per cent successful (35 dB/60 dB). Since Holcomb and Goodhill do not correct preoperative bone conduction for the Carhart notch, there can be instances when an operation turns out to have been more than 100 per cent successful.

It should be emphasized that the Holcomb and Goodhill method of computing the success of an operation tells only how successful the surgeon has been in eliminating the air-bone gap. It was designed as a practical and reasonable way for surgeons to report the success of their particular techniques on a series of patients. Thus a surgeon might report in a paper or article that with technique A he achieved an average of 90 per cent success with a series of 100 patients, whereas with technique B his average success with another series of 100 patients was only 84 per cent. The success or failure of an operation so far as a particular patient is concerned depends on many factors that cannot be quantified into a formula. If he hears appreciably better following the operation, then for him the operation was a success, and if he does not hear appreciably better, the operation was unsuccessful. Of course, in most cases there would be a high correlation between the patient's report of degree of success and the percentage of the air-bone gap that was eliminated, but this would not necessarily be true.

Sometimes the elimination of the air-bone gap, while resulting in a 100 per cent "successful" operation, will have a deleterious effect on a patient's speech discrimination. Rosenberg pointed out this possibility in regard to stapes mobilization surgery, and it is true also for stapedectomy.[9] Consider the following example.

	PREOPERATIVE Hearing Levels in dB		POSTOPERATIVE Hearing Levels in dB	
	AC	BC (corrected)	AC	BC
500	60	0	0	0
1000	55	10	10	10
2000	65	45	45	45

[9] Philip E. Rosenberg, "Audiometric Considerations in Stapes Mobilization Surgery," *Journal of Speech and Hearing Disorders*, Vol. 24 (February, 1959), pp. 21-24.

It can be seen that the operation in this case was 100 per cent successful, since the air-bone gap was completely eliminated. But let us compare this patient's preoperative and postoperative speech audiometric results.

	PREOPERATIVE	POSTOPERATIVE
SRT	54 dB	10 dB
Discrimination	96%	80%

While the operation resulted in an improvement in SRT to within 10 dB of audiometric zero, it *reduced* the discrimination score by 16 per cent. So while this patient no longer needs amplification, he still has a disability of hearing in the operated ear because of his discrimination loss. The impairment in discrimination has probably resulted from the tilting of the air-conduction curve postoperatively. The patient's preoperative air-conduction curve was flat and his discrimination was excellent, at supra-threshold levels of course. It will be recalled from Chapters 5 and 6 that speech discrimination is related to the shape of the air-conduction curve through the speech frequencies. The more this curve "tilts" toward the high-frequency end, the more speech discrimination is likely to be impaired. Knowing what can happen to speech discrimination following a "successful" operation, the otologist may decide against an operation in a case where the preoperative bone-conduction curve is sharply tilted. At least he should explain to the patient what is likely to occur with speech discrimination if the air-bone gap is completely eliminated, so that the patient approaches the operation with full realization that he may develop a discrimination problem postoperatively.

A patient's preoperative discrimination scores are thought to give a good indication of his "cochlear reserve." In considering the suitability of a candidate for surgery in cases of otosclerosis, therefore, his discrimination ability as demonstrated in speech audiometry should be evaluated as well as his air-bone gap. Other things being equal, the patient who has a high pre-operative discrimination score in the ear to be operated will probably be more likely to experience a "successful" operation—from both his and the surgeon's point of view—than the patient whose preoperative discrimination score is relatively low.

TESTS FOR DETERMINING THE PRESENCE OF FUNCTIONAL OR NONORGANIC HEARING PROBLEMS

Usually, the responses of a patient in the testing situation represent his best performance, but every audiologist will sooner or later meet a patient who, for some reason, fails to give responses on hearing tests consistent with his actual hearing levels. The test results, therefore, reflect a hearing loss that does not exist, or exaggerations of the seriousness of an actual impairment. It is not surprising, perhaps, that the incidence of functional or nonorganic hearing problems is greatest in instances where the patient is receiving, or may be eligible to receive, some type of monetary payment as compensation for hearing impairment.

The problem of nonorganic or functional hearing loss was discussed in Chapter 3. Reference was made then to the two types of loss that can be termed functional—hysterical or conversion deafness, and-malingering. The first type is marked by the fact that the patient himself believes that he has a genuine loss, or he believes that the moderate loss he may have is really a serious one. He is not trying to "fool" anyone, and he is perfectly willing to cooperate in a test situation. The malingerer, on the other hand, knows what the true status of his hearing is, and he definitely is trying to deceive the examiner. His attitude during a hearing test may be one of suspicion and belligerence. Nevertheless, he has to "cooperate" in the test situation in order to maintain his role of a hearing-handicapped individual. This type of problem is frequently referred to in the literature as "pseudohypoacusis," or feigned hearing loss. For the sake of convenience, all hearing problems of a psychological character will be referred to as "functional" losses, to distinguish them from genuine organic impairments.

It is the psychiatrist's and not the audiologist's responsibility to differentiate between functional losses due to hysteria or conversion and those which represent malingering on the part of the patient. The differentiation is not possible on the basis of test results, in any event. It is the audiologist's responsibility to recognize a functional loss, or a functional overlay on an actual loss, and to determine what the patient's actual hearing levels are. Detection of functional hearing loss requires astute observation of the patient's behavior and speech by the examiner, correlation of test results to check on their consistency, and administration of special tests which are designed specifically to disclose the presence of functional factors. The reader who is interested in the psychological profiles of individuals with functional hearing loss as well as otological and audiological evaluations of such individuals is referred to a comprehensive study performed in the San Francisco Veterans Administration Hospital.[10]

Observation of Patient's Behavior

Frequently clues to functional loss can be detected from observing the patient's behavior before, during, and after the test, for its consistency with the amount of hearing impairment that he presumably has. While talking with the patient, note whether he seems to be experiencing any difficulty in hearing or understanding you. Check to see how closely he is watching you as you speak. A person with a genuine hearing loss of serious extent will watch speakers carefully in order to benefit from lipreading. Try talking to the

[10] Ira M. Ventry and Joseph B. Chaiklin, eds., "Multidiscipline Study of Functional Hearing Loss," *Journal of Auditory Research*, Vol. 5 (July, 1965), pp. 179-272.

patient occasionally when your head is turned and he can't see your face. At times, speak softly and rapidly, being careful to do so naturally, however.

A patient's own speech is a valuable index to his hearing impairment. If a patient claims to be severely or profoundly hard-of-hearing, yet speaks with a well-controlled voice and good articulation (enunciation), there is reason to be suspicious of the extent of his loss. It is possible for a genuinely hard-of-hearing patient to learn control of his voice and diction, but as a general rule the presence of a significant hearing impairment is betrayed by its effect on the patient's voice and speech.

Consistency of Test Results

We have seen in previous chapters that a patient's hearing level for speech can be predicted from the pure-tone audiogram by averaging the hearing levels at the speech frequencies. Also, we have seen that the configuration of the pure-tone audiogram gives an indication of the speech-discrimination difficulties that the patient can be expected to demonstrate on the speech tests. Thus we can examine a patient's pure-tone audiogram and make a rough estimate of how he will perform on the speech test. If the actual speech-test results vary significantly from those which would be predicted from the patient's pure-tone audiogram, there is reason to suspect that functional factors may be operating. For example, suppose that a patient presents a relatively flat sensori-neural loss of approximately 60 dB. You would expect that he would have a speech-reception threshold in the neighborhood of 60 dB with perhaps some loss of speech discrimination. Now suppose that this patient instead turns out to have an SRT of only 30 dB and 100 per cent discrimination. Then it is obvious that factors in addition to organic hearing loss are operating. On the other hand, assume that this patient should present poorer speech-test results than would be predicted from the pure-tone audiogram. Perhaps his SRT turns out to be 80 dB instead of the 60 dB that was predicted, or his discrimination score is close to zero. Again, it is obvious that psychological factors are operating. Before concluding that a patient is demonstrating a functional loss, however, you must make certain that the differences between the predicted and the obtained speech results are not a function of improperly calibrated equipment, or of other explainable factors, such as the patient's unfamiliarity with the English language.

One characteristic of the patient with functional loss, whether of the conscious or of the unconscious variety, is that he may have difficulty in demonstrating the same degree of loss on repeated tests. This is particularly true of the pure-tone tests. Therefore, if a functional loss is suspected, it is wise to administer more than one pure-tone test to the patient and to compare the results. Naturally, the greater the interval is between the test, the more difficulty the patient will experience in trying to present a consistent picture. If possible, it is advisable to schedule the patient for tests on different days, rather than giving him two or three tests on the same day. As a general rule, if the patient is unable to duplicate his test results within plus or minus 10 dB on successive tests, the tester should suspect the presence of functional loss. It should be emphasized, however, that consistency from test to retest does not, of itself, rule out the possibility that the loss is functional. With practice, a patient may become skilled in selecting the proper loudness level at which to cease responding. If there is other evidence that the patient's responses may not be representative of his actual hearing levels, then the fact that he is able to present a consistent picture from test to retest should not rule out the possibility of a functional hearing problem.

Figures 7-1, 7-2, and 7-3 illustrate the resolution of a functional hearing loss in a series of tests performed in a three day period. The patient was a veteran claiming compensation for a service-incurred hearing problem. In Figure 7-1 the patient presents a pure-tone audiogram illustrative of a profound hearing loss, presumably of the mixed type, since there is some air-bone gap. Note, however, the variation in threshold at 1000 Hz obtained with repeated testing. The speech test results are significantly better than the pure-tone findings. From the pure-tone audiogram one would have predicted that the patient's speech thresholds would be at hearing levels around 80 dB in each ear, and with as severe an air and bone-conduction hearing loss as this patient's pure-tone audiogram reveals it is unlikely that he would have very good discrimination. The examining audiologist was alerted by these discrepancies, and his own observations of the patient's behavior, to the presence of a functional hearing loss. Following are his edited comments on this first examination:

Conditioning schedule [for GSR test] could not be completed, since part of the time he moved his head, arms, and legs, and the remainder of the time he would appear to drowse.

During the voluntary tests the patient assumed a very strained expression of concentration (cocking his head to one side and squinting) about 10 dB lower than his responses to the tones. He would move his hand and finger up very slowly as if he were uncertain that he was hearing the tones.

The following results suggest the presence of a functional overlay: (a) discrepancies of 10–25 dB in test-retest thresholds at 1 kHz [1000 Hz], (b) discrepancies of 30–40 dB between the SRT's and PTA's [pure-tone averages].

The patient is to be rescheduled for further testing.

Figure 7-2 shows the test results obtained two and a half weeks later, after the patient had been hospitalized for additional observation and testing. Preceding this second examination the patient was counseled concerning the discrepancies noted in his initial tests. The pure-tone results shown in Figure 7-2 are considerably different from those obtained in the first examination. Repeated testing at 1000 Hz shows continuing discrepancies, particularly in the right ear. Bone conduction is markedly better than air conduction.

AUDIOMETRIC EXAMINATION

REASON FOR REFERRAL	NAME OF REFERRING STATION
Compensation Exam	Regional Office

AIR CONDUCTION

EXAMINER'S INITIALS	RIGHT							LEFT						
	125	250	500	1000	2000	4000	8000	125	250	500	1000	2000	4000	8000
		70	90	80	90	NR	NR		75	75	85	90	95	NR
				95							75			
				70							75			
MASKING LEVEL IN OPPOSITE EAR														

BONE CONDUCTION

EXAMINER'S INITIALS	RIGHT							LEFT						
	125	250	500	1000	2000	4000	8000	125	250	500	1000	2000	4000	8000
		NR	NR	55	60	NR			NR	NR	55	NR	NR	
MASKING LEVEL IN OPPOSITE EAR														

GALVANIC SKIN RESPONSE

EXAMINER'S INITIALS	RIGHT							LEFT						
	125	250	500	1000	2000	4000	8000	125	250	500	1000	2000	4000	8000

SPEECH AUDIOMETRY / SUMMARY PURE TONE AUDIOMETRY

EXAMINER'S INITIALS	SPEECH RECEPTION THRESHOLD					ITEM	DISCRIMINATION SCORE (PB MAX.)					AVERAGE LOSS		
	1	2	3	4	5		1	2	3	4	5	EAR	TWO FREQ.	THREE FREQ.
RIGHT EAR	46					RIGHT EAR	88					RIGHT		
						LIST								83
LEFT EAR	34					LEFT EAR	84					LEFT		
FREE FIELD						LIST								80

RIGHT EAR CONSISTENCY	WEBER TEST	LEFT EAR CONSISTENCY

REMARKS

PATIENT'S LAST NAME—FIRST NAME—MIDDLE INITIAL	AGE	CLAIM NO.
KAC	45	C-

NAME OF EXAMINING STATION OR CLINIC	SIGNATURE OF EXAMINING AUDIOLOGIST OR PHYSICIAN	DATE OF EXAMINATION
VA Hospital	LRK	7/20/62

Figure 7-1. Results obtained in initial examination of patient with functional hearing problem.

AUDIOMETRIC EXAMINATION

REASON FOR REFERRAL	NAME OF REFERRING STATION
Compensation Re-examination	Regional Office

AIR CONDUCTION

EXAMINER'S INITIALS	RIGHT							LEFT						
	125	250	500	1000	2000	4000	8000	125	250	500	1000	2000	4000	80C0
		45	40	50	55	95	NR		35	35	45	55	95	NR
				65							40			
				35							40			
MASKING LEVEL IN OPPOSITE EAR														

BONE CONDUCTION

EXAMINER'S INITIALS	RIGHT							LEFT						
	125	250	500	1000	2000	4000	8000	125	250	500	1000	2000	4000	8000
		15	15	10	15	NR			15	15	10	20	NR	
MASKING LEVEL IN OPPOSITE EAR														

GALVANIC SKIN RESPONSE

EXAMINER'S INITIALS	RIGHT							LEFT						
	125	250	500	1000	2000	4000	8000	125	250	500	1000	2000	4000	8000
				10							10			

SPEECH AUDIOMETRY / SUMMARY PURE TONE AUDIOMETRY

EXAMINER'S INITIALS	SPEECH RECEPTION THRESHOLD					ITEM	DISCRIMINATION SCORE (PB MAX.)					AVERAGE LOSS		
	1	2	3	4	5		1	2	3	4	5	EAR	TWO FREQ.	THREE FREQ.
RIGHT EAR	22					RIGHT EAR	98					RIGHT		43
						LIST								
LEFT EAR	30					LEFT EAR	94					LEFT		43
FREE FIELD						LIST								

RIGHT EAR CONSISTENCY	WEBER TEST	LEFT EAR CONSISTENCY

REMARKS

PATIENT'S LAST NAME—FIRST NAME—MIDDLE INITIAL	AGE	CLAIM NO.
KAC	45	C-

NAME OF EXAMINING STATION OR CLINIC	SIGNATURE OF EXAMINING AUDIOLOGIST OR PHYSICIAN	DATE OF EXAMINATION
VA Hospital	JTZ	8/7/62

Figure 7-2.   Results obtained in re-examination of patient with functional hearing problem.

Speech thresholds are still much lower than would be predicted from pure-tone results. The primary evidence that this patient still is not responding voluntarily at levels approaching his actual thresholds, however, is the GSR test results at 1000 Hz in each ear. The conditioned GSR test as a special test for functional hearing loss will be discussed in detail in the next section. Following are the examining audiologist's comments on the re-examination:

Prior to today's tests, patient was counseled re test differences noted on 7/20/62. The intratest and intertest differences noted today indicate that the functional problem was *not* resolved. Further testing is planned. The patient does not wear a hearing aid and appears to have little difficulty hearing and understanding normal conversational speech. No speech or voice problems were noted.

Two days later this patient was re-examined, and the results are shown in Figure 7-3. The first test administered was the pure-tone air-conduction test. The patient maintained his "loss" for this test. Next a conditioned GSR test was administered, indicating that the patient's hearing was normal through the speech frequencies except at 2000 Hz in the left ear, where his hearing level was 30 dB. It is interesting to note that GSR testing confirmed the presence of losses in both ears at frequencies higher than 2000 Hz. Following the GSR test the patient was counseled again concerning the discrepancies in his responses, and then the pure-tone air-conduction test was repeated. This time the patient responded voluntarily at near-normal levels except at those frequencies where evidently his hearing problem was organically based. Bone-conduction tests and speech audiometric tests were in reasonable agreement with the air-conduction findings. It should be explained that the audiometric results shown in Figures 7-1, 7-2, and 7-3 were all based on the ASA-1951 standard for audiometric zero and a 29 dB SPL calibration for speech audiometric zero. The audiologist had this to say on the final examination:

Following GSR the patient was counseled at length re test differences noted at previous tests. The post-counseling results suggest that the bilateral functional problem has been resolved. The post-counseling pure-tone and speech results obtained today appear to be valid estimates of this patient's hearing acuity.

Another clue to the presence of a functional hearing loss is when a patient who claims to have unilateral impairment fails to demonstrate "shadow hearing" at the expected level. Consider, for example, the test results shown in Figure 7-4. The patient presents a pure-tone air-conduction and bone-conduction picture of near-normal hearing in the right ear and almost a total loss of acuity in the left ear. In the case of an organic unilateral hearing problem, one would expect to obtain a shadow curve by air conduction in the poor ear that would differ from the hearing levels of the good ear by 50–60 dB and, without masking, the bone-conduction hearing levels of the poor ear

AUDIOMETRIC EXAMINATION

REASON FOR REFERRAL	NAME OF REFERRING STATION
Compensation--Second re-examination	Regional Office

AIR CONDUCTION

EXAMINER'S INITIALS	RIGHT							LEFT						
	125	250	500	1000	2000	4000	8000	125	250	500	1000	2000	4000	8000
			30	45	45	70				30	45	55	80	
Post-counseling			5	10	5	75			0	-10	5	30	80	
MASKING LEVEL IN OPPOSITE EAR														

BONE CONDUCTION

EXAMINER'S INITIALS	RIGHT							LEFT						
	125	250	500	1000	2000	4000	8000	125	250	500	1000	2000	4000	8000
		5	10	0	5	NR			5	5	5	35	NR	
MASKING LEVEL IN OPPOSITE EAR		·												

GALVANIC SKIN RESPONSE

EXAMINER'S INITIALS	RIGHT			3 KC				LEFT			3 KC			
	125	250	500	1000	2000	4000	8000	125	250	500	1000	2000	4000	8000
		0	5	-5	50				-5	5	30	60		

SPEECH AUDIOMETRY

EXAMINER'S INITIALS	SPEECH RECEPTION THRESHOLD					ITEM	DISCRIMINATION SCORE (PB MAX.)					SUMMARY PURE TONE AUDIOMETRY AVERAGE LOSS		
	1	2	3	4	5		1	2	3	4	5	EAR	TWO FREQ.	THREE FREQ.
RIGHT EAR	-4					RIGHT EAR	98					RIGHT		7
						LIST								
LEFT EAR	-10					LEFT EAR	88					LEFT		8
FREE FIELD						LIST								

RIGHT EAR CONSISTENCY	WEBER TEST	LEFT EAR CONSISTENCY

REMARKS

PATIENT'S LAST NAME—FIRST NAME—MIDDLE INITIAL	AGE	CLAIM NO.
KAC	45	C-
NAME OF EXAMINING STATION OR CLINIC	SIGNATURE OF EXAMINING AUDIOLOGIST OR PHYSICIAN	DATE OF EXAMINATION
VA Hospital	LRK	8/9/62

Figure 7-3.   Final results obtained in case of patient with functional hearing problem.

AUDIOMETRIC EXAMINATION

REASON FOR REFERRAL	NAME OF REFERRING STATION
Compensation Exam	Regional Office

AIR CONDUCTION

EXAMINER'S INITIALS	RIGHT							LEFT						
	125	250	500	1000	2000	4000	8000	125	250	500	1000	2000	4000	8000
			20	15	10					90	95	95		
Post-counseling	15	15	15	10	25			NR	95	95	95	NR		
MASKING LEVEL IN OPPOSITE EAR	------None------------------							--------None----------------						

BONE CONDUCTION

EXAMINER'S INITIALS	RIGHT							LEFT						
	125	250	500	1000	2000	4000	8000	125	250	500	1000	2000	4000	8000
		0	-10	5	10	30			NR	NR	NR	NR	NR	
MASKING LEVEL IN OPPOSITE EAR	-------None----------------							------None--------------						

GALVANIC SKIN RESPONSE

EXAMINER'S INITIALS	RIGHT							LEFT						
	125	250	500	1000	2000	4000	8000	125	250	500	1000	2000	4000	8000
			10	10	5					20	20	35		

SPEECH AUDIOMETRY / **SUMMARY PURE TONE AUDIOMETRY**

EXAMINER'S INITIALS	SPEECH RECEPTION THRESHOLD					ITEM	DISCRIMINATION SCORE (PB MAX.)					AVERAGE LOSS		
	1	2	3	4	5		1	2	3	4	5	EAR	TWO FREQ.	THREE FREQ.
RIGHT EAR	4					RIGHT EAR	92					RIGHT		13
						LIST								
LEFT EAR	70	(no masking AD)				LEFT EAR	70					LEFT		93
FREE FIELD						LIST								
RIGHT EAR CONSISTENCY		WEBER TEST						LEFT EAR CONSISTENCY						

REMARKS

PATIENT'S LAST NAME—FIRST NAME—MIDDLE INITIAL	AGE	CLAIM NO.
PSJ	50	C-
NAME OF EXAMINING STATION OR CLINIC	SIGNATURE OF EXAMINING AUDIOLOGIST OR PHYSICIAN	DATE OF EXAMINATION
VA Hospital	RFT	9/14/62

Figure 7-4.   A case of unilateral functional hearing loss.

should approach rather closely those of the good ear. The differences in speech test scores obtained without masking of the right ear (AD) in this instance are fairly close to what one expects in a true organic unilateral impairment. In the case of this patient, conditioned GSR test results revealed that there was only a mild loss in the left ear (through the speech frequencies, at least), but even after the patient was counseled following the GSR test he persisted in his failure to respond except at extremely high hearing levels when the stimuli were applied to the left ear. Incidentally, in this case the GSR findings were verified by pure-tone and speech Stenger test results. The Stenger test is one of the special tests for functional hearing loss that will be described in the next section.

In the preceding illustration, the lack of a shadow curve, particularly by bone conduction, was a clear indication of a functional hearing loss. If more proof were needed that this patient's ears were in fact both close to normal limits of sensitivity, his bone conduction in each ear could have been checked while occluding the other ear with an earphone, as suggested by Thompson and Denman.[11] If ears are essentially normal in sensitivity, occluding an ear causes the bone-conducted signal to refer to that ear, as in the Weber test. If this patient's left ear were occluded while retesting the right by bone, he probably would have given no response for the low frequencies, because he would have been aware of hearing them in his left or supposedly impaired ear. On the other hand, if the right ear were occluded while testing bone conduction on the left, the patient might have responded to the low frequencies, because the occlusion would have referred them to the right or good ear. The higher frequencies are of no use in checking the occlusion effect, because their thresholds are not affected by occlusion.

Special Tests for Functional Hearing Impairment

The purpose of administering special tests designed to identify functional loss in a patient is to confirm or reject impressions which have been obtained through observation of the patient's behavior and through an examination of the patient's consistency on routine tests. For proper administration, however, most special tests for functional loss require special equipment or at least modifications of standard test equipment. For this reason, the average examiner has to depend primarily on his subjective evaluations of the patient's behavior, both in and out of the testing situation, in judging whether or not he is dealing with a functional loss. If more complete testing facilities are available in hearing centers or clinics, the audiometrist can refer the patients whom he suspects of manifesting functional loss to one of them for the special tests described below.

The special tests to be described have developed from clinical necessity—

[11] Gary Thompson and Marie Denman, "The Occlusion Effect in Unilateral Functional Hearing Loss," *Journal of Speech and Hearing Research*, Vol. 13 (March, 1970), pp. 37-40.

the need to identify patients with functional loss or functional overlay. For the most part, these tests evolved from the observations of astute clinicians that patients with functional loss tended to respond in unusual ways to pure-tone and speech stimuli. Until recently, there has been little attempt to evaluate the validity and efficiency of these tests through carefully designed and controlled research studies. In 1963 an extensive interdisciplinary research study begun in 1959 was completed at the Veterans Administration Hospital in San Francisco. As a part of this study, various special tests for functional hearing loss were evaluated on experimental and control groups. The general findings of this study, including the evaluations of the special tests, have been reported by Chaiklin and Ventry.[12] Before making clinical use of the tests to be described here, the reader is advised to familiarize himself with the findings on test validity and efficiency reported by these investigators. In making a determination as to whether or not a given patient demonstrates functional hearing loss or a functional overlay on an organic hearing problem the audiologist must avoid depending too strongly on the results of any single test. Instead, he must correlate all information obtainable —case history, otological findings, observations of the patient's behavior, the results of routine pure-tone and speech audiometric tests, and the results of special tests—before arriving at a diagnosis.

Lombard or Voice-Reflex Test. This test is based on the fact that we monitor our own voices through the sensation of hearing. If we are speaking in a noisy environment, we unconsciously increase the intensity of our voice to compensate for the masking effect of the noise. In the Lombard test, the patient is given some material to read while a masking noise is fed into earphones which he is wearing. The examiner then observes fluctuations in the intensity of the patient's voice as he increases and decreases the level of the masking noise that the patient is hearing. The result of the test is positive if the patient's voice does become more intense when the masking is increased. The level of masking at which the patient's voice becomes noticeably more intense should be noted. That level is then compared with the degree of supposed hearing loss the patient has. If his voice is affected when the level of the masking is less than the degree of the supposed hearing loss, it is evident that the patient is actually hearing at lower levels than he admits on routine testing. The result of the Lombard test is negative if the patient's voice remains at the same intensity regardless of the fluctuations in the level of the masking noise within the limits of the supposed hearing loss. The Lombard test is usually administered only in cases of bilateral functional loss.

The limitations of the Lombard test are: (1) The test is not standardized to the point where it is known with certainty at just what level of masking in

---

[12] Joseph B. Chaiklin and Ira M. Ventry, "Functional Hearing Loss," James F. Jerger, ed., *Modern Developments in Audiology* (New York, Academic Press, 1963), Chap. 3, pp. 76-125. Ventry and Chaiklin, *op. cit.*

relation to the threshold the voice reflex begins. With this test, therefore, an accurate measure of the patient's true threshold is not assured. The only result obtainable is a gross judgment that the patient's intensity of voice increases when the level of masking reaches a certain point; that point can then be compared with the patient's supposed threshold. If the reflex occurs at levels of intensity less than the supposed threshold, it is apparent that the supposed threshold is in error, but it is not possible to say by how much it is in error. (2) A sophisticated patient, so far as testing is concerned, can learn to control the intensity of his voice even in the presence of an extremely intense masking noise. The Lombard test, then, can be "beaten" by a patient who is aware of the purpose of the test and who knows the responses that are expected. Attempts have been made to objectify and to quantify the Lombard test,[13] but since other tests are superior in their ability to determine organic thresholds, it is doubtful if the Lombard will ever be used for more than a rough screening test.

Stenger Test. When both ears are stimulated by a tone of the same frequency but of differing sensation level in each ear, an individual with normal hearing or with an equal bilateral hearing loss is aware of hearing the tone only in the ear in which it is louder. This phenomenon is the basis of the Stenger test. The test is useful in determining the genuineness of a patient's claim that one ear is impaired. The test requires either a two-channel audiometer or an audiometer in which the signal can be divided between the ears and its intensity be independently controlled in each ear.

Before the Stenger test is given, measures of the patient's supposed hearing loss should be obtained through standard audiometric techniques. Thus the examiner has a record of the patient's "thresholds" at each frequency in both the good and the "poor" ear. If the interaural difference between the patient's admitted thresholds at any frequency is at least 20 dB, the use of the Stenger test could be considered. Ventry and Chaiklin report that the efficiency of the Stenger test is highest when the admitted thresholds of the patient differ interaurally by more than 40 dB.[14] Suppose, for the sake of illustration, that the patient has yielded threshold measurements at 1000 Hz of 5 dB in the right ear and 50 dB in the left ear. You have reason to believe that the hearing in the left ear is better than the patient has admitted and you decide to administer the Stenger test. First, you would introduce the 1000-Hz tone to the good ear at a hearing level of 10 or 15 dB. The patient reports that he hears the tone, for he has previously admitted to

---

[13] Daryle L. Waldron, "The Lombard Voice Reflex Test: An Experimental Study," unpublished Ph.D. dissertation, Stanford University, 1960.

Clair N. Hanley and Donald G. Harvey, "Quantifying the Lombard Effect," *Journal of Speech and Hearing Disorders,* Vol. 30 (August, 1965), pp. 274-277.

[14] Ventry and Chaiklin, *op. cit.,* p. 201.

a threshold of 5 dB in that ear. Now, without disturbing the level of the tone in the patient's right ear, introduce the tone in the left ear, gradually increasing its intensity until it exceeds the level of the same tone in the right ear. When the sensation level of the tone becomes about 10 dB greater in the left ear than it is in the right ear, the patient will have the sensation of hearing it only in the left ear. When the patient becomes aware that he is hearing the tone in his allegedly poor ear at a level lower than his admitted threshold, he will usually report that he no longer hears the tone. He does not realize that the tone is still present at a suprathreshold level in his good ear. If the patient reports that he no longer hears the tone when it is presented at any level below the admitted threshold of the "poor" ear, the result of the Stenger test is "positive," that is, indicative of a functional loss. The examiner knows that the actual threshold in the "poor" ear is no greater than the hearing level at which the patient ceased responding. On the other hand, if the patient reports that he hears the tone while the level of the signal to the poor ear is being increased up to the point of his admitted threshold, the result of the Stenger test is "negative," that is, it gives no indication to the examiner that a functional problem is present. It should be noted that methods of administering the Stenger test may differ somewhat from examiner to examiner. Some clinicians will withdraw the signal from the good ear when the patient is reporting he hears, in order to make sure that it is the signal in the good ear to which he is responding. If the patient continues to respond after the signal in the good ear has been withdrawn, then obviously he is hearing the tone in his "poor" ear. In performing the Stenger test, it is preferable to interrupt the signals to the earphones while the hearing-level controls are being adjusted.

Sometimes the Stenger test is ineffective because the patient has pronounced diplacusis, that is, he hears a tone of a given frequency differently in each ear. If this should be so, he may be aware of the presence of the tone in his good ear when the level of presentation in the "poor" ear is at a higher sensation level. So even if negative Stenger results have been obtained with pure tones, the test should be repeated with speech stimuli, if the difference in SRT between the ears is at least 20 to 25 dB. When the auditory signal is speech instead of pure tones the test is called the "modified" or speech Stenger test. The manner of administering and interpreting the speech Stenger test is the same as that described for the pure-tone Stenger test. Spondee words are used, and the patient is asked to repeat each word. The signal is directed initially only to the good ear at a level at which he can repeat the words with almost 100 per cent accuracy (usually 5 to 10 dB sensation level). After the patient has repeated several words correctly, the examiner directs the speech signal also to the "poor" ear and gradually increases its intensity until the hearing level of the signal in the "poor" ear is higher than it is in the good ear. If, as the intensity of the speech signal is increased in the "poor" ear, the patient ceases to repeat the spondee words at any hearing level below his admitted SRT in that ear, the result of the speech Stenger test is positive, since the patient is still receiving the speech signal at a suprathreshold level in his good ear. As was the case with the pure-tone Stenger test, the efficiency of the speech Stenger procedure is greater in instances where the apparent interaural difference in sensitivity is large.

Shifting-voice Test. This test is a special modification of the speech Stenger and is useful in disclosing cases of assumed unilateral hearing loss. The examiner keeps talking informally to the patient, asking him questions and giving him instructions to carry out, while shifting the output of the speech audiometer from one ear to the other. Occasionally spondees will be inserted which the patient will be asked to repeat. The patient is instructed to indicate in which ear he is hearing the examiner by pointing to the appropriate earphone. Johnson, Work, and McCoy suggest that this manner of testing is suitable also in the case of patients with bilateral losses characterized by only a slight difference in admitted threshold between the ears.[15] They suggest starting this procedure with the level slightly above the admitted threshold in the better ear and slightly below in the poorer ear. Pressure is kept on the patient to make immediate responses to the spondee words or to the questions or directions given him, so that he has no time to consider in which ear he is hearing and at what level. In the course of the testing, the intensity of the signal is independently varied in each ear. Occasionally, a large change in intensity can be made, but usually the changes are slight. The object of this testing method is so to confuse the patient that he "gives himself away" by responding at levels that are below those which he has previously admitted. Of course the patient with an actual hearing loss will be able to respond only when the speech signal is above his threshold in either ear, and his responses will be consistent regardless of the manipulations of the examiner; the individual with a functional loss, or a functional overlay on an actual loss, on the other hand, will respond inconsistently on the shifting-voice test.

A similar confusion technique involving pure tones instead of speech has been proposed by Nagel, who calls his method RRLJ for "rapid random loudness judgments."[16] The patient is asked to make rapid judgments as to the ear in which he hears the tone more loudly, as the examiner skips around frequencies, randomly varying the intensity and the order of tonal presentations to the two ears. Should the patient report that a tone below his admitted threshold is louder, it is evidence of nonorganicity. Both of these confusion techniques tax the examiner's manual dexterity and concentration in controlling signal presentations and monitoring the patient's responses.

[15] Kenneth O. Johnson, Walter P. Work, and Gordon McCoy, "Functional Deafness," *Annals of Otology, Rhinology, and Laryngology*, Vol. 65 (March, 1956), p. 165.

[16] Robert F. Nagel, "RRLJ—A New Technique for the Noncooperative Patient," *Journal of Speech and Hearing Disorders*, Vol. 29 (November, 1964), pp. 492-493.

Delayed Auditory Feedback Test. In 1950 and 1951, Lee[17] and Black[18] reported that many normal speakers would experience changes in their speech similar to stuttering when they heard themselves through earphones under various conditions of delay. The delay is produced by modifying a tape recorder in such a way that the tape is carried over a spindle and makes a loop between the cutting head and a monitoring head. The spindle is adjustable for different-sized loops, thus producing different amounts of time lag, or delay, between the cutting and monitoring heads.

By varying the position of the spindle, and thus the amount of time lag, a critical degree of "delay" in hearing one's speech can be attained that will have distressing effects principally on the rhythm and rate of that speech, but also to some extent on the intensity. For most people who are susceptible to delayed feedback, a delay of 0.1 to 0.2 second has the most devastating effects. The changes that occur in an individual's speech under the influence of the delayed "feedback," or "side-tone," as it is also called, are often quite pronounced.

The delayed-feedback principle can serve as a test for functional loss by having some means of controlling the intensity of the signal that reaches the patient's earphones. If preliminary speech testing discloses that a patient has a presumed loss of, say, 60 dB, the hearing level of the patient's voice in the earphones as he monitors his own speech in the delayed auditory feedback test would be set at 30 to 40 dB. If the patient's speech deteriorates under the influence of the delayed feedback, this would be evidence that he is actually hearing his own voice through the earphones at a level considerably less than that of his presumed hearing loss. One change in the patient's speech which can be measured quantitatively in the delayed auditory feedback test is the rate. A patient is given several paragraphs of material to read. He reads the material aloud two or three times while wearing the earphones but with no signal in the phones. Each time that he reads the material the examiner times the reading with a stop watch. He then computes the average time of the reading when the patient has no signal in the earphones. This is the base for comparing the patient's rate of reading under the conditions of feedback. Then feedback is introduced, and the patient's reading is timed again. Each time a different hearing level of feedback is employed, another timing is obtained. The effect of the feedback is usually to cause a slowing down of the rate of reading, although occasionally a patient will markedly increase his rate, apparently in an attempt to "beat" the test. In either event, the examiner notes the hearing level of the feedback at the point that the patient's rate of reading changes substantially from his base time with no signal in the phones. It has been found that, on the average, delayed

17 Bernard S. Lee, "Some Effects of Side-Tone Delay," *Journal of the Acoustical Society of America,* Vol. 22 (September, 1950), pp. 639-640.

18 John W. Black, "The Effect of Delayed Side-Tone upon Vocal Rate and Intensity," *Journal of Speech and Hearing Disorders,* Vol. 16 (March, 1951), pp. 56-60.

feedback affects a person's reading rate when it is heard at a level of 20 to 40 dB above his threshold.[19] Some individuals, however, will be affected when the feedback occurs at a lower sensation level than 20 dB, and some are able to endure feedback at high sensation levels without any observable effects on their speech.

All during the test the patient's speech is being recorded on the tape, thus providing a permanent record of how his speech has changed owing to the delayed feedback. If the patient actually has a hearing loss, his speech patterns will not be changed by a delay in feedback which occurs at any intensity less than the amount of his hearing loss or usually at any intensity which is less than 20 dB above his threshold. The delayed auditory feedback test can serve as a check for binaural or monaural functional loss. When the feedback is directed to only one ear, the contralateral ear should be masked.

Gibbons and Winchester have reported a technique for administering the delayed auditory feedback test as a screening test for functional hearing loss when voluntary SRT's suggest a unilateral hearing impairment.[20] While the subject reads aloud a passage of simple prose, the delayed feedback is fed to one earphone at a level of 60 dB above the SRT of the better ear, while a complex masking noise is delivered to the other earphone at a level of 80 dB above the SRT of the better ear. The reading is precisely timed with a stop watch. Next the signals in the two earphones are reversed and the subject reads another passage of the same number of syllables while he is timed again. If there is a pronounced difference in reading time between the two conditions of the test, the presumption is that there is a real difference in acuity between the ears. If, however, the reading times for the two conditions are approximately equal, it would appear that there was no substantial difference in acuity between the ears. Norms for this test have been developed at the Audiology and Speech Pathology Service, Veterans Administration Outpatient Clinic, Los Angeles.[21]

Because generally the delayed feedback of speech does not affect an individual at threshold levels of intensity, it cannot be used as a test to determine organic thresholds. Rather, it is useful as a means of detecting the presence of functional loss, although a negative test result does not necessarily rule out the possibility of a functional loss.

Ruhm and Cooper have reported a delayed auditory feedback procedure that can determine thresholds for pure tones within 5 to 10 dB of their

[19] Clair N. Hanley and William R. Tiffany, "An Investigation into the Use of Electro-Mechanically Delayed Side Tone in Auditory Testing," *Journal of Speech and Hearing Disorders,* Vol. 19 (September, 1954), pp. 367-374.

[20] Edward W. Gibbons and Richard A. Winchester, "A Delayed Sidetone Test for Detecting Uniaural Functional Deafness," *A.M.A. Archives of Otolaryngology,* Vol. 66 (July, 1957), pp. 70-78.

[21] "The Unilateral Delayed Sidetone Test," unpublished report (June, 1959), Audiology and Speech Pathology Service, Veterans Administration Outpatient Clinic, Los Angeles.

actual levels.[22] The subject is asked to tap out a pattern of four taps, pause, and two taps with his index finger on a spring steel key which causes a variation in output voltage of a strain gauge and at the same time triggers a pure-tone signal in a single earphone worn by the subject. The subject keeps repeating the tapping pattern while he hears the pure tone in synchrony with his tapping key. Then a delay circuit is suddenly activated, so that the pure-tone signal in the earphone lags behind the actual key tapping. Under the influence of the delay the subject's tapping performance deteriorates. The effects can be observed and heard by the examiner and can be analyzed more completely on a graphic record of the subject's responses. Ruhm and Cooper validated their test, called DFA for "delayed feedback audiometry," on normals, veterans with organic hearing losses, and veterans with functional components in their hearing losses.[23] There are obvious advantages of this technique as a test for functional hearing loss, provided the instrumentation can be simplified so that it becomes practical for use as a clinical tool.

Galvanic Skin Response (GSR)

One of the most useful special tests in cases of functional hearing loss is the conditioned galvanic skin response test (GSR), frequently referred to also as the electrodermal response test (EDR) or electrodermal audiometry (EDA). The primary advantage of the test is that it makes possible the measurement of a patient's threshold with a high degree of validity and reliability provided a careful, systematic methodology is employed. The limitation of the test is that it requires the patient to be conditioned to a noxious stimulus (electrical shock), and it is not possible in every case to establish conditioning or to maintain conditioning throughout the test. Investigators with extensive clinical experience in administering the GSR test report that it can be successfully administered to about 80 per cent of adult male patients.[24] While the test is usually given with pure tones as the auditory stimuli, techniques have been suggested for utilizing GSR with speech audiometry.

The principle of GSR has been employed for many years in psychological research, but it is only since World War II that it has been used as a method for testing hearing. Bordley, Hardy, and Richter;[25] Doerfler;[26] and Bordley

---

[22] Howard B. Ruhm and William A. Cooper, Jr., "Low Sensation Level Effects of Pure-Tone Delayed Auditory Feedback," *Journal of Speech and Hearing Research,* Vol. 5 (June, 1962), pp. 185-193.

[23] Howard B. Ruhm and William A. Cooper, Jr., "Delayed Feedback Audiometry," *Journal of Speech and Hearing Disorders,* Vol. 29 (November, 1964), pp. 448-455.

[24] Chaiklin and Ventry, *op. cit.,* p. 106.

[25] John E. Bordley, William G. Hardy, and C.P. Richter, "Audiometry with the Use of Galvanic Skin-resistance Response; a Preliminary Report," *Bulletin of Johns Hopkins Hospital,* Vol. 82 (1948), p. 569.

[26] Leo G. Doerfler, "Neurophysiological Clues to Auditory Acuity," *Journal of Speech and Hearing Disorders,* Vol. 13 (Sept., 1948), pp. 227-232.

and Hardy[27] made the initial reports on GSR audiometry. The skin of an individual has a resistance to the flow of electric current. As this resistance increases, the amount of current that can flow across the skin decreases, and vice-versa. Under circumstances of quiet and relaxation, an individual's skin resistance remains relatively constant. Stimuli that excite any kind of emotional response, however, will cause the resistance of the skin to decrease. The increased flow of current resulting from this resistance drop may be amplified and displayed on a graphic recorder. The technique of utilizing the skin response in hearing testing is to condition the patient to respond to sound as an emotion-producing stimulus. This is done by pairing the test stimulus from an audiometer with a mild electric shock, but strong enough to produce momentary discomfort. The shock is sufficient to induce an emotional response, which causes a momentary drop in skin resistance. During the conditioning process, a spurt of tone and an almost-simultaneous shock are presented to the patient, alternated in a random fashion with the presentation of tone alone. When conditioning has been achieved, the presentation of tone alone will cause a drop in skin resistance as the patient anticipates the unpleasantness of the shock that might occur. Once the patient has been satisfactorily conditioned to tones above his voluntary thresholds, the "sampling" process begins: attempts to specify the minimum hearing levels at which consistent GSR's can be obtained. Conditioning is maintained by random *reinforcements*, that is, presenting the tone and shock together as in the conditioning process.

Conditioned GSR audiometry requires carefully-controlled procedures at every step if it is to yield valid and reliable results. Without such control, errors in diagnosis may be made, and an examiner's interpretation of the test might be colored by his subjective impressions of the patient. At the Veterans Administration Hospital in San Francisco a set of procedures for administering and interpreting the results of conditioned GSR audiometry with adult patients has evolved which will be described in the following paragraphs. These procedures are designed to minimize the factor of subjective evaluation of the test results. They draw upon the research results with GSR audiometry reported by Stewart,[28] Doerfler and McClure,[29] Meritser and Doefler,[30]

[27] John E. Bordley and William G. Hardy, "A Study in Objective Audiometry with the Use of a Psychogalvanometric Response," *Annals of Otology, Rhinology, and Laryngology,* Vol. 58 (Sept., 1949), pp. 751-760.

[28] Kenneth C. Stewart, "Some Basic Considerations in Applying the GSR Technique to the Measurement of Auditory Sensitivity," *Journal of Speech and Hearing Disorders,* Vol. 19 (June, 1954), pp. 174-183.

[29] Leo G. Doerfler and Catherine T. McClure, "The Measurement of Hearing Loss in Adults by Galvanic Skin Response," *Journal of Speech and Hearing Disorders,* Vol. 19 (June, 1954), pp. 184-189.

[30] Clay L. Meritser and Leo G. Doerfler, "The Conditioned Galvanic Skin Response Under Two Modes of Reinforcement," *Journal of Speech and Hearing Disorders,* Vol. 19 (September, 1954), pp. 350-359.

Aronson *et al.*,[31] and Hind *et al.*[32] Some of the clinical procedures to be described were reported by Chaiklin, Ventry, and Barrett.[33] For the remainder, the writer is indebted to one of these authors.[34]

The equipment used at the San Francisco Veterans Administration is standard: a Grason-Stadler Psychogalvanometer and an Allison Laboratories audiometer. The equipment and the examiner are situated outside the test room occupied by the patient, to whom pick-up and shock electrodes have been attached. The two pick-up electrodes are placed on the pads of the index and ring fingers of the left hand, and the two shock electrodes are similarly placed on the right hand. The testing is performed monaurally through earphones, although during the conditioning procedure, tone may be presented binaurally through the phones.

A conditioning schedule is followed, specifying a randomized presentation of "events," consisting of tone alone or tone and shock, with the auditory signal presented at a level of 10 dB above the previously determined voluntary threshold at the frequency being tested. If the tonal presentations are binaural, then the level would be set 10 dB above the binaural threshold. Tone and shock in combination (reinforcement) are presented about 40 per cent of the time. Intervals of 30, 45, or 60 seconds, randomly mixed, are used between events to give time for the patient's skin resistance to stabilize following a response. The graphic recorder on the Psychogalvanometer gives a continuous record of the current flow between the pick-up electrodes. The stylus of the recorder automatically marks the onset of the tone or the combined tone and shock. Conditioning continues until the patient gives "acceptable" GSR responses to three successive presentations of tone alone (although some reinforcements may have intervened). An "acceptable" response is defined as one having a *latency* of between 1.5 and 3.5 seconds, that is, occurring within this time interval following the start of the tonal presentation, a minimum magnitude of 1 mm (deviation from the baseline on the recording), and a minimum slope from the baseline of 45°. Of course the magnitude and slope of the response are dependent on the speed of the graphic recorder, and the sensitivity setting of the Psychogalvanometer. The specific criteria for magnitude and slope of the recorded response might not apply, therefore, in different clinical settings. The latency criterion, however, is the most important one by which to judge the acceptability of a response, and it is

[31] A. E. Aronson, J. E. Hind, and J. V. Irwin, "GSR Auditory Threshold Mechanisms: Effect of Tonal Intensity on Amplitude and Latency Under Two Tone-Shock Intervals," *Journal of Speech and Hearing Research,* Vol. 1 (September, 1958), pp. 211-219.

[32] J. E. Hind, A. E. Aronson, and J. V. Irwin, "GSR Auditory Threshold Mechanisms: Instrumentation, Spontaneous Response, and Threshold Definition," *Journal of Speech and Hearing Research,* Vol. 1 (September, 1958), pp. 220-226.

[33] Joseph B. Chaiklin, Ira M. Ventry, and Lyman S. Barrett, "Reliability of Conditioned GSR Pure-Tone Audiometry with Adult Males," *Journal of Speech and Hearing Research,* Vol. 4 (September, 1961), pp. 269-280.

[34] Personal communications from Dr. Joseph B. Chaiklin.

independent of recorder speed and sensitivity of the Psychogalvanometer.

Once the conditioning criterion has been met, threshold "sampling" is commenced. Tone is presented monaurally, but it is alternated between the ears. In other words, threshold sampling proceeds simultaneously for the two ears. The purpose of this alternation is to obtain threshold information on each ear under the same degree of patient conditioning. The validity of the measurements on the two ears is thus kept equivalent. During the sampling procedure, a randomized schedule of events is followed as in conditioning, and reinforcement occurs at a 40 per cent rate. The first event in threshold sampling involves a tonal presentation (with no shock) at zero-dB hearing level. If no response occurs, the intensity of the tone is increased 10 dB and it is presented again. Additional 10-dB increases are made until a response is obtained or the patient's voluntary threshold is reached. If the next event on the schedule is a presentation of tone without shock, the tone is switched to the opposite ear and decreased to zero-dB hearing level. Again intensity is increased in 10-dB steps until a response occurs or the level of the patient's voluntary threshold is reached. If, however, the next event on the schedule calls for the simultaneous presentation of tone and shock, this event would be presented before switching to the opposite ear and starting another ascending series. Following a response, the procedure is always to move to the next event on the schedule, and if that event is a presentation of tone alone, the signal is reduced to zero-dB hearing level and switched to the opposite ear. If, early in the sampling, it appears that the patient's thresholds are actually fairly high, then increases of intensity in 20-dB steps may be made for the first one or two presentations in an ascending series.

In each ascending series a *control* event is inserted. A control event consists in going through the motions of presenting a stimulus, so that the marker on the recorder shows a tonal presentation was made, but the tone is not actually presented. A patient's GSR shows random changes throughout a record. If a random change occurs within the acceptable latency period following presentation of a tonal stimulus, it may erroneously be judged as a response to the stimulus. The use of control events is a check on the rate of occurrence of random responses and thus on the validity of the test. If a "response" occurs to a control event, then obviously that "response" is spurious, since no auditory stimulus was presented to the patient. Random GSR responses may occur when a patient coughs, breathes deeply, makes a muscular movement, or sometimes for no apparent reason. If there are few or no significant GSR changes noted in conjunction with control events, the examiner assumes adequate validity of his test. On the other hand, if many responses occur to control events, the entire record must be discarded and the test declared invalid.

At the beginning of a sampling series the examiner notes on the paper of the graphic recorder the frequency being tested. Then each event is labeled as it occurs: hearing level of the presentation, ear under test, control event. Such extraneous occurrences as coughs, sighs, and movements of the patient are also noted on the recorder paper adjacent to the responses they produced. The sampling procedure is continued until the threshold criterion has been met in each ear. Then the audiometer is switched to another frequency and sampling is continued in the same manner. If the patient maintains his conditioning at an adequate level, the test can continue until threshold sampling has been completed for all the frequencies to be tested (usually only 500, 1000, and 2000 Hz). But if the patient's GSR responses to tone *extinguish*, that is, disappear, the test must be discontinued until conditioning has been re-established, usually at a different time. GSR testing is fatiguing to patients (and examiners), and rarely is it possible or advisable to prolong a test beyond an hour at one sitting. Since good GSR results are dependent on an optimal arousal state of the patient, it is good practice to remove the earphones and allow the patient to rest every fifteen minutes during the test.

Decisions regarding the patient's threshold require the application of rigid criteria to an analysis of the test record. Threshold is usually defined as the lowest hearing level at which three responses were obtained out of five presentations. If the record shows a number of "false alarm" responses to control events, the criterion of acceptability should be four responses out of four presentations. On the other hand, if the validity of the test is high as judged by the presence of very few "responses" to control events, it may be permissible to accept two responses out of four presentations as the criterion for threshold. In no case should threshold judgments be made if fewer than 50 per cent responses are recorded at a particular hearing level. In conventional audiometry we insist on the application of at least a 50 per cent response criterion, and certainly in GSR testing we should hold at least to this standard. Judgments of threshold from GSR testing are made by analyzing the permanent record of the test, applying the response criteria previously mentioned: latency, magnitude, and slope angle. Any audiologist applying these criteria should be able to analyze a record and determine the patient's threshold at the frequencies tested, if the examiner has marked the record clearly during the progress of the test.

A word should be said concerning reinforcement and level of the shock. Research evidence has demonstrated that the best reinforcement is obtained when the shock occurs approximately one-half second after the onset of the tone.[35] The time of the occurrence of the shock in relation to the tone can be controlled automatically on the Grason-Stadler Psychogalvanometer. A one-second duration of the tonal stimulus is usually regarded as the most desirable. The level of the shock is important, too, both in achieving proper conditioning and in keeping the patient cooperative. The shock should be unpleasant but not painful. In setting the level of the shock, the examiner asks

[35] Charles A. Tait, Richard F. Dixon, and Joseph B. Chaiklin, "Effects of Two CS-US Intervals on Conditioning and Response Decay in Electrodermal Audiometry," *Journal of Speech and Hearing Research*, Vol. 10 (September, 1967), pp. 570-577.

the patient to report when shock becomes "distinctly unpleasant." The patient is then asked if he can tolerate a shock of greater strength. If he agrees, then the shock is increased until the patient reports he cannot tolerate it at any greater strength. Unless the patient is "coaxed" to accept a higher level, the initial setting at which the patient reported the shock was unpleasant may be too low to achieve or to maintain conditioning. It is poor practice— and inhumane—for the examiner to set the level of the shock without consulting the patient. It should be pointed out that for some patients any level of shock is terrifying, and in some cases it may be impossible to obtain the patient's cooperation for the conditioned GSR test.

The Veterans Administration has specified that in every compensation examination in which a compensable disability would result from accepting the patient's voluntary thresholds a GSR test must be performed at one frequency in each ear. If this "screening" procedure reveals a functional hearing loss, then GSR testing should be performed for all the speech frequencies in each ear. The Veterans Administration rating schedule allows a disability rating to be based on GSR test results, if these are the only valid threshold measurements that can be obtained. Ordinarily, as mentioned in the preceding chapter, the Veterans Administration bases disability ratings on an adaptation of the SAI concept, that is, on speech test results, but pure-tone test results—including GSR measurements—are acceptable for rating purposes in exceptional cases.

Earlier in this section it was mentioned that there have been some attempts to develop conditioned GSR testing in conjunction with speech stimuli. Ruhm and Carhart[36] evolved a procedure that depended upon establishing a conditioned response to a particular spondaic word. During the conditioning procedure, the subject received a shock each time the "key" word was presented in company with other "neutral" spondaic words. After conditioning had been established, threshold sampling proceeded, with the key word inserted among neutral words at various hearing levels sampled. The conditioned GSR speech threshold was defined as the lowest hearing level to which the subject gave a GSR response that met the investigator's criteria for acceptability. Ruhm and Carhart reported excellent validity and reliability for this method of assessing SRT.

Chaiklin[37] employed a different procedure for obtaining speech threshold by conditioned GSR testing. For the speech stimulus he used a phrase, "Now you hear me," on a tape loop. He followed a 40 per cent reinforcement conditioning schedule and the same criteria for determining the subject's conditioning and acceptability of responses during the sampling procedure that have previously been described for pure-tone GSR audiometry. While

[36] Howard B. Ruhm and Raymond Carhart, "Objective Speech Audiometry: A New Method Based on Electrodermal Response," *Journal of Speech and Hearing Research,* Vol. 1 (June, 1958), pp. 169-178.
[37] Joseph B. Chaiklin, "The Conditioned GSR Auditory Speech Threshold," *Journal of Speech and Hearing Research,* Vol. 2 (September, 1959), pp. 229-236.

there were statistically significant differences between what Chaiklin termed the "conditioned GSR auditory speech threshold" and voluntary speech thresholds with normal-hearing subjects, the majority of his subjects had GSR thresholds within ± 5 dB of their voluntary SRT's as determined by spondee words.

Although there have been some reports in the literature concerning the use of conditioned GSR speech audiometry with patients who present functional hearing loss problems, at the present writing the emphasis in GSR testing is on pure-tone evaluation.

Doerfler-Stewart Test

One of the earliest tests devised as a screening instrument to detect the presence of functional hearing loss was the Doerfler-Stewart (D-S) test, which was developed at an Army aural rehabilitation center during World War II.[38] This test examines a patient's ability to respond to spondee words in the presence of a masking noise. The test is performed binaurally through earphones, and the speech signal and masking noise are mixed and varied in intensity in relation to each other. The theory of the test is that, if a patient has a functional loss, the masking noise will interfere with his ability to judge the level at which he should no longer be able to "hear" the test material. Conclusions as to whether or not a patient exhibits a functional loss are based on an analysis of the relationships among the patient's SRT; his "noise interference level," that is, the level of the masking noise at which he ceases to repeat spondee words; and his "noise detection threshold." Procedures and norms for the test have been described by Doerfler and Epstein,[39] and in the first edition of this book. Doerfler and Epstein recommended that the D-S test be given as an initial screening test for functional hearing loss in all cases involving compensation. If the results of the test are positive, the examiner is then alerted to the possibility that the patient does have a functional hearing loss and should employ other special tests, such as GSR, to verify the patient's thresholds. The specific test procedures and norms will not be described here, inasmuch as there is now some question concerning the efficiency of this test as a means of detecting the patient with functional hearing loss.[40]

TESTS FOR IDENTIFYING SITE OF LESION

Hearing impairments are designated as conductive, sensori-neural, or mixed on the basis of an inspection of air- and bone-conduction hearing levels obtained in routine pure-tone audiometry. Identifying an impairment as

---

[38] Leo G. Doerfler and Kenneth Stewart, "Malingering and Psychogenic Deafness," *Journal of Speech Disorders,* Vol. 11 (September, 1946), pp. 181-186.

[39] Leo G. Doerfler and Aubrey Epstein, The Doerfler-Stewart (D-S) Test for Functional Hearing Loss, unpublished monograph submitted to the Veterans Administration, 1956.

[40] Ventry and Chaiklin, *op. cit.,* pp. 201-210.

sensori-neural does not say anything about the location of the pathological condition producing the impairment except that it is not in the outer or the middle ear. The term sensori-neural implies that the site of the lesion may be in the sensory end organ (the cochlea), in the auditory nerve, or in both. Ever since Dix, Hallpike, and Hood reported that cochlear involvements could be differentiated from retrocochlear pathology on the basis of noting the presence (cochlear) or absence (retrocochlear) of the recruitment of loudness,[41] there has been great interest on the part of otologists and audiologists in developing tests that would assist in the determination of site of lesion in cases of sensori-neural impairment. If these tests were in any way indicative of cochlear involvement, there was a tendency to say that they were tests of recruitment on the assumption that all cochlear involvements demonstrated recruitment.

In the late 1940's and early 1950's considerable interest developed in the use of difference limen for intensity tests as substitutes for binaural and monaural loudness-balance tests, the "classical" tests for determining the presence of recruitment.[42] Difference limen tests provoked theoretical arguments as to whether they measured recruitment of loudness or some other manifestation of cochlear dysfunction that may or may not be related to the recruitment phenomenon.[43] More recently the emphasis has been placed on the development of tests that yield information concerning the site of lesion in cases of sensori-neural impairment, and the question as to whether or not a particular test result represents the presence of "recruitment" has been considered irrelevant. Jerger sums up this point of view:

From the standpoint of differential diagnosis the important consideration is not recruitment but site of lesion. Recruitment tests (that is, loudness balance methods) are of value to the extent that they predict site of lesion successfully. The most meaningful criterion to apply to other tests involving other phenomena is not whether they predict recruitment but whether they predict site of lesion. If they do, then they are of value whether they predict recruitment or not.[44]

[41] M. R. Dix, C. S. Hallpike, and J. D. Hood, "Observations upon the Loudness Recruitment Phenomenon with Especial Reference to the Differential Diagnosis of Disorders of the Internal Ear and VIIIth Nerve," *Journal of Laryngology and Otology*, Vol. 62 (November, 1948), pp. 671-686.

[42] E. Lüscher and J. Zwislocki, "A Simple Method for Indirect Monaural Determination of the Recruitment Phenomenon (Difference Limen in Intensity in Different Types of Deafness)," *Acta Otolaryngologica*, Supplement 78 (1949), pp. 156-168.

P. Denes and R. F. Naunton, "The Clinical Detection of Auditory Recruitment," *Journal of Laryngology and Otology*, Vol. 64 (July, 1950), pp. 375-398.

James F. Jerger, "A Difference Limen Recruitment Test and Its Diagnostic Significance," *Laryngoscope*, Vol. 62 (December, 1952), pp. 1316-1332.

James F. Jerger, "DL Difference Test: Improved Method for Clinical Measurement of Recruitment," *A.M.A. Archives of Otolaryngology*, Vol. 57 (May, 1953), pp. 490-500.

[43] Ira J. Hirsh, T. Palva, and A. Goodman, "Difference Limen and Recruitment," *A.M.A. Archives of Otolaryngology*, Vol. 60 (November, 1954), pp. 525-540.

[44] James F. Jerger, "Recruitment and Allied Phenomena in Differential Diagnosis," *Journal of Auditory Research*, Vol. 2 (1961), p. 151.

Jerger has also made the point that it is unwise if not impossible to make decisions regarding the site of lesion on the basis of any single test. Instead, one must view the results of a battery of tests in order to predict with any degree of assurance whether a given patient presents a sensori-neural involvement of a cochlear or a retrocochlear type, or presents a central auditory disorder. We shall now discuss some of the tests that have been found to be most useful in such a battery.

Tests for Recruitment

While historically tests for recruitment have been used to differentiate between cochlear and retrocochlear sensori-neural impairments, Jerger[45] has presented evidence that determining the presence or absence of recruitment as an indication of site of lesion may be misleading, since in some cases of cochlear lesions in his experimental group no recruitment could be demonstrated, while some patients with acoustic neurinomas did show recruitment. In Jerger's opinion, other tests may be more accurate for determining the site of lesion than tests for recruitment.

Regardless of its diagnostic significance—and it seems to be of most usefulness in identifying cases of Ménière's syndrome and vascular disturbances of the cochlea—the presence of recruitment may be a limiting factor in a patient's ability to benefit from amplification. For example, a patient who has a greatly compressed dynamic range of hearing may find it impossible to utilize a hearing aid, because when the aid's volume control is turned to the point where speech can be heard, the intensity peaks of speech may be uncomfortably loud. Thus from the standpoint of planning for rehabilitative procedures, if not for purposes of medical diagnosis, it is important to ascertain whether or not a patient with a sensori-neural type impairment does have recruitment.

Alternate Binaural Loudness-Balance Test. This test was first described by Fowler.[46] Briefly, the test consists of comparing the hearing levels at which a pure tone sounds equally loud to both ears of a patient, and it is useful only when there is a monaural impairment or when a patient presents a picture of one relatively normal ear and one ear with some degree of sensori-neural impairment. The test requires an audiometer with which the examiner can present pulses of a tone of the same frequency but different hearing level to each ear of a patient. If such an audiometer is not available, a separate audiometer may be used with each ear. The test is performed, of course, through earphones.

The method of administering the test is as follows. Threshold measurements are obtained for both ears at all frequencies. The frequencies that show at

45 *Ibid.,* pp. 148 and 149.
46 E. P. Fowler, "Marked Deafened Areas in Normal Ears," *Archives of Otolaryngology,* Vol. 8 (1928), pp. 151-155.

least a 20-dB loss in the poor ear may then be balanced for loudness in the good ear. Choose one frequency at which to begin the loudness balancing. Increase the intensity of this frequency until it is 20 dB above the threshold of the good ear, and present the tone briefly to the good ear. Then, leaving the hearing-level control for the good ear at that setting, change the hearing-level control for the poor ear until an intensity of about 20 dB above the threshold of the poor ear is obtained. Present the tone briefly to the poor ear, and ask the patient to tell you whether the tone in the poor ear is louder or softer than the one which he heard in the good ear. Switch the tone from good to poor ear several times, changing the intensity in the poor ear as necessary until the patient tells you that the tones are equally loud. In other words, the patient must balance the loudness of the tone in the poor ear to the fixed loudness of the tone which is 20 dB above threshold in the good ear. Note the hearing level of the tone in the poor ear when loudness balance is achieved. Then increase the intensity of the tone in the good ear by another 20 dB, and again vary the intensity of the tone in the poor ear until the patient tells you that he has balanced the loudness. Again make note of the hearing level of the tone in the poor ear. Continue in this fashion, increasing the intensity of the tone in the good ear by 20 dB each time and finding the hearing level of the tone in the poor ear necessary to obtain a sensation of equal loudness, until the intensity limits of the audiometer have been reached. The same procedure is then followed for each of the other frequencies to be balanced.

Figure 7-5 illustrates the usual manner of recording the results of the binaural loudness-balance test. The points of equal loudness in the good and the poor ear are connected by lines which straddle the frequency being balanced. The points on the audiogram for the good (right) ear appear at intervals 20 dB apart, starting at threshold; the points for the poor ear are marked at whatever hearing level was required to balance loudness. If the lines connecting the points of equal loudness remain essentially parallel throughout the course of the test at a specific frequency, no recruitment has been demonstrated, since an equal increment of intensity results in an equal increment of loudness in each ear. However, if the lines tend to converge on the poor ear, indicating that increments of loudness in the poor ear are not proportional to the increments of increasing intensity, the presence of recruitment is demonstrated. The graph of equal loudness at each frequency is called a *laddergram*. In Figure 7-5, for purposes of illustration, no recruitment is evidenced at the frequency of 500 Hz, since the lines connecting the points of loudness balance are parallel throughout. At 1000 Hz there is some recruitment, although "incomplete," because the sensation of loudness in the poor ear does not ever equal the loudness in the good ear. At 2000 Hz the recruitment is "complete," that is, the loudness of the tone in the poor ear equals the loudness in the good ear at maximum intensity levels. The laddergram at 4000 Hz illustrates "hyper-recruitment." As the intensity increases above threshold, a point is reached at which the sensation of loudness in the

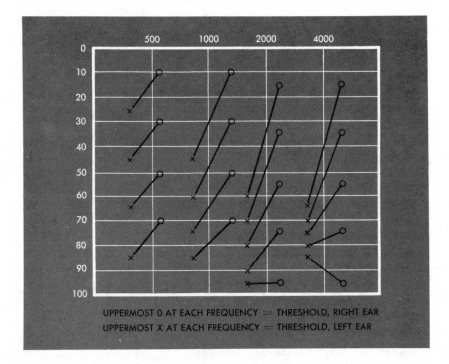

Figure 7-5.   Binaural loudness balance at four frequencies.

poor ear exceeds that in the good ear, although a difference of some 40 dB existed between the ears at threshold levels. One must be careful not to make conclusions regarding the presence or absence of recruitment or differentiating one degree of recruitment from another, unless the differences in hearing level on which the conclusions are based are greater than the allowable limits of reliability of pure-tone testing, in other words, greater than ± 5 dB.

When administering the binaural loudness-balance test, it is essential that the presentations of tone in each ear be very brief. If the tone is prolonged at above-threshold levels, there is danger of fatiguing the ears, thus invalidating the loudness-balance results. It is best if the tone is alternated between the good and the poor ear with pulses of no longer than one second's duration. In Figure 7-5, the growth of the loudness sensation has been studied at intervals of 20-dB intensity in the good ear. The selection of the interval of intensity is purely arbitrary; it could as well be 10 dB or 30 dB. As a matter of fact, the presence of recruitment can be disclosed by having the patient perform a loudness balance only at maximum intensity at each frequency. Then only the top and bottom "rungs" of the laddergram would be drawn. Of course the complete laddergram, as shown in Figure 7-5, gives information concerning the *growth* of the sensation of loudness which would not be obtained if loudness were balanced only at threshold and at maximum intensity. With some patients, recruitment may be most pronounced at the first step above threshold. With others, there may be a "delayed" recruitment that does not become evident until hearing levels considerably above threshold are reached. Thus it is important to observe the growth of loudness throughout the patient's range of hearing in the impaired ear.

The procedure for administering the alternate binaural loudness-balance test described here calls for using fixed intensity in the good ear and variable intensity in the poor ear until loudness balance is achieved at any given step on the laddergram. Jerger and Harford administer the test by putting the fixed intensity in the poor ear and varying the intensity in the good ear, but they report that either method yields the same results.[47] Their rationale for reversing the "traditional" procedure is that conclusions regarding the presence of absence of recruitment, or the degree of recruitment found, can be based on fewer judgments, since it is seldom possible to exceed the threshold of the poor ear by more than 40 dB—2 "steps" in the alternate binaural loudness-balance test. Jerger and Harford also recognize only two degrees of recruitment: partial (incomplete) and complete. While it may be difficult to rationalize the existence of hyper-recruitment on any theoretical neurological basis, it is a frequent clinical finding in patients with Ménière's syndrome or a vascular disturbance of the cochlea; therefore, the classification "hyper-recruitment" has clinical usefulness.

Monaural Loudness-Balance Test. In bilateral sensori-neural impairment in which the higher frequencies are more severely impaired than the lower ones, it is possible to administer a monaural loudness-balance test. In this test, first suggested by Reger,[48] the loudness at the impaired frequencies is compared with the loudness of a normal frequency at threshold and at set intervals above threshold. The procedure is the same in principle as for the ABLB test. The standard (normal) frequency is increased in intensity in 20-dB steps above threshold. The patient is instructed to balance the loudness of the test frequency to the loudness of the standard frequency at each step. The points of equal loudness are then connected to form a laddergram. Each frequency to be evaluated is then compared in this manner with the frequency that has been selected as the standard.

The usefulness of the monaural loudness-balance test is that it is not necessary for the patient to have one good ear with which to compare a poor ear in order to obtain a measure of recruitment. The test can be performed in either ear in the case of a bilateral impairment. Of course the patient must

[47] James F. Jerger and Earl R. Harford, "Alternate and Simultaneous Binaural Balancing of Pure Tones," *Journal of Speech and Hearing Research,* Vol. 3 (March, 1960), p. 20.
[48] Scott N. Reger, "Differences in Loudness Response of the Normal and Hard-of-Hearing Ear at Intensity Levels Slightly Above the Threshold," *Annals of Otology, Rhinology, and Laryngology,* Vol. 45 (December, 1936), pp. 1029-1039.

have normal or relatively normal hearing for at least one frequency, so that this frequency can serve as the standard to which the sensation of loudness at other frequencies is compared. The primary disadvantage of the monaural loudness-balance test is that it is a difficult task for a patient to match the loudness of two tones of different frequency. The greater the separation of the tones in frequency, the more difficult the task becomes. The patient may need considerable practice in balancing loudness at different frequencies before the examiner can place reliance in his judgments.

Temporal Summation or Integration. Psychoacousticians have long been interested in the effects of stimulus duration on auditory sensitivity for pure tones. According to Harris, ". . . for careful studies at threshold, Hughes first showed the regularity of the trading relation between audibility and duration, popularly known now as the phenomenon of temporal integration."[49] As the duration of tonal bursts is decreased from 500 msec (milliseconds) to 10 msec, the normal ear requires increased intensity to make the tone audible. At some frequencies the normal ear's threshold will shift 12 to 13 dB over this range of durations.[50] On the other hand, the recruiting ear will demonstrate significantly lesser degrees of threshold shift with decreasing duration.[51] Thus the measurement of threshold shift obtained by varying duration of the signal holds promise as another clinical technique for determining the presence of recruitment. Wright has proposed a "tracking" technique with the Békésy audiometer (to be described later in this chapter) to evaluate threshold at various short durations and has demonstrated that recruiting ears can be differentiated from normal and from conductively impaired ears by this technique.[52] Wright and Cannella have also shown that in cases of mixed impairment, it is the amount of sensori-neural loss that determines the degree of abnormal threshold-duration function.[53]

By comparing "time thresholds" and loudness balance data on ears demonstrating recruitment, Miskolczy-Fodor developed a rationale and method for translating time thresholds into loudness functions and thus measuring degrees of recruitment in terms of variations of time thresholds

[49] J. W. Hughes, "The Threshold of Audition for Short Periods of Stimulation," in J. Donald Harris, ed., *Forty Germinal Papers in Human Hearing* (Groton, Connecticut, *The Journal of Auditory Research* 1969), pp. 43-46.

[50] J. Zwislocki, "Theory of Temporal Auditory Summation," *Journal of the Acoustical Society of America,* Vol. 32 (August, 1960), p. 1053.

[51] H. N. Wright, "Clinical Measurement of Temporal Auditory Summation," *Journal of Speech and Hearing Research,* Vol. 11 (March, 1968), pp. 118-124.

[52] H. N. Wright, "The Effect of Sensori-Neural Hearing Loss on Threshold-Duration Functions," *Journal of Speech and Hearing Research,* Vol. 11 (December, 1968), pp. 842-852.

[53] H. N. Wright and F. Cannella, "Differential Effect of Conductive Hearing Loss on the Threshold-Duration Function," *Journal of Speech and Hearing Research,* Vol. 12 (September, 1969), pp. 607-615.

from normal values. A time threshold is the minimum pulse length in msec that a subject can maintain the audibility of a tone, measured at sensation levels of 1 to 6 dB.[54]

Most Comfortable and Uncomfortable Loudness Level. A simple, although not very reliable, means of determining the presence of recruitment is to obtain two points on the pure-tone audiogram at above-threshold levels. One of these points is termed the patient's most comfortable loudness level (MCL), and the other is called the patient's uncomfortable loudness level (UCL). These measures can be secured while the patient is being given a standard pure-tone audiometric test. If the patient has a sensori-neural loss, the examiner can then ask the patient to tell him at which point, as the intensity of a tone is increased, the patient finds it most comfortable to listen, and again the examiner can find the point at which the tone becomes uncomfortably loud for the patient as the intensity is increased. For each frequency thus tested, there will be three points marked on the audiogram: first, the patient's threshold for that tone; second, the level at which the patient reported that the tone was most comfortable to listen to; and, third, the level at which the tone became intolerably loud. These points will tend to be relatively close together for the patient who presents recruitment, whereas with the patient with no recruitment the points may be spread far apart. As a matter of fact, the patient who has no recruitment should be able to tolerate the full intensity at each frequency without experiencing physiological discomfort.

The range from threshold to MCL to UCL may vary at different frequencies. A patient who has a typical sensori-neural loss, showing greater losses for the higher frequencies, would be expected to show the presence of recruitment at the higher frequencies where the loss is greatest. At the lower frequencies, where his hearing is more normal, the recruitment should be negligible or absent. The interpretation of the degree of recruitment present by this method requires experience on the part of the examiner in having examined many audiograms of patients both with and without recruitment. There is no quantification of results; the examiner must rely on his clinical experience to judge the severity of the recruitment. Also, the judgment of most comfortable loudness of a pure tone is a difficult one for a patient to make reliably. A number of trials may show a wide spread of judgments. It is best to average the results of several trials, some with ascending intensity and some with descending intensity. The method of comparing threshold, MCL, and UCL is useful only as a gross indication of the presence of recruitment.

Where speech audiometric equipment is available, the MCL and UCL for speech may be obtained in the same manner as with pure tones. As was

[54] F. Miskolczy-Fodor, "Relation Between Loudness and Duration of Tonal Pulses. 1. Response of Normal Ears to Pure Tones Longer Than Click-Pitch Threshold," *Journal of the Acoustical Society of America*, Vol. 31 (August, 1959), pp. 1128-1134; "III. Response in Cases of Abnormal Loudness Function," *ibid.*, Vol. 32 (April, 1960), pp. 486-492.

mentioned in Chapter 6, the MCL is obtained by asking the patient to report the point above his threshold at which speech is most comfortably loud. Although spondee words may be used for this determination, it is preferable to use running speech. The UCL for speech is obtained in the tolerance test, as the loudest speech which the patient can tolerate is his threshold of discomfort. A patient who is unable to tolerate speech at a hearing level of 90 dB or less may have some degree of recruitment. The presence of recruitment may be indicated also when the patient's SRT, his MCL, and his tolerance level for speech are relatively close together or, in other words, when his dynamic range is compressed. The speech audiogram form in Figure 6-4 has space for recording MCL and dynamic range. A patient will experience difficulty in making reliable judgments of MCL for speech as well as for pure tones. Determining the presence of recruitment from an evaluation of speech audiometric results requires considerable clinical experience, and at best only general observations of the patient's loudness function can be obtained.

SISI Test

As was mentioned earlier in this section, there was a period during the late 1940's and early 1950's when tests of the difference limen became popular as a means for determining the presence or absence of "recruitment." Many psychological experiments in the field of sensation and perception have been performed to measure *difference limens* or *limena*. A difference limen (DL) in any sensory process is defined as a *just noticeable difference* (jnd) in whatever aspect of the sensation is under investigation. Thus, so far as hearing is concerned, the DL for frequency is the amount of change in frequency required to produce a jnd in pitch, or the DL for intensity is the amount of change in intensity required to produce a jnd in loudness. Most of the work with DL's in clinical hearing tests has been concerned with measuring the size of the DL for intensity.

Lüscher and Zwislocki described a DL test that was administered at a sensation level of 40 dB. It involved the presentation of a tone that "wobbulates" in intensity, that is, varies in intensity so the patient hears intensity beats. The examiner then reduces the wobbulation gradually until the patient reports the tone sounds "steady." The amount of intensity variation occurring at the point at which the patient signals the tone is no longer fluctuating is his DL. An "abnormal" DL is one that is smaller than the minimum value within the range of the norms established by Lüscher and Zwislocki.[55]

Denes and Naunton developed a test that compares the size of a patient's DL's at sensation levels of 4 and 44 dB. In determining the size of the DL at each sensation level they use two separate tones of the same frequency, one tone held constant in intensity and the other varied. These tones are presented to the patient's ear alternately. In the beginning the tones are of equal inten-

55 Lüscher and Zwislocki, *op. cit.*

sity, but as the test progresses one tone is varied until the patient reports he can detect a difference in intensity between the tones. The amount by which the intensity of the variable tone differs from the tone of constant intensity at this point is the patient's DL. Denes and Naunton were not interested in the absolute size of a patient's DL's, but only in the *difference* in the value of the DL's at the two sensation levels. They determined that normal ears had fairly wide differences, with the DL at 4 dB sensation level being greater than the DL at 44 dB ,whereas the ear with abnormal DL functioning was able to detect about as small increments of intensity at 4 dB as at 44 dB. Denes and Naunton reported a range of norms for difference limen differences.[56]

Jerger experimented with two different tests based on the DL for intensity. He first employed a technique similar to that described by Lüscher and Zwislocki, except that he presented the tone at a sensation level of 15 dB, and he started with a steady tone, gradually introducing intensity changes until the patient reported the tone was fluctuating in intensity.[57] Later Jerger developed a difference-limen-difference (DLD) test similar to that described by Denes and Naunton. He compared the size of a patient's DL at sensation levels of 10 and 40 dB and used a single wobbulating tone for determining the size of the DL's.[58]

Because of clinical findings that the results of DL tests could not always be correlated with the presence or absence of recruitment as determined with loudness-balance techniques, and because of apparent lack of reliability (repeatability of results) in DL testing, little emphasis was placed on the clinical significance of "abnormal" DL's until Jerger and his co-workers reported in 1959 their experience with a new procedure that was satisfactorily reliable and could be administered with a greater degree of objectivity than was previously possible in DL testing. By this time, Jerger was interested in test results that shed light on the site of lesion, instead of attempting to develop a different technique for assessing the presence or absence of recruitment. The new test was christened "SISI" for the words, "short-increment sensitivity index."[59]

The SISI test consists of superimposing brief bursts of 1-dB intensity increments on a sustained tone presented at a sensation level of 20 dB at each frequency to be tested. The test is administered monaurally through earphones. The patient is instructed to report any "jumps in loudness" he detects while listening to the sustained tone for a period of about two minutes. The apparatus used makes possible the presentation of an intensity increment every five seconds. Each increment has a rise time of 50 msec, a duration at

[56] Denes and Naunton, *op. cit.*

[57] Jerger, "A Difference Limen Recruitment Test and Its Diagnostic Significance," *op. cit.*

[58] Jerger, "DL Difference Test: Improved Method for Clinical Measurement of Recruitment," *op. cit.*

[59] James Jerger, Joyce Lassman Shedd, and Earl Harford, "On the Detection of Extremely Small Changes in Sound Intensity," *A.M.A. Archives of Otolaryngology,* Vol. 69 (February, 1959), pp. 200-211.

full strength of 200 msec, and a decay time of 50 msec. The size of the increment can be zero dB, 1 dB, or 5 dB, depending on the choice of the examiner, although the test is scored only on the percentage of 1-dB increments correctly identified by the patient. During the test, twenty 1-dB increments are presented. If the patient pushes his signal button for five of the twenty 1-dB increments, his sensitivity index is 25 per cent. In all, 28 increments are presented in a series. The first five increments presented are 5 dB in size in order to provide the patient a noticeably intense increment to which to respond. The next five increments are 1 dB in size. If the patient responds to three or more of these, the size of the sixth increment is set at zero dB as a "control presentation" for checking on the validity of the test. If the patient responds to two or less of the first five 1-dB increments, the size of the sixth increment is set at 5 dB to enable him once again to respond positively. After the tenth and fifteenth presentations of 1-dB increments, the following increment is set either at zero dB or 5 dB, depending on whether or not the patient responded to the majority of the preceding five 1-dB increments. As mentioned before, only the responses to the twenty 1-dB increments are scored. If the patient signals during a control presentation (increment of zero dB), the examiner discards the test as being invalid. In such a case the patient is probably responding to the rhythmic presentation of increments instead of to an increase in intensity. If the patient does not respond to a 5 dB increment, it is necessary to stop the test and reinstruct the patient as to his task, since a 5-dB increment should be a noticeable increase in intensity for any patient.

The results of the SISI test can be reported as percentages scored at each frequency, or they can be graphed on a "SISI-gram," which has frequency on the abscissa and percentages ascending from zero to 100 per cent on the ordinate. Jerger *et al.* reported the following ranges of SISI scores (in percentages) at the frequencies of 1000 and 4000 Hz for a group of 75 patients with various medical diagnoses[60]

	No. Cases	*1000 Hz*	*4000 Hz*
conductive	21	0–15	0–15
noise-induced	9	0–40	95–100
Ménière's	8	70–100	95–100
presbycusis	34	0–100	0–100
retrocochlear	3	0	0

Jerger *et al.*[61] have the following comments about their results.

... In general, purely conductive losses yield very low scores, while losses presumed to be localized in the sensory structure of the inner ear tend to show very high scores. Values between these extremes are infrequent. When they do occur, they are observed most commonly in presbycusis. ... Presbycusis appears to be a clinical entity in which the SISI score is quite unpredictable.

60 *Ibid.,* p. 208.
61 *Ibid.,* pp. 203-206.

The spread of SISI scores in cases of presbycusis suggested that presbycusis may be either sensory or neural in nature, or that it may be due to a combination of sensory and neural factors. In other words, there apparently is no single pathology that is characteristic of the hearing impairments associated with aging.

Since its first description, the SISI test has been widely used in a number of clinics and is now a valuable part of the test battery used to yield information regarding site of lesion. Many audiometers either have built-in SISI units or provide for the use of a separate SISI unit as an accessory. While some authors have suggested minor variations in test procedure such as shortening the test to ten presentations or varying the sensation level at which the test is presented, there is agreement that the SISI is useful (although not 100 per cent effective) in differentiating cochlear from VIIIth-nerve lesions.[62] Owens suggests that the SISI test reflects recruitment and is duplicative with the ABLB test. He prefers the SISI, however, because it can be used in cases of bilateral impairment, it appears to provide a more precise, objective measure than the ABLB, and it is easier for the patient to perform.[63]

With the development and clinical acceptance of the SISI test, interest in the clinical application of DL tests was rekindled. In a comprehensive survey of the literature and reporting of psychophysical experimental data on the loudness discrimination function, Harris suggests that the variability in test results and lack of reliability from examiner to examiner reported in previous clinical trials of DL for intensity measures may have been due to improper test administration rather than to any inherent defect of the tests themselves. He points out that the examiner must instruct the patient carefully in the task he is to perform and must be willing to "train" the patient in taking the test. With careful methodology, the examiner can obtain valid and reliable results in DL testing, according to Harris, who suggests also that the different kinds of psychophysical judgments required of patients in the Lüscher and Zwislocki test and in the Denes-Naunton test may be getting at different kinds of aural pathologies.[64] Whether or not these and other tests of the DL for intensity are revived for clinical use, the SISI test exists as a quick and reliable means of obtaining information of diagnostic significance through one technique of DL testing.

[62] Phillip A. Yantis and Robert L. Decker, "On the Short Increment Sensitivity Index (SISI Test), *Journal of Speech and Hearing Disorders*, Vol. 29 (August, 1964), pp. 231-246.

Elmer Owens, "The SISI Test and VIIIth Nerve Versus Cochlear Involvement," *Journal of Speech and Hearing Disorders*, Vol. 30 (August, 1965), pp. 252-262.

Earl R. Harford, "Clinical Application and Significance of the SISI Test," in A. Bruce Graham, ed., *Sensorineural Hearing Processes and Disorders* (Boston, Little, Brown and Company, 1967), pp. 223-233.

[63] Elmer Owens, "The SISI Test and Recruitment of Loudness by Alternate Binaural Loudness Balance," *Journal of Speech and Hearing Disorders*, Vol. 30 (August, 1965), pp. 263-268.

[64] J. Donald Harris, "Loudness Discrimination," *Journal of Speech and Hearing Disorders*, Monograph Supplement No. 11 (February, 1963), pp. 24-32.

Békésy Audiometry

Békésy developed and Reger improved and produced an audiometer by means of which a patient could administer his own hearing test.[65] This instrument consists of a pure-tone oscillator, the controls of which are driven by small electric motors and chain or gear drives. The frequency selector control covers a range from the lowest frequency to be tested to the highest in a steady progression. The hearing-level control or attenuator is driven by an instantly reversible electric motor, the direction of rotation of which is determined by a push button operated by the patient. When the button is held down, the hearing-level control rotates counterclockwise, decreasing the intensity of the signal. When the button is released, the control rotates in a clockwise direction, thus increasing the intensity. The patient is instructed to push the button when he hears the signal and keep it depressed as long as he continues to hear the signal; then to release it. The audiometer is connected with an X-Y recorder that traces the patient's audiogram as a series of vertical oscillations of the marking pen along the horizontal dimension of frequency. Figure 7-6 shows a conventional Békésy audiogram. Some information regarding the size of the patient's DL at threshold levels can be obtained by an inspection of the vertical excursions of the pen which, depending on the rate of attenuation employed (dB change per second), may cover a range of from 8 to 12 dB or more for a normal ear. An abnormal DL for intensity at threshold would be indicated by narrower excursions of the pen, such as those occurring for frequencies above 2000 Hz in Figure 7-6.

In addition to the conventional tracing shown in Figure 7-6, it is also possible to obtain "fixed-frequency" tracings with Békésy audiometers—that is, to sample a patient's threshold at any given frequency for a period of time, usually not exceeding four minutes. In Figure 7-7, fixed-frequency tracings are shown for three frequencies for the same patient whose conventional tracing was shown in Figure 7-6. A red and a blue pen are supplied with the X-Y recorder, so that different-colored tracings may be obtained for the right and left ears. The examiner may choose to present the stimulus as a continuous tone, or as a periodically interrupted or pulsing tonal signal. Tracings for continuous and interrupted signals for the same ear can be compared by using one color for continuous and the other for interrupted.

[65] Georg von Békésy, "A New Audiometer," *Acta Otolaryngologica*, Vol. 35 (1947), pp. 411-422.

Scott N. Reger, "A Clinical and Research Version of the Békésy Audiometer," *Laryngoscope*, Vol. 62 (December, 1952), pp. 1333-1351.

Figure 7-6. Conventional Békésy audiogram tracing for one ear.

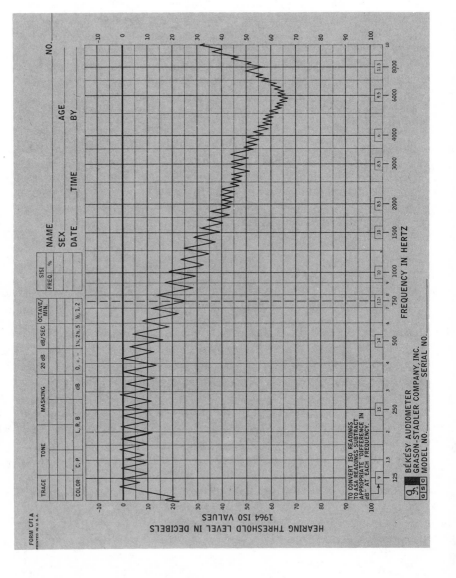

184

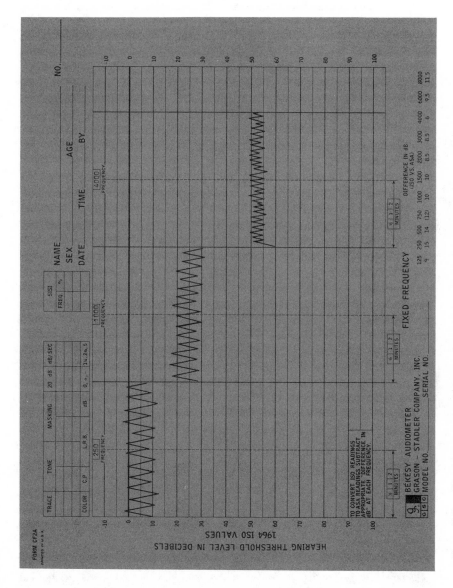

Figure 7-7. Fixed-frequency Békésy audiogram tracings for the frequencies of 250, 1000, and 4000 Hz.

While the Békésy audiometer yields some information regarding size of the DL for intensity as we have seen, the primary advantage of the test method so far as determining site of lesion is concerned lies in the comparison of thresholds obtained with continuous versus periodically interrupted signals, both in conventional and in fixed-frequency tracings. The comparison of thresholds obtained with continuous versus interrupted tone reveals that some patients demonstrate much higher (poorer) thresholds with the tone presented continuously. Lierle and Reger reported that when a patient who had an acoustic neurinoma was asked to trace threshold with a Békésy audiometer at a fixed frequency for a period of twenty minutes the threshold steadily became higher, while little difference in threshold occurred when patients with cochlear involvements performed this same task.[66] Jerger, Carhart, and Lassman confirmed the results reported by Lierle and Reger that excessive threshold "adaptation" occurs within a three-minute period in cases of VIIIth-nerve tumors when tonal stimulation at fixed frequencies is continuous, but they reported that the "adaptation" effect was not observed in these patients when the tonal stimulus was pulsed (three interruptions per second) instead of being continuous. In contrast, patients with sensori-neural losses of cochlear origin showed slight "adaptation" effects that did not increase with time through the three minutes of threshold tracing at fixed frequencies.[67]

Subsequently, Jerger analyzed conventional and fixed-frequency Békésy tracings obtained with continuous and periodically interrupted tone ($2\frac{1}{2}$ interruptions per second) on 434 patients seen over a period of three years at the Northwestern Medical School Hearing Clinic. From this analysis he described four basic types of Békésy audiograms. All but 16 of the 434 audiograms analyzed could be classified as one of the four types.[68] The type I audiogram shows no essential difference in thresholds obtained with continuous versus interrupted tone in either conventional or fixed-frequency tracings. The type II audiogram is the same as the type I for frequencies below 1000 Hz. Above 1000 Hz, the continuous tracing drops below (shows higher thresholds than) the interrupted tracing to a slight degree but usually differs from the interrupted tracing by no more than 20 dB. The tracing narrows in vertical range for the higher frequencies when the tone is continuously presented, but not when it is interrupted. In fixed-frequency presentations, the tracings obtained with continuous and interrupted tones are the same for frequencies below 1000 Hz. At 1000 Hz and at higher frequencies, however, the tracing for continuous

---

[66] Dean M. Lierle and Scott N. Reger, "Experimentally Induced Temporary Threshold Shifts in Ears with Impaired Hearing," *Annals of Otology, Rhinology, and Laryngology,* Vol. 64 (March, 1955), pp. 263-277.

[67] James Jerger, Raymond Carhart, and Joyce Lassman, "Clinical Observations on Excessive Threshold Adaptation," *A.M.A. Archives of Otolaryngology,* Vol. 68 (November, 1958), pp. 617-623.

[68] James Jerger, "Békésy Audiometry in Analysis of Auditory Disorders," *Journal of Speech and Hearing Research,* Vol. 3 (September, 1960), pp. 275-287.

tone drops below that for interrupted tone within the first minute by from 5 to 20 dB and then remains stable for the remainder of the three-minute period of stimulation.

In the type III audiogram, the tracing obtained with continuous tone drops below that for interrupted tone beginning with very low frequencies. As the test with conventional tracing continues, the gap between the thresholds for continuous and interrupted tone widens markedly until the maximum intensity limit of the audiometer is reached, perhaps at as low a frequency as 1000 Hz. There is no difference, however, in the vertical range of the tracing between continuous and interrupted tone. In the fixed-frequency presentations, the tracing obtained with interrupted tone remains horizontal for the three-minute period, while the tracing for continuous tone almost immediately begins a sharp decline and descends rapidly to the intensity limit of the audiometer. Fixed-frequency tracings show this same relationship between continuous and interrupted tone for all frequencies.

The type IV audiogram resembles the type II in that there is a constant difference between the tracings obtained with continuous and with interrupted tone, except that this difference (up to 20 dB) occurs for lower frequencies as well as for 1000 Hz and higher frequencies. There may or may not be some narrowing of vertical range of the tracing for continuous tone at the higher frequencies. The fixed-frequency tracings demonstrate a constant difference between the tracings for continuous and for interrupted tone at all frequencies. So the type IV is distinguished from the type II in that the difference in tracing between continuous and interrupted tone is noted for frequencies below 1000 Hz, and the type IV is distinguished from the type III in that there is no increase in the gap between tracings for continuous and for interrupted tone with the progress of time.

Jerger compared the Békésy audiogram type—for the 418 patients whose audiograms could be classified—with the otological diagnosis for each patient and drew some conclusions regarding the relationship between Békésy audiogram type and presumed site of lesion.

... In lesions of the middle ear (otosclerosis, otitis media) the type I tracing predominates. In cochlear lesion (Ménière's, noise-induced) the type II tracing predominates although some fall into the type I category. No Ménière's case ever showed a type III tracing. In eighth nerve lesion (acoustic neurinoma) type III and type IV tracings predominate. No acoustic neurinoma ever gave a type II tracing.[69]

Subsequent to the publication of Jerger's 1960 article defining four types of Békésy audiograms, Jerger and Herer described a type V Békésy, which was characterized by poorer threshold hearing levels when the signal was interrupted than when it was continuous—just the opposite result to what would be expected. They suggested that the type V Békésy might be

___

[69] *Ibid.,* p. 284.

associated with functional hearing loss.[70] Others have found the type V Békésy to be useful as a screening test for nonorganicity, particularly if the interval between pulses is lengthened[71] and if only separations between continuous and interrupted tracings in excess of 5 to 6 dB are accepted as indicators of a type V Békésy.[72]

Owens analyzed Békésy results with 92 patients having cochlear lesions, 20 patients with retrocochlear lesions, and 2 patients having mixed cochlear and retrocochlear lesions. He feels that the conventional or sweep-frequency definition of the type II Békésy audiogram needs revising, and he suggests the following rewording: "In cochlear lesions the 'C' tracing may drop below 'I' at any point in the frequency range (250–4000 Hz), typically with concomitant narrowing; it then characteristically remains essentially parallel to 'I,' but occasionally may rejoin 'I.' " Broadening Jerger's definition of type II in effect eliminates his type IV, which Owens found was not characteristic of any of the VIIIth-nerve cases in his series. Owens prefers the fixed-frequency Békésy analysis to the sweep frequency. He reported that 23 per cent of his patients with cochlear lesions demonstrated type I instead of type II tracings, but generally they were the patients with milder losses. Of the patients with retrocochlear lesions due to VIIIth-nerve tumors, all demonstrated type III tracings. The patients with combined cochlear and retrocochlear involvements yielded type II Békésy tracings and reacted on recruitment and SISI tests in a manner typical of those with cochlear pathology, leading Owens to suggest that the presence of a cochlear lesion may mask the presence of an accompanying VIIIth-nerve lesion.[73]

Békésy audiometry is becoming increasingly popular, and it can be anticipated that with the passage of time the information obtained with this flexible instrument will become increasingly important in assisting the otologist and audiologist to a determination of the site of lesion.

Tone Decay

Various investigators have noted that some patients have difficulty maintaining audibility for a tone presented at threshold. In fact the basis for the recommendation in Chapter 5 that the examiner utilize tonal pulses rather than continuous tone for seeking threshold was the recognition that patients might adapt to a steady tone, requiring increases in intensity to keep the tone audible. Hood termed this phenomenon "perstimulatory

70 James Jerger and Gilbert Herer, "Unexpected Dividend in Békésy Audiometry," *Journal of Speech and Hearing Disorders,* Vol. 26 (November, 1961), pp. 390-391.

71 Karl W. Hattler, "Lengthened Off-Time: A Self-Recording Screening Device for Nonorganicity," *Journal of Speech and Hearing Disorders,* Vol. 35 (May, 1970), pp. 113-122.

72 Norma Trozzo Hopkinson, "Type V Békésy Audiograms: Specification and Clinical Utility," *Journal of Speech and Hearing Disorders,* Vol. 30 (August, 1965), pp. 243-251.

73 Elmer Owens, "Békésy Tracings and Site of Lesion," *Journal of Speech and Hearing Disorders,* Vol. 29 (November, 1964), pp. 456-468.

fatigue."[74] Other terms most frequently used to describe this phenomenon are abnormal adaptation and tone decay.

Carhart proposed a "tone decay test" and reported that patients with Ménière's syndrome and patients with other types of sensori-neural disorders demonstrated tone decay on this test. Carhart's procedure involved presenting a continuous tone at a patient's previously determined threshold hearing level and checking the patient's response with a stopwatch. If the patient maintains the tone at an audible level for sixty seconds, the test result is negative: there is no tone decay. If the patient "loses" the tone short of sixty seconds, the examiner increases the intensity by one or more 5-dB steps until the patient again signals that he hears the tone. The timing then commences anew. Additional increases in intensity are made if necessary until a hearing level is reached at which the patient can respond to the tone for a full sixty seconds. The amount of tone decay is expressed as the dB change from original threshold to the final hearing level required to meet the sixty-second criterion.[75]

A modification of the tone decay test that shortens the time required for administration was suggested by Philip Rosenberg in a paper read at the 1958 convention of the American Speech and Hearing Association.[76] The patient is presented a tone at threshold and the examiner starts his watch. When the patient signals that he can no longer hear the tone, the examiner increases the intensity by one or more 5-dB steps, but without stopping the watch. The test is continued for only one minute at each frequency. Tone decay is expressed as the dB shift in threshold that occurred in one minute. Green reported that the degree of threshold shift may be related to the instructions given the patient. If the patient is instructed to respond only as long as he can hear the tone with its original tonality, he may exhibit considerably more tone decay than if he is allowed to respond to any signal heard. In other words, Green believes that in disorders involving the VIIIth-nerve a tone may change to noise, and unless the patient is specifically instructed to respond only to *tone*, it may appear that he has little or no tone decay. He calls the test in which the patient is instructed to respond only to tone the modified tone decay test (MTDT).[77]

While abnormal adaptation is characteristic of patients with VIIIth-nerve lesions, patients with cochlear disorders exhibit tone decay as well, which confuses the problem of differential diagnosis. Owens reported tone decay results with 53 patients diagnosed as Ménière's cases and

[74] J. D. Hood, "Studies in Fatigue and Auditory Adaptation," *Acta Otolaryngologica,* Supplement 92 (1950), pp. 26-56.

[75] Raymond Carhart, "Clinical Determination of Abnormal Auditory Adaptation," *Archives of Otolaryngology,* Vol. 65 (1957), pp. 32-39.

[76] David S. Green, "The Modified Tone Decay Test (MTDT) as a Screening Procedure for Eighth Nerve Lesions," *Journal of Speech and Hearing Disorders,* Vol. 28 (February, 1963), pp. 31-32.

[77] *Ibid.,* p. 32.

18 patients with VIIIth-nerve lesions. He employed a test method described by Hood,[78] which permitted the patient to rest for up to sixty seconds after each fading of the tone before the next 5-dB increment was introduced. The test continued until a level was reached at which the patient could sustain the tone for one minute, or until at least four intensity increments had been presented. The test was started at a sensation level of 5 dB instead of at threshold. Owens reported that all but 12 of the 53 Ménière's patients showed tone decay at one or more frequencies. The decay was more prevalent at 4000 Hz than at other frequencies. In the VIIIth-nerve group, all but one showed tone decay at two or more frequencies. Owens suggests that the cochlear and VIIIth-nerve groups can be differentiated by the number of frequencies showing decay, and by the rapidity of the decay between intensity increments. Those with cochlear lesions showed a reduced rate of decay as intensity increased, whereas those with VIIIth-nerve lesions showed the same rapid rate of decay at each intensity increment.[79] In a subsequent study, Owens found that patients presenting rapid rate of decay demonstrated Békésy type III tracings, but that patients whose decay rate slowed down with increasing intensity were characterized by Békésy type II tracings. In cases of equivocal tone decay results, the type of Békésy audiogram could be predicted from an ABLB test for recruitment. Patients demonstrating recruitment subsequently yielded type II audiograms. If there was no recruitment, the type III audiogram would occur.[80]

The advantage of the tone decay test is its simplicity. No special equipment is required other than an audiometer and a watch. The high correlation between the tone decay test and the Békésy comparison of interrupted and continuous tone suggests that if one does not have access to a Békésy audiometer he may still classify patients as to presumed Békésy types II and III on the basis of tone decay tests, following Owen's criteria of differentiation of cochlear and retrocochlear results, and being guided by the ABLB test in cases of equivocal tone decay results.

Other Tests

Comparison of Alternate and Simultaneous Balancing of Pure Tones. One of the items in the test battery proposed by Jerger and his associates for use in differentiating between cochlear and retrocochlear sensori-neural involvements is a comparison of intensities required for (1) balancing the loudness of pure tones when the signal is presented alternately to the good and poor ear, and (2) achieving a median-plane localization of the tone when the signal is presented simultaneously to the good and the

[78] J. D. Hood, "Auditory Fatigue and Adaptation in the Differential Diagnosis of End-Organ Disease," *Annals of Otology, Rhinology and Laryngology,* Vol. 64 (1955), pp. 507-518.

[79] Elmer Owens, "Tone Decay in VIIIth Nerve and Cochlear Lesions," *Journal of Speech and Hearing Disorders,* Vol. 29 (February, 1964), pp. 14-22.

[80] Elmer Owens, "Békésy Tracings, Tone Decay, and Loudness Recruitment," *Journal of Speech and Hearing Disorders,* Vol. 30 (February, 1965), pp. 50-57.

poor ear.[81] In both types of presentation, the duration of the stimulus is one second. We have already discussed the alternate binaural loudness-balance test as a measure for determining the presence of recruitment in unilateral sensori-neural loss. In the simultaneous binaural balance test the patient's task is to localize the signal in the midline, that is, in the center of his head, by varying the intensity in one ear while keeping the intensity in the opposite ear constant. As mentioned earlier, Jerger and Harford follow the procedure of keeping the signal at constant intensity in the poor ear and varying the intensity on the good ear in performing the alternate binaural loudness-balance test. They follow the same procedure in simultaneous balancing. Without going into the details of Jerger and Harford's findings in various experiments with normal ears, conductively-impaired ears, masked normal ears, and ears with unilateral sensori-neural impairment, it can be reported that they found the two types of balancing procedures do not yield equivalent results. They say, ". . . equal loudness cannot be inferred from median-plane localization. The two types of judgment are apparently independent and not interchangeable."[82] Since these two procedures are not inter-changeable, it follows that in recruitment testing by binaural loudness balancing the signal must always be presented alternately to the good and poor ear.

Jerger and Harford noted different relationships between the results of the two types of balancing with "recruiting" and "non-recruiting" ears with unilateral sensori-neural impairment. With recruiting ears (pre-sumed cochlear involvement) the simultaneous matching procedure re-quires approximately equal hearing levels at both ears, whereas with non-recruiting ears a higher hearing level is required on the poor ear in order to achieve a midline localization. With both recruiting and non-recruiting ears, more intensity at the poor ear is required for the simultaneous match than for the alternate loudness balance. The difference in intensity required at the poor ear for the two kinds of judgments is greater for the non-recruiting ear than for the recruiting ear. It thus appears that a com-parison of the interaural intensity relations required for loudness balancing and for median-plane localization may contribute valuable information regarding the site of lesion in cases of unilateral sensori-neural impairment.

There is some evidence also that patients who have lesions in central auditory pathways will exhibit abnormal interaural intensity relations affecting their ability to perform the loudness balance task. Median-plane localization may or may not demonstrate an abnormality, apparently depending on the nature and extent of the central nervous system lesion. Cortical or subcortical lesions apparently exert subtle effects on auditory perception that cannot be detected through routine audiological procedures. Thus a patient with a lesion in one temporal lobe, for example, may have normal pure-tone and speech thresholds and normal speech discrimination.

[81] Jerger and Harford, *op. cit.*
[82] *Ibid.*, p. 28.

It is only when his auditory system is forced to perform difficult tasks that abnormalities become apparent. Unlike unilateral peripheral hearing impairments in which a lesion in the left cochlea or the left auditory nerve produces abnormal test results in the left ear, a central auditory disorder is manifested by abnormal functioning of the contralateral ear. Thus a lesion in the left temporal lobe would affect the ability of the right ear to perform complex auditory functions. It will be remembered from Chapter 2 that, because of decussations of the ascending auditory pathways at subcortical levels, there is representation of both ears in both temporal lobes. Apparently this bilateral representation in the auditory cortex is sufficient to enable both ears to respond to simple auditory stimuli even though the auditory pathway or auditory cortex on one side of the brain is damaged. But as the auditory tasks increase in complexity, the presence of the central nervous system lesion is revealed by an inability of the contralateral ear to perform at the same level as the ipsilateral ear. Also, there may be deficiencies noted in the performance of auditory tasks that demand binaural integration, for example, localizing the source of a sound in space.

Jerger has shown with the alternate binaural loudness-balance test that some patients with central auditory lesions require considerably more intensity in the ear contralateral to the lesion in order to balance loudness with the ipsilateral ear at suprathreshold levels, although the two ears have the same threshold sensitivity for the tonal stimulus.[83]

Speech Discrimination Tests. There is little information yielded by speech discrimination tests that will assist the clinician to determine whether a particular unilateral sensori-neural impairment is of a cochlear or a retrocochlear origin. Both Ménière's syndrome and acoustic neurinoma, for example, may produce discrimination scores that are markedly poorer than would be predicted from the degree and configuration of the pure-tone loss. The clinician must depend on the SISI test, Békésy audiometry, the tone decay test, and binaural balance tests to differentiate cochlear from retrocochlear involvements. Nor will the results of speech discrimination tests performed in routine speech audiometry give an indication of a disorder of the central auditory system, as we have just mentioned in the preceding section. When speech discrimination tasks are increased in complexity, however, by filtering or masking procedures, the ear contralateral to the central auditory lesion will perform more poorly than the ipsilateral ear.

Patterning his procedures after those developed in Italy by Bocca and his associates,[84] Jerger developed what he called "distorted speech tests" that consisted of PB word lists recorded on magnetic tape and presented to the patient either through a low-pass filter, or at a "faint" level of intensity.

[83] James F. Jerger, "Observations on Auditory Behavior in Lesions of the Central Auditory Pathways," *A.M.A. Archives of Otolaryngology*, Vol. 71 (May, 1960), pp. 797-806.

[84] E. Bocca, "Clinical Aspects of Cortical Deafness," *Laryngoscope*, Vol. 68 (March, 1958), pp. 301-309.

The filter passed frequencies below 500 Hz. Filtered PB words were presented to the patient at a sensation level of 45 dB. The "faint" level was established empirically to produce approximately 50 per cent correct responses, and it varied, depending on the patient, between sensation levels of 5 and 15 dB. Six distorted speech tests were presented to the patient in the following order:

1. Left ear: low-pass filtered
2. Right ear: faint unfiltered
3. Combined (left ear: low-pass filtered; right ear: faint unfiltered)
4. Right ear: low-pass filtered
5. Left ear: faint unfiltered
6. Combined (right ear: low-pass filtered; left ear: faint unfiltered).[85]

These tests were administered to three patients whose neurological diagnoses were (1) left temporal glioblastoma, (2) left temporal epilepsy, and (3) left frontal meningioma. In routine speech audiometry, the first two patients demonstrated equally good speech discrimination scores in each ear (88 and 92 per cent for the first patient, and 90 and 98 per cent for the second patient). There were marked differences in the scores obtained on the two ears, however, when the speech was distorted by filtering or by making it "faint." The right ear in each case (contralateral to the temporal lobe lesion) performed much more poorly than the left ear. When the distorted conditions were presented binaurally in combination the speech discrimination scores were affected equally by conditions 3 and 6. The third patient demonstrated poor discrimination scores in each ear in routine speech audiometry (74 and 60 per cent), and both ears were affected equally by low-pass filtering. No data were reported for other conditions of speech distortion. The third patient presumably demonstrated more diffuse central nervous system involvement than the other two patients, although in his case the alternate binaural loudness-balance test revealed disturbed intensity relations in the ear contralateral to the cortical lesion.[86]

In a study of sixteen patients with Parkinsonism, Jerger et al. compared the auditory performance of the patients with age-matched control subjects.[87] In routine pure-tone and speech-audiometric tests there were essentially no differences in the performance of the experimental and control groups. Two difficult listening tasks were demanded of the subjects, however, that did reveal differences in performance between the patients with Parkinsonism of the post-encephalitic and arteriosclerotic types and the control subjects. Five patients whose Parkinsonism was classified as "idiopathic" did not differ in their performance on the difficult listening tasks from their matched controls. The tasks involved first, listening to low-pass filtered PB words in each

85 Jerger, "Observations on Auditory Behavior in Lesions of the Central Auditory Pathways," op. cit., p. 798.

86 Ibid., p. 804.

87 J. Jerger, M. Mier, B. Boshes, and G. Canter, "Auditory Behavior in Parkinsonism," Acta Otolaryngologica, Vol. 52 (December, 1960), pp. 541-550.

ear separately as in the study by Jerger referred to in the preceding paragraphs, and, second, listening binaurally to PB words while 0.5 second bursts
of thermal noise at a level 20 dB higher than the speech was alternated between the ears. This latter procedure was dubbed the "SWAMI" test
(speech with alternating masking index). While differences in performance
between right and left ears were not noted for any of the experimental subjects,
their mean right and left ear discrimination scores on the filtered-speech test
were lower than the mean scores for the control subjects, and their scores
on the SWAMI test were likewise lower (by the same amount as on the
filtered-speech test) than the scores for the control subjects. Incidentally,
while the performance of control subjects was affected by low-pass filtering
(although not as much, of course, as for experimental subjects), their
performance was relatively unaffected in the SWAMI test. Jerger *et al.* say:

> . . . through either earphone singly the words are virtually unintelligible. The
> periodic noise bursts effectively mask all or part of most of the words. Listening
> through both earphones, however, the listener experiences a unique illusion in
> which bursts of noise are localized in the ears, but the words are heard in the center
> of the head. It is as if the brain literally "fuses" the word-fragments from each ear
> into a single unitary image. As a result, the words are easily understood by normals
> and the discrimination score is quite good (90–100%).[88]

Bocca and Calearo[89] and Bocca[90] emphasize the advantage of using
sentences rather than isolated words in evaluating central auditory disorders.
They believe that the effect of a central lesion can best be observed by noting
interference with understanding the meaning of sentences, since it is the
function of the higher centers to integrate and give form to the acoustic
signals processed by the peripheral structures. Under normal conditions of
communication, speech messages (i.e., sentences) are understood with a
minimum of difficulty because of the abundance of neural pathways (intrinsic
redundancy) and the multiple cues contained in the speech signal (extrinsic
redundancy). Central lesions reduce intrinsic redundancy, but understanding
may still occur because of extrinsic redundancy. When extrinsic redundancy
is reduced by introducing frequency or time distortions in the speech signal,
communication breaks down. Thus while the reduction of either intrinsic or
extrinsic redundancy may not seriously affect the perception of speech, the
combined effects of the reduction of both kinds of redundancy may be disas-
trous. Bocca and Calearo utilize various kinds of distorted speech (sentence)
tests: filtered speech, time compressed (i.e., "speeded up") speech, swinging
speech, and interrupted speech. In cases of unilateral central lesions, the

88 *Ibid.*, p. 547.

89 E. Bocca and C. Calearo, "Central Hearing Processes," in James Jerger, ed., *Modern
Developments in Audiology* (New York, Academic Press, 1963), pp. 337-370.

90 Ettore Bocca, "Distorted Speech Tests," in A. Bruce Graham, ed., *Sensorineural Hearing
Processes and Disorders* (Boston, Little, Brown and Company, 1967), pp. 359-370.

ear contralateral to the lesion shows greater involvement; in diffuse central lesions, both ears will demonstrate reduced performance. The authors believe that their tests will differentiate between brain stem and cortical lesions, because ". . . responses to interrupted and swinging speech are more impaired than those to filtered or time-compressed speech, when brain stem or midbrain lesions are present, while the contrary is true with cortical pathology."[91]

Another speech test for detecting central auditory dysfunction, but one that utilizes words instead of sentences, is the Staggered Spondiac Word Test (SSW) described by Katz.[92] In this test, the patient is presented a list of paired tape-recorded spondee words, each pair of which partially overlaps; i.e., the second syllable of the first spondee is superimposed on the first syllable of the second spondee. The first spondee is directed to one ear, while the second spondee is directed to the other ear. The presentation is at a sensation level of 50 dB in each ear. The pairs of spondees are chosen so that the first syllable of the first spondee and the second syllable of the second spondee, if combined, would form a third spondee. The paired spondees are spoken with a slight pause between the syllables. The stimulus presentation can be described best in an example:

	Time Sequence		
	1	2	3
Right Ear	up	stairs	
Left Ear		down	town

The patient is instructed to repeat all the words he hears in a group. The "normal" response is to repeat the two basic words—in the above example, "upstairs" and "downtown." If the overlapping syllables interfere with each other, the patient may repeat only the combination word, "uptown." Or he may demonstrate errors in one or both of the competing syllables.

The order in which the ears are stimulated is alternated, so that with every other group the left ear would receive the first syllable of the first word. The examiner keeps track of errors on each syllable and then totals the errors occurring in each of eight conditions: right noncompeting, right competing, left competing, left noncompeting, left noncompeting, left competing, right competing, right noncompeting. In the first four conditions the right ear was stimulated first, while in the second four conditions the left ear was stimulated first. The raw scores are converted into percentage of errors for deriving an ear score, a condition score, and a total score. Katz has described scores that are characteristic of normal hearing, peripheral disorders, central nonauditory disorders, and central auditory disorders.[93] An analysis of ear

[91] *Ibid.*, p. 366.

[92] Jack Katz, "The Use of Staggered Spondaic Words for Assessing the Integrity of the Central Auditory Nervous System," *Journal of Auditory Research,* Vol. 2 (1962), pp. 327-337.

[93] Jack Katz, "The SSW Test: An Interim Report," *Journal of Speech and Hearing Disorders,* Vol. 33 (May, 1968), pp. 132-146.

performance is apparently most meaningful in pointing to the existence of a central auditory disorder, the presumed lesion being in the cerebral hemisphere contralateral to the ear with the poor score.

Impedance Measurements. Thus far in this section we have dealt with tests for determining the site of the lesion in cases of sensori-neural and central impairments. Progress is also being made in differentiating the site of pathology in cases of conductive impairment by measurement of the acoustic impedance at the eardrum. According to Zwislocki:

> When acoustic waves enter the ear canal, the eardrum is exposed to sound pressure and vibrates with an amplitude and phase that depend on the acoustic impedance resulting from the mechanical properties of the middle and, in part, inner ear. The most important factors are: the compliance and mass of the eardrum, the acoustic impedance of the middle-ear cavities, the coupling between the eardrum and the ossicular chain, the mass of the malleus and incus, the compliance of the ligaments and muscles holding the ossicular chain in place, the compliance of the incudostapedial joint, the compliance of the cochlear windows, and the acoustic impedance at the entrance to the cochlea. In all elements, motion is accompanied by friction.[94]

Thus, at the risk of oversimplifying a complex concept, it can be said that the acoustic impedance at the eardrum is a function of the *resistance* resulting from friction of the movable structures of the middle ear, the *mass* of these structures, and the *compliance,* or degree of stiffness, of ligaments, muscles, joints, and membranes.

Using an "acoustic bridge" invented by Schuster in the 1930's, Metz reported impedance measurements made on normal and impaired ears.[95] Zwislocki extended Metz's work and developed improved instrumentation for obtaining acoustic impedance measurements at the eardrum.[96] The Zwislocki acoustic bridge, produced commercially by the Grason-Stadler Company, enables an examiner to obtain measurements of compliance and resistance by adjusting a variable impedance until it matches the impedance of the ear being measured. Balance is achieved when a probe tone reflected from the eardrum is canceled by a tone of opposite phase that is controlled by the matching impedance in the bridge. The examiner monitors the signal through a stethoscope and "tunes" the bridge until the interaction of the reflected tone and the variable tone results in a null. The resistance and compliance values required to achieve the null are then read on the calibrated controls of the instrument. Measurements are made at some or all of the

94 J. Zwislocki, "An Acoustic Method for Clinical Examination of the Ear," *Journal of Speech and Hearing Research,* Vol. 6 (December, 1963), pp. 306-307.

95 O. Metz, "The Acoustic Impedance Measured on Normal and Pathological Ears," *Acta Otolaryngologica,* Supplement 63 (1946).

96 J. Zwislocki, "Acoustic Measurement of Middle Ear Function," *Annals of Otology, Rhinology, and Laryngology,* Vol. 70 (1961), pp. 599-607.

following frequencies produced by a commercial audiometer: 125, 250, 500, 750, 1000, and 1500 Hz.

Impedance measurements on normal ears and on ears with conductive impairments have been reported by Feldman[97] and by Zwislocki and Feldman.[98] These investigators report that stapes fixation (otosclerosis) and ossicular discontinuity can be identified and differentiated by characteristic alterations from normal impedance values. The impedance bridge can be used also to determine the presence or absence of the acoustic reflex. Since the reflex is bilateral, a noise of sufficient intensity to induce the reflex can be introduced to one ear after the bridge has been balanced on the other ear. If a reflex occurs, the stiffness of the ossicular chain is altered, causing the null to disappear and requiring a rebalancing of the bridge. The absence of an acoustic reflex may be indicative of a middle-ear pathology.

Other models of impedance bridges are now commercially available, and it can be anticipated that impedance measurements will become increasingly important in the differential diagnosis of middle-ear pathologies.

Interpretations of Test Batteries

In the introductory paragraphs to this section dealing with tests for identifying the site of lesion, the statement was made that rather than placing dependence on any single test, the clinician should view the results of a test battery before deciding whether a particular sensori-neural disorder is cochlear or retrocochlear. It is the composite picture that is important in assigning patients to one or the other diagnostic category.

From the various site of lesion tests that have been discussed in this section we can construct a chart partially modeled after that given by Jerger.[99] Table 7-1 shows the test results that classically would differentiate sensory from neural impairments. While any single test may have an atypical result in a particular instance, it is unlikely that all the tests in the battery would yield atypical results. It must be kept in mind, however, that some sensori-neural impairments are truly combined sensory and neural involvements, and it should be expected that in such cases the results of tests designed to identify *the* site of lesion would yield equivocal results. Shapiro and Naunton[100] agree with Owens [101] that when a patient has both cochlear and VIIIth-nerve pathology the audiologic signs will point to a cochlear lesion. In other words, the cochlear signs seem to dominate the retrocochlear signs so that the presence

[97] Alan S. Feldman, "Impedance Measurements at the Eardrum as an Aid to Diagnosis," *Journal of Speech and Hearing Research*, Vol. 6 (December, 1963), pp. 315-327.

Alan S. Feldman, "Acoustic Impedance Studies of the Normal Ear," *Journal of Speech and Hearing Research*, Vol. 10 (June, 1967), pp. 165-176.

[98] Jozef J. Zwislocki and Alan S. Feldman, "Acoustic Impedance of Pathological Ears," *ASHA Monographs*, No. 15 (January, 1970).

[99] James F. Jerger, "Hearing Tests in Otologic Diagnosis," *Asha*, Vol. 4 (May, 1962), p. 143.

[100] Irving Shapiro and Ralph F. Naunton, "Audiologic Evaluation of Acoustic Neurinomas," *Journal of Speech and Hearing Disorders,* Vol. 32 (February, 1967), p. 34.

[101] Owens, "Békésy Tracings and Site of Lesion," *op. cit.,* pp. 466-467.

of the VIIIth-nerve problem may go undetected. Matkin *et al.*, on the other hand, cite two cases of Ménière's disease whose audiologic signs changed from cochlear to retrocochlear immediately following a partial sectioning of the VIIIth-nerve. Of course in these cases there was no confusion of test results prior to surgery.[102]

Table 7-1. Test results typical of sensory and neural impairments

	Sensory (Cochlear)	*Neural (Retrocochlear)*
Tests for recruitment (alternate binaural loudness balance or monaural loudness balance)	incomplete, complete, or hyper-recruitment	no recruitment
SISI test (4000 Hz)	95-100%	0%
Békésy audiometry	Type II	Types III or IV
Tone decay test	slight to moderate decay; less decay at higher sensation levels	marked decay; same rate of decay at each sensation level
Simultaneous binaural balance (median-plane localization)	approximately equal hearing levels in both ears at point of balance.	greater hearing level at poorer ear at point of balance

We would like to think that audiologic testing can clearly differentiate between cochlear and VIIIth-nerve involvements, and it is true that the more unified the results of a test battery the more confidence the clinician can place in his prediction of site of lesion. Nevertheless, tests—even test batteries—may be fallible, as Johnson[103] and Shapiro and Naunton[104] have pointed out in discussing misleading and contradictory tests results on patients whose retrocochlear pathology has been confirmed by surgery. One needs reminding occasionally that hearing testing is but one part of the diagnostic process, and one needs to keep searching for ways to make the test batteries more definitive. In the meantime, since both Ménière's syndrome and VIIIth-nerve tumors typically result in unilateral sensori-neural hearing losses and disproportionately poor speech discrimination, the clinician should administer some or all of the site-of-lesion tests to all patients presenting these audiometric symptoms.

TESTING CHILDREN

Thus far in the chapters dealing with evaluation of hearing we have been concerned with patients whose physical and mental maturity make

102 Noel D. Matkin, William R. Hodgson, R. Carhart, and Tom W. Tillman, "Audiological Manifestations of Acute Neural Lesion in Cases with Ménière's Disease," *Journal of Speech and Hearing Disorders*, Vol. 30 (November, 1965), pp. 370-376.

103 E. W. Johnson, "Auditory Test Results in 110 Surgically Confirmed Retrocochlear Lesions," *Journal of Speech and Hearing Disorders*, Vol. 30 (November, 1965), pp. 307-317.

104 Shapiro and Naunton, *op. cit.*, pp. 29-35.

possible their involvement in the test situation as active participants, and, except for those individuals who manifest functional hearing problems, the examiner depends on the patient's positive responses to the presence or absence of test stimuli in determining threshold. In other words, the usual testing situation involves a patient who is capable of responding to the test stimuli introduced, whether they be pure tones or speech, who can understand and follow instructions, and who cooperates with the examiner. With such patients, certain standard procedures have evolved to insure test reliability, for example, the ascending method of arriving at threshold in pure-tone audiometry; and certain test materials such as spondee words and PB word lists have been agreed upon. When the examiner is confronted by a small child whose hearing he must evaluate, many of the "rules" of hearing testing must be modified or abandoned. The child may or may not be able to understand and follow instructions. He may not be capable of responding to auditory stimuli in an adult fashion, and his cooperation may be almost completely lacking—at least in the initial stages of the test procedure. Frequently, the examiner must make up the rules of the game as he proceeds and exercise every bit of ingenuity he can muster in order to obtain some information concerning the child's hearing. Of course there are many young children who can be examined easily and accurately with minimum modification of adult testing procedures, but the examiner must be prepared to meet the challenge of assessing the hearing of youngsters who are difficult to test. It is hoped that the suggestions contained in this section will help the examiner to meet that challenge successfully.

The Neonate and Infant

With the increasing importance of hearing conservation programs in the schools (see Chapter 8), there has developed the realization that many children whose hearing impairments are discovered in school testing programs might have been helped medically and socially had their hearing problems been identified at an earlier age. At how early an age is it feasible to attempt an assessment of hearing? The answer to this question is that with proper examination methods some information concerning the integrity of the hearing mechanism can be obtained with infants of only a few hours of age. As the infant's nervous system begins to mature during the first year of life, more definitive information concerning his hearing can be obtained. Methods of assessing the hearing of infants have been known for several years, but it is only recently that they have begun to be applied to any extent in this country.

The Ewings in England pioneered hearing examination techniques for use with infants. In 1958 they reported procedures they had developed and used over a period of twenty years.[105] The pioneer work in the United

[105] Irene R. Ewing and Alex W. G. Ewing, *New Opportunities for Deaf Children* (London, University of London Press Ltd., 1958).

States in the area of assessing the hearing of infants was done collaboratively by Johns Hopkins University School of Medicine and the Maryland State Department of Health—both located in Baltimore. In 1959 the Baltimore group reported test procedures based on the Ewing test battery, and the results of a pilot study that utilized these procedures with 327 infants from three to fifty-two weeks of age, 111 infants from ten to twenty-nine weeks of age, and 107 newborn infants.[106]

While the Ewings agree that deafness or profound hearing loss can be ruled out by observing the responses of babies of a few days of age to intense sound, they tend to dismiss the testing of the neonate as being too crude to yield significant information. They report cases of infants of very tender age who apparently did not respond to sound at all but who subsequently—say at age seven or eight months—demonstrated normal hearing abilities. The Ewings prefer to concentrate their attention on infants of seven months of age and older. The Baltimore group reported reasonably good success in eliciting positive responses from newborn infants with a specially constructed wooden "clacker." This consists of two pieces of wood fastened together with a screen-door spring hinge. When the top piece is raised to a 90 degree angle with the lower piece and then released, a very brief sound of broad spectrum results (reported as a sound level of 64 dB with the "B" weighting network of a sound-level meter at a distance of 12 feet). The duration of the sound is estimated as 5 msec.

The response of a newborn infant to such a sound is a startle or Moro's reflex, which is a contraction of the limbs and the neck muscles. Sometimes an eye blink occurs simultaneously with the general muscular activity that characterizes the Moro's reflex. The Baltimore group obtained "satisfactory" responses to the clacker in about 90 per cent of the newborn infants with whom it was tried. Of course a response to a stimulus of this intensity and spectrum does not rule out some hearing impairment, but it does indicate that the infant is not deaf. Failure of the newborn infant to respond to the clacker may or may not indicate a hearing impairment. In any event the infant who does not respond should be studied closely as he matures over the next few weeks or months to discover whether his hearing is impaired, or whether he presents some neurological or other deficit that could have accounted for his failure to respond. Hardy, Dougherty, and Hardy suggest that pediatricians should be able to utilize this technique of hearing "evaluation" to advantage with newborn infants in the hospital nursery.[107]

Downs and her colleagues at the University of Colorado Medical Center have focused attention on the auditory screening of newborn infants in the

---

[106] Janet B. Hardy, Anne Dougherty, and William G. Hardy, "Hearing Responses and Audiologic Screening in Infants," *Journal of Pediatrics,* Vol. 55 (September, 1959), pp. 382-390.
[107] *Ibid.,* p. 390.

hospital nursery.[108] As a result of Downs's work, there are available on the market several electronic devices designed for auditory screening in the nursery. These are hand-held, battery-powered instruments that generate a warbling pure tone of 3000 Hz or a narrow band of noise centered at 3000 Hz and possibly also a wide-band noise. The output is variable from 70 to 100 dB SPL when delivered through a loudspeaker held a few inches from the infant's ear. Downs selected the frequency of 3000 Hz for screening so that infants with sloping hearing losses could be identified when they might be missed by a test tone of lower frequency. She recommends 90 dB SPL as the criterion intensity for general use "because it is the lowest level that will consistently produce responses when presented to normal infants in the noise levels common to nursery situations."[109] A sound pressure level of 90 dB at 3000 Hz is equal to a hearing level of 82.5 dB according to the ANSI–1969 standard. Downs gives precise instructions for administering the test, observing the infant's behavior, judging whether or not a response occurred, and recording the intensity of the response on a 1-5 scale. The number 5 on the scale is reserved for a Moro's response. Downs reports also on her experience with training volunteers as observers and examiners, and she recommends their use. Infants who are screened as not responding to the test should be evaluated by an audiologist, if at all possible while they are still in the nursery. If the results are still equivocal, the infant should be rescheduled for testing when he is three to four weeks of age, preferably in an audiology clinic.

At the present writing there is disagreement as to the desirability of conducting widespread auditory screening in hospital nurseries. Downs reports that the incidence of "deafness" discovered in the Denver program is at least one in 2000 infants, or 0.05 per cent. She reports that "false positive" results are found in 1½ per cent of the population tested, although among the false positives are infants later discovered to have nonauditory CNS involvements.[110] Silverman and Davis, quoting from the proceedings of a 1964 Canadian conference on the young deaf child, suggest that because of the low yield a widespread screening program of newborns may be economically indefensible. Also they question the validity and reliability of infant screening tests, saying, "The number of 'false positives' and the number of cases missed, which are both rather high, must be considered; the former will cause unfounded anxiety, and the latter will give a false sense of security

108 Marion P. Downs and Graham M. Sterritt, "Identification Audiometry for Neonates: A Preliminary Report," *Journal of Auditory Research,* Vol. 4 (April, 1964), pp. 69-80.

Marion P. Downs, "Testing Hearing in Infancy and Early Childhood," in Freeman McConnell and Paul H. Ward, eds., *Deafness in Childhood* (Nashville, Tenn., Vanderbilt University Press, 1967), pp. 25-33.

Marion P. Downs, "Organization and Procedures of a Newborn Infant Screening Program," *Hearing and Speech News,* Vol. 35 (March, 1967), pp. 27-36.

109 *Ibid.,* p. 29.

110 Downs, "Testing Hearing in Infancy and Early Childhood," *op. cit.,* p. 26.

and thus delay later recognition of an auditory impairment."[111] Ling *et al.* pointed out variables in the testing situation that affect the validity of screening tests of newborn infants and concluded that without more definitive studies of "stimulus, response, and observer variables . . . newborn screening programs will continue to be assumption-ridden, time-consuming, and highly inefficient."[112]

With infants from three to fourteen weeks of age, the Baltimore group use some of the articles and procedures suggested by the Ewings for older infants, plus some items of their own selection. In addition to the clacker used with newborns, these include a doorbell, a tonette, a xylophone, a squeaker, three rattles (low, middle, and high frequency), voiceless consonants *sss* and *kkk*, voice, crumpling tissue paper, and a spoon stirring in a cup. As checked with a sound-level meter, these stimuli all produced sound levels of around 40 dB, with the exception of the squeaker (50 dB), and the bell and clacker (60 dB). These sound levels cannot be translated into *hearing* levels on the basis of the information reported. We can only say that the hearing levels of these sounds would be less than their sound levels.

The testing is performed by two examiners while the infant's mother, seated in a chair, holds the baby in her lap. The room in which the testing is performed should be reasonably quiet. One examiner sits in a low chair or kneels in front of the mother and baby, holding toys, puppets, dolls, and so forth, to attract the visual attention of the infant, while the other examiner introduces auditory stimuli behind the chair in which the mother is seated. The examiner in back holds a noisemaker to either side of the infant, well outside its peripheral vision. The infant should be supported under the arms and held away from the mother's body, so it is free to move its head or its body from side to side. The examiner in front serves as an observer to evaluate the infant's responses to the auditory stimuli produced by the examiner in back. Following a response, he must regain the infant's visual attention.

Infants in the three to fourteen weeks age group may respond by turning the head to seek the source of the sound (the response that is characteristic of older infants); they may exhibit "eye responses" such as turning the eyes, widening the eyes, and making searching movements with the eyes; they may exhibit Moro's reflex with or without an accompanying eye blink, or a body "jump" or general muscular activity; or they may indicate by cessation of muscular activity, cessation of crying, or waking from a dozing or sleeping state, that they are aware of the auditory stimulus. The most common response, especially to the stimuli of greater intensity, is Moro's reflex or a

[111] S. R. Silverman and H. Davis, "Hard-of-Hearing Children," in Hallowell Davis and S. Richard Silverman, eds., *Hearing and Deafness* (New York, Holt, Rinehart and Winston, 1970), p. 428.
[112] Daniel Ling, Agnes H. Ling, and Donald C. Doehring, "Stimulus, Response, and Observer Variables in the Auditory Screening of Newborn Infants," *Journal of Speech and Hearing Research*, Vol. 13 (March, 1970), p. 17.

partial Moro's reflex. A surprising number of infants in this age group respond by head turning or eye responses, however. A "streamlined" version of the test, consisting of the voiceless consonants, the "middle" rattle, and voice, representing high, middle, and low frequency ranges, respectively, can be given in about two minutes. If the infant does not respond, then additional items should be introduced. If the infant still does not respond, he should be scheduled for a retest, and as he matures he should be periodically re-examined.

The same test procedures are followed with infants between fifteen and thirty weeks of age, and between thirty-one and fifty-two weeks of age. In the former group, the predominant responses are turning the head toward the source of the sound, and eye responses. Moro's reflex occurs infrequently except in response to the more intense stimuli. Because infants in the latter age group should all be sufficiently mature to turn the head toward the sound, they are required to respond in this fashion in order to pass the test. Furthermore, the head must be turned at least 45 degrees before the response is accepted.

As was mentioned earlier, the Ewings concentrate their efforts on infants beyond the age of seven months. The physical arrangements for the test are the same as described by the Baltimore group. The Ewings insist on obtaining the head turning response, requiring that the infant look directly at the source of the sound before accepting his response. If the infant merely looks up and appears to be listening, or if he turns his eyes and head toward the sound but does not look directly at the sound source, he is not considered to have passed the test, since infants of seven months should demonstrate the ability to localize sound "automatically." The Ewings stress the importance of using "quiet" sound stimuli for the test. For infants from seven to nine months of age they employ two "high-pitched" sounds (opening a small ball of crumpled tissue paper and "gently" shaking a high-pitched rattle), and two "low-pitched" sounds (metal teaspoon stirred quietly in the bottom of a china cup and low-pitched rattle). The child must localize all these sounds on both left and right sides in order to pass the screening test. According to the Ewings, the spoon and cup item is a sound of special interest to the infants, because it should suggest feeding time. It is interesting to note that the Baltimore group found the tissue crumpling and the spoon and cup sounds to be their least effective test stimuli. Murphy has reported the successful use of pure tones with infants in this age range. He checks the infant's localizing ability first with rattles and then substitutes a "telephone" connected to an oscillator for the rattles. He reports that localizing responses may be obtained at hearing levels as low as 40 dB for the frequencies from 400 to 6000 Hz.[113]

With infants from ten to fifteen months of age, the Ewings depend

[113] K. P. Murphy, "Ascertainment of Deafness in Children," *Audecibel,* Vol. 15 (Summer, 1966), pp. 89-93.

primarily on speech sounds to attract the baby's attention. The examiner calls the infant's name quietly and sings quietly at a distance of 5 to 6 feet, and he (or she) utters the voiceless consonants *sss, ppp, ttt, kkk* "naturally and rhythmically" at 3·feet from either ear. If the infant does not respond to these speech stimuli, then the test items used with younger infants are introduced.

Both the Ewings and the Baltimore group stress that their tests are screening tests—not diagnostic tests or tests designed to yield threshold information. The purpose of the testing is to detect infants whose responses to sound are not typical for their age, so that they may be more carefully tested in the audiology clinic, or observed for signs of neurological or intellectual deficits. The younger the infant, the more gross the screening procedure. Failure of an infant to respond to any but intense stimuli—for example, the clacker—may indicate the presence of a hearing impairment, or it may mean only that the child is not yet sufficiently mature to be interested in less intense sounds. On the other hand, the infant who does respond appropriately to the various "quiet" stimuli employed is demonstrating that he does not have any serious impairment in either ear.

While the techniques of screening infants described here may appear to be simple, the success of these methods depends on the skill of both examiners and their experience in working together. Hardy, Dougherty, and Hardy believe that with some special training, nurses in "a clinic setting," for example, a well-baby clinic, will be able to perform these screening tests adequately with infants from thirty to fifty-two weeks of age. The screening of infants from three to thirty weeks of age, however, requires much more skill in evaluating the subtle responses the infant makes to quiet sounds. About the testing of this younger age group, these investigators say, "It [the test] appears to be a useful diagnostic and research tool but because of the complexity of the responses obtained probably not applicable as a screening device on a general pediatric and public health level."[114] Ling *et al.* go a step further, saying,

Many programs using localization responses, derived from the original work of Ewing, have proved to have high levels of reliability and validity with children from about five months of age. These programs have the advantage of detecting deafness arising postnatally. There appears to be no advantage to the infant from detection of deafness in the first few months. Parents are often quite unable to accept a diagnosis of sensory defect before they have had time to develop a relationship with their child. They are, therefore, likely to frustrate very early efforts at training through hostility both to the baby and to the clinicians who press the immediate use of hearing aids.[115]

The Young Child

Children between the ages of twelve and twenty-four months will probably need to be evaluated on the basis of the tests described for the infant,

114 Hardy *et al., op. cit.*
115 Ling *et al., op. cit.,* p. 16.

although some of the children in this age group will cooperate adequately in at least a portion of the testing situations now to be described. Since the Ewing-type test gives only a general indication of the child's hearing abilities, it is desirable as soon as possible to administer a more formal hearing test in order to determine the child's thresholds with greater accuracy. This means that calibrated audiometric equipment must be employed. If suitable modifications of audiometric procedures are utilized, including in most instances the help of a trained observer or test assistant, the examiner can often obtain valid and reliable threshold measurements on children as young as twenty-four months. Not infrequently, however, more than a single testing period will be required before satisfactory measurements can be achieved. The difficult task is in winning the child's confidence so he will cooperate in the testing situation. For example, the child must be willing to accept earphones before the examiner can obtain threshold information on the ears individually. Many very young children refuse to permit the earphones to be placed on their heads. The examiner should be firm with the child and simply take for granted that the child will wear the earphones. In many cases, such a positive attitude on the part of the examiner is sufficient to convince the child that he has no choice but to accept the earphones. If the child believes he can get his own way by putting up a protest, then of course he will refuse to accept the earphones. The examiner who approaches the young child with obvious trepidation will likely meet the resistance he anticipates, much like the salesman who asks the customer, "You wouldn't like to subscribe to this magazine, would you?" Sometimes it is helpful if the examiner, or someone else in the room, wears earphones for a short time prior to placing them on the child's head.

There will be occasions, however, when no amount of firmness or cajolery will enable the examiner to accomplish his task of getting the child to wear earphones. The examiner must exercise fine judgment in such cases, because to persist in forcing the earphones on the child may destroy completely any chance for establishing rapport with him at that time or in future testing sessions. The examiner, therefore, must know when to compromise. An acceptable compromise for both patient and examiner may be to hold one earphone to the child's ear instead of having him wear the headset. It may be necessary, however, for the examiner to forego completely the use of earphones and be content—at that time—to secure such information as he can through the use of sound-field procedures. Eventually, however, the answer to the question as to whether or not an impairment exists in either ear will require testing with earphones and perhaps also with a bone-conduction vibrator. If the examiner can keep from alienating the child, sooner or later he will succeed in obtaining the measurements he seeks.

In many cases, the examiner is more likely to succeed if the child's mother is not in the test room, but frequently the mother's presence is a help rather than a hindrance. If the examiner has made the decision to invite the mother into the test room and this decision turns out to have been a mistake he probably cannot then ask the mother to leave without upsetting the child and perhaps also the mother. When he schedules the child for a re-examination he will suggest to the mother that he would prefer this time to try working with the child alone.

If the mother is to be present during the examination, it is perhaps best that she sit slightly to the side and behind the child. Care should be taken that no one is sitting between the child and any loudspeakers which are to be used in the hearing evaluation. The child should be given no reason to look toward loudspeakers unless he is aware of a sound originating from them. Usually it is good practice to inform the parent before entering the room that she is not to speak or take part in the procedure unless requested to do so. The aim usually is to keep the mother out of the situation as much as possible but still make use of her presence in the room as a comfort to the child.

A skilled test assistant can be a great help to the examiner in working with a small child. Some of the testing procedure will require the examiner to be outside the test room. The assistant stays in the room with the child and, hopefully, keeps the child interested and happy while the examiner is operating the test equipment in the control room. The assistant serves also to supplement the examiner's observations of the child's reactions to the stimuli presented. Ideally, there should be communication from the examiner to the assistant by means of an amplifying system, so that the assistant can receive instructions through an earphone and be kept informed as to what the examiner is doing and plans to do. The assistant can signal with a nod or shake of the head whether or not a response was observed, and since the examiner will be monitoring the talk-back system, the assistant can speak to the examiner whenever necessary.

The examiner will usually wish to begin the test by observing the child's reactions to speech and various noises introduced by sound-field through the microphone circuit of the speech audiometer. The child's responses to such signals are perhaps facilitated if, before any stimuli are presented, he is allowed to play quietly for a period of five to ten minutes, during which time no one speaks in the room and care is taken to present only toys that do not make any significant amount of noise. In this situation the child is more likely to respond when low-intensity signals are presented through the loudspeaker than if these signals are introduced into an already noisy environment. The examiner may also attempt to observe the child's responses to pure-tone signals presented through a loudspeaker, but a more complex signal, such as speech or noise, is more likely to evoke an observable response.

For whatever group of signals is presented, an ascending intensity technique is usually most appropriate. The examiner should note each stimulus presented and rate the child's responses in some systematic fashion. For instance, a scale ranging from zero to 3 might be used to indicate the examiner's confidence in the child's response to a particular stimulus. A score of zero indicates "no observable response," and a score of 3 indicates "a definite response," such as a startle reaction, or pointing toward the loudspeaker. Scores of 1 and 2 indicate less definite responses. This system of recording results obtained is valuable when the examiner is re-examining a child and trying to recall what results were obtained on previous examinations.

After the examiner has exhausted the possibilities of observing the child's response to stimuli presented through loudspeakers, he may enter the test room and, working with the child directly, attempt to make more precise measurements. We shall now discuss more specifically the modifications of conventional speech and pure-tone audiometric procedures that may be found useful in evaluating a child's hearing.

Modifications of Speech Audiometry. Initially, the examiner is interested in noting the child's reactions to speech stimuli—words, sentences, individual speech sounds, and noises made with the speech mechanism—when these are presented by sound-field through the microphone circuit. The test assistant and the child will usually be seated at a child's table across from each other. The assistant will be showing the child some toys, trying to interest him in a game or puzzle, or otherwise keeping him reasonably quiet and occupied. The examiner can watch the child through the window between the control and test rooms, and the assistant will also be in a good position to evaluate the child's reactions whenever a stimulus is presented. Any indication that the child is aware of the stimulus should be noted and rated as to confidence as suggested above. Responses may consist of interruption of a task, head movements trying to locate the sound, attempts to imitate the stimulus, interruption of vocal play, or eye responses—widening of the eyes, searching movements, or, when an intense sound occurs, an eyeblink. If two loudspeakers are available, the examiner can alternate the signal between them to see if the child appears to be aware of the differing sources of the sound within the test room.

One of the first stimuli the examiner should employ is whispered speech —saying the child's name, for example. Starting with zero hearing level, the examiner gradually increases the intensity of the whispered signal until he or the test assistant notes a response. Whispered speech emphasizes high frequencies. If the child responds to whispering at relatively low hearing levels, the examiner knows that the child's hearing for speech is adequate, or that he is not dealing with a serious impairment of hearing. In such a case the examiner may wish to proceed immediately to the pure-tone evaluation of the child's hearing, or he may decide to observe the child's responses to other stimuli.

If the child does not respond to whispered speech at any hearing level, the examiner may next try saying the child's name aloud, starting at zero hearing level and gradually increasing the intensity until a response is noted, or maximum intensity is reached. Other words than the child's name may, of course, be used. If no response is noted when the intensity is gradually increased, the examiner may elect to attempt to elicit a startle response by suddenly introducing a word at a high hearing level. The examiner should warn the test assistant of his intention, so the assistant does not give a startle response that attracts the child's attention.

In place of words or sentences, the examiner may use individual speech sounds in order to determine, for example, whether there is any difference in the child's responses to voiced and voiceless sounds. Or he may make noises with his vocal mechanism such as tongue clicks or perhaps animal noises. He may also employ various noisemakers—rattles, whistles, a drum, and so forth. He may present pulses of masking noise. Also music may be introduced by using the phonograph or tape circuit of the speech audiometer. Whatever stimulus is used, a useful technique that provides a positive response for the examiner to evaluate is to pair the auditory signal with a rewarding visual stimulus. Reddell and Calvert have described such a procedure in which a hollow plastic toy animal is illuminated by a bulb mounted inside it whenever the examiner presses a button. The toy is mounted to the side of the child, so he has to turn his head to look at it. In preliminary trials the child is taught by the test assistant to look at the animal when an intense sound stimulus is presented. When he looks, the examiner presses the button that illuminates the animal. When the child is conditioned, then the examiner reduces the stimulus intensity to below the child's threshold. He presents the test stimulus, gives the child time to respond, and then presents the stimulus at a 10 dB greater intensity. Each time the child responds appropriately by turning to look at the animal, the examiner reinforces the response activity by illuminating the animal. Reddell and Calvert call their procedure CA-VR for Conditioned Audio-Visual Response Audiometry.[116] Their technique was suggested by one developed in Japan called COR for Conditioned Orientation Reflex.[117] The basic difference between the two techniques is that with COR the examiner is evaluating the child's localizing behavior, since two hollow plastic toys are used—one on each of a pair of speakers. With CA-VR, there is no attempt to assess localizing ability. The technique is designed only to assist the examiner by giving the child an interesting way to respond. CA-VR may be utilized while testing through earphones or with a bone-conduction vibrator as well as in a sound-field.

As soon as the examiner is satisfied that he has obtained all the information he needs from the speech audiometer, or all the information he

116 Rayford C. Reddell and Donald R. Calvert, "Conditioned Audio-Visual Response Audiometry, *The Voice* (Journal of the California Speech and Hearing Association), Vol. 16 (May, 1967), pp. 52-57.

117 Tokuro Suzuki and Yoshio Ogiba, "Conditioned Orientation Reflex Audiometry," *A.M.A. Archives of Otolaryngology*, Vol. 74 (1961), pp. 84-90.

can get, he will proceed to the next stage in the examination, the evaluation of the child's responses to pure tones. Before leaving the control room to begin direct work with the child in the test room, the examiner may check the child's responses to pure tones presented by sound-field. At this point in the examination the examiner is not attempting to get precise threshold measurements but only a general idea of the hearing levels at various frequencies at which some overt response of the child is noted.

With children who are old enough or mature enough to respond to directions, and who have sufficient understanding of language, more refined techniques of speech audiometry may be employed. Special methods of applying speech audiometry for children have been described by Keaster,[118] by Sortini and Flake,[119] and by Siegenthaler, Pearson, and Lezak.[120] These methods require that the child point to an object or picture of an object when directed to do so by the examiner. Before the test, the objects or pictures are shown to the child to make sure that he recognizes them or knows their names. Then the examiner, using the microphone circuit of the speech audiometer, asks the child to hold up an object or to point to a picture. A test assistant may or may not be needed in this situation, depending on the maturity and cooperativeness of the child.

By starting the procedure at a hearing level at which the child can respond and then gradually decreasing the intensity until the child fails to respond, the examiner can ascertain the child's threshold for speech. Initially the presentations would probably be made by sound-field. Monaural speech thresholds can be determined in a similar fashion by having the child use earphones. If some of the objects or pictures have similar names that are easily confused, such as "bus" and "gun," or "knife" and "light," it is possible to gain some information as to whether the child has speech-discrimination problems.

Ross and Lerman have standardized a picture identification test for obtaining discrimination scores with young hearing-impaired children who have limited vocabularies. Their final evaluation of the test was made with 61 children ranging in age from four years, seven months to thirteen years, nine months. Twenty-four of the subjects were enrolled in a school for the deaf. Ross and Lerman call their test WIPI for Word Intelligibility by Picture Identification.[121]

118 Jacqueline Keaster, "A Quantitative Method of Testing the Hearing of Young Children," *Journal of Speech Disorders*, Vol. 12 (June, 1947), pp. 159-160.

119 A. J. Sortini and C. G. Flake, "Speech Audiometry Testing for Preschool Children," *Laryngoscope*, Vol. 63 (October, 1953), pp. 991-997.

120 Bruce M. Siegenthaler, Jack Pearson, and Raymond J. Lezak, "A Speech Reception Threshold Test for Children," *Journal of Speech and Hearing Disorders*, Vol. 19 (September, 1954), pp. 360-366.

121 Mark Ross and Jay Lerman, "A Picture Identification Test for Hearing-Impaired Children," *Journal of Speech and Hearing Research*, Vol. 13 (March, 1970), pp. 44-53. (This test may be obtained from Stanwix House, Inc., 3020 Chartiers Avenue, Pittsburgh, Pennsylvania 15204.)

Children with greater language sophistication can be tested with the speech audiometer in a similar manner to adults. Special lists of spondees and phonetically balanced words have been compiled specifically for children, using a more restricted vocabulary than the adult lists. The Appendix to this book contains word lists suitable for speech audiometric testing of young children.

Modifications of Pure-tone Audiometry. Special techniques are required to achieve pure-tone threshold measurements on very young children, and as has been mentioned previously, it frequently is necessary to spend more than one testing session with a child before satisfactory results can be achieved. If the purpose of the examination is to determine whether or not a significant hearing impairment exists, then the sound-field procedures described above should be sufficient. But if the purpose is to rule out the possibility of even a slight impairment in either ear, then the examiner must aim to obtain monaural thresholds at least by air conduction and probably also by bone conduction.

Very young children have to be trained to respond in some positive manner when they are aware of hearing pure tones. This requires the presence of the examiner in the test room with the child. The examiner sits at a small table opposite the child and operates the audiometer. It is advisable to use a portable audiometer which can be placed at the end of the table or on a chair next to the table, so it does not intrude between the examiner and the child.

Initially, the examiner may place the earphones on the table between him and the child. Turning the frequency selector to 4000 Hz he presents a brief burst of tone that is clearly audible to him, while he observes the child for any reaction. If the child does respond, he lowers the intensity and presents the tone again, continuing in this way until the child no longer gives evidence that he is aware of the tone. If the child does not respond to the initial presentation of the 4000 Hz tone, the examiner increases the intensity and presents it again, continuing until the child responds or until the maximum output of the audiometer is reached. If the child responds to any of these presentations, the examiner knows the approximate level of his binaural hearing. Since the earphones are placed between the child and the examiner, the sound pressure at the child's ears should be about the same as it is at the examiner's ears. The tone selected for this initial screening is 4000 Hz, because if the child responds at this frequency the chances are good that he does not have a significant hearing impairment. As we shall see in the next chapter, a screening test for use in schools has been devised on the principle that any significant hearing impairment will have a 4000 Hz component. If the child does not give any evidence of hearing the 4000 Hz tone at any level, it may or may not be indicative of a hearing loss. The initial screening procedure is meaningful only if the child does respond.

Next, the child must be trained to make a positive, unequivocal response when he hears a tone. Usually the response that is easiest for the young child to make is to place a block in a box, a smaller cup in a larger cup, a smaller wooden circle on a larger wooden circle in building a "Christmas tree" toy, or some similar definite motor act. The examiner's problem is to teach the child to wait for a tone to be heard before performing the required motor act. The child will usually want to complete the "game" without waiting for an auditory event to occur at each step.

A convenient and clinically useful method of teaching him to wait for an auditory event before responding is to condition him with tactile sensations from a bone-conductor vibrator that he holds in his hand. The examiner sets the audiometer frequency selector at 500 Hz and the hearing-level control at maximum for bone conduction. Then, supposing that he is using a nest of plastic cups for the objects the child is to manipulate, he hands the first cup to the child. He presents a brief signal from the audiometer that the child feels through the vibrator and then guides the child to a response, helping the child to place the cup on the table. The examiner hands the child the next cup, holds the child's hand so he will not immediately put this cup in the first one, and then presents another signal through the vibrator and guides the child to making his "response." After three or four such guided responses, the examiner tries handing a cup to the child and seeing if the child will voluntarily wait until he feels the tactile signal before responding. If necessary, the examiner will continue guiding the child's hand until the child has learned to perform the task correctly himself. When the child does respond appropriately, the examiner compliments him by gesture, expression, and words of praise, so the correct response is reinforced by reward in the form of approval from the examiner. There are distinct advantages in using a non-auditory stimulus for this training procedure, particularly when the examiner has no idea of the child's hearing levels. Otherwise, the examiner might be attempting to develop a response to a tone of a frequency outside the child's hearing range, or, if earphones are in place, in a "dead" ear. In addition, with a non-auditory stimulus, the examiner has the opportunity to correct the child's mistakes before audition is tested as well as to see whether or not the child possesses the maturity and inclination to respond to this type of testing technique. A similar tactile conditioning procedure with a bone-conduction vibrator was described by Thorne.[122]

When the child has learned to respond appropriately to tactile stimuli, the examiner places earphones on the child and indicates to the child by word and gesture that he is to listen through the earphones for a signal and then repeat the activity of building the nest of cups that he has just successfully accomplished. If necessary, the examiner will guide the child

[122] Bert Thorne, "Conditioning Children for Pure-tone Testing," *Journal of Speech and Hearing Disorders,* Vol. 27 (February, 1962), pp. 84-85.

to making responses when tones are presented, until the child is able to handle the task by himself. Care must be taken to alter the intervals between tonal presentations so the child does not learn to respond to a rhythm pattern. The first tone to present in the test is usually 500 Hz, since even deaf children will probably have some sensitivity at this frequency. The hearing level at which this tone is presented will depend on the information regarding the child's hearing the examiner has already obtained through the sound-field procedures described earlier. Or if no information has been obtained, the examiner will have to experiment with levels, seeking a level that is high enough for the child to obtain a sensation of hearing, but not so high that he will be startled or perhaps frightened. Once the child has responded appropriately, the examiner will decrease intensity in successive presentations, seeking the minimum hearing level at which the child responds.

When threshold in each ear has been established by this procedure at 500 Hz, the frequency is changed to 2000 Hz and threshold in each ear is determined in similar fashion. Then threshold measurements are made at 1000 Hz, and if time permits and the child's cooperation continues at a satisfactory level, other frequencies can be tested as the examiner considers desirable. The reason for testing at 2000 Hz after obtaining thresholds at 500 Hz is to get information on the highest of the speech frequencies while the child is still cooperating. In case the test must be discontinued before responses to all the speech frequencies have been obtained, the examiner will have a better notion of the child's hearing abilities for speech from the frequencies of 500 and 2000 Hz than from 500 and 1000 Hz.

If the air-conduction testing reveals some hearing loss, the examiner will wish to obtain information on the child's hearing by bone conduction. The same procedures can be followed for bone-conduction testing. It must be remembered that, regardless of the vibrator placement, it is the response of the better ear by bone conduction that is being assessed. With a very young child it is obviously not possible in most cases to utilize masking procedures. The examiner must be prepared to switch tasks for the child to perform whenever there is an indication that the child's interest is waning. As was mentioned previously, the test of a very young child may frequently require several sessions, particularly if there is a problem in gaining his cooperation or getting him to accept the earphones. If the child can be taught to respond to auditory stimuli by performing a positive motor act when he hears and holding off performing the act until he does hear, the examiner can use the same technique to obtain speech detection thresholds with the speech audiometer. These speech detection thresholds can be compared with pure-tone thresholds as a check on test reliability. It is even possible to use this type of response to observe improvement of the speech detection threshold with a hearing aid.

Adaptations of pure-tone testing technique may be required also with somewhat older children. Since pure tones are not inherently interesting to children, their attention may have to be maintained by means of procedures that make the testing situation a game. Various play-audiometry procedures and "gadgets" to make the testing situation enjoyable have been described in the literature.[123] The important thing to remember in testing children, however, is that no ingenious procedure or fascinating gadget will substitute for a skillful examiner who "has a way" with children. And the more skillful the examiner is, the less he will have to depend on complicated special instrumentation to accomplish his testing goals.

In summary, here are some guiding principles that the examiner of young children should keep in mind.

1. Obtain first information which is easiest to obtain. Getting the child to accept earphones may be a major hurdle. The following observations in a sound-field can be made before earphones are introduced and may be sufficient to establish a tentative diagnosis:

    a. gross response to complex stimuli.

    b. gross response to pure tones.

    c. thresholds for pure tones.

    d. threshold of speech detection.

    e. estimates of speech discrimination.

2. Obtain first that information which is most meaningful. It is short-sighted to spend time trying to obtain thresholds at 8000 Hz, for example, when it may be much more important to sample the child's bone-conduction hearing.

3. Perform tests as rapidly as possible without sacrificing accuracy. A child of two and a half years of age cannot be expected to yield accurate responses to pure tones for long periods. An experienced examiner, using 10-dB steps on the audiometer, can obtain approximations of threshold at 500, 1000, and 2000 Hz in each ear by both air and bone conduction in ten to fifteen minutes, once the child has been trained to respond consistently to auditory stimuli. A more accurate audiogram can be obtained in later testing sessions.

4. Avoid asking the child to perform motor acts that are difficult for him. For example, do not insist he place a block on a peg if this is frustrating for him. Switch to a simpler type of response, such as dropping the block on the floor when he hears the tone. Also do not inject irrelevant mental tasks into the testing situation, such as sorting sizes, colors, and so forth.

---

[123] M. R. Dix and C. S. Hallpike, "The Peep Show: A New Technique for Pure Tone Audiometry in Young Children," *British Medical Journal*, Vol. 2 (1947), pp. 719-723.

F. R. Guilford and C. O. Haug, "Diagnosis of Deafness in the Very Young Child," *A.M.A. Archives of Otolaryngology*, Vol. 55 (February, 1952), pp. 101-106.

Edgar L. Lowell, Georgina Rushford, Gloria Holversten, and Marguerite Stoner, "Evaluation of Pure Tone Audiometry with Preschool Age Children," *Journal of Speech and Hearing Disorders*, Vol. 21 (September, 1956), pp. 292-302.

David S. Green, "The Pup-Show: A Simple, Inexpensive Modification of the Peep-Show," *Journal of Speech and Hearing Disorders*, Vol. 23 (February, 1958), pp. 118-120.

John J. O'Neill, Herbert J. Oyer, and James W. Hillis, "Audiometric Procedures Used with Children," *Journal of Speech and Hearing Disorders*, Vol. 26 (February, 1961), pp. 61-66.

5. Always obtain complete history information including a description from the parent of the child's speech and hearing abilities. Such information may help to validate your hearing measurements, or perhaps may shed a completely different light on your estimations of the problem.

6. Whenever possible, make your own observations of the child's "speech" and vocal characteristics. With some children who are unresponsive to you, observations of the child and mother alone in the test room might be made through the window while you monitor the talk-back system.

7. Be on the lookout for indications of other communicative problems, such as mental retardation, emotional disturbances, central auditory problems, and so forth. Remember, these may exist in combination and with or without peripheral hearing impairment.

Neurophysiological Methods

It would be most convenient if it were possible to secure an adequate measure of a child's hearing levels by some means not dependent upon the child's cooperation and voluntary reponses. In recent years, there have been attempts to devise tests that would depend upon neurophysiological clues rather than upon voluntary responses from the patient. The two most popular methods are (1) *electroencephalography* (EEG), or as it is sometimes called when applied to hearing measurements, *electroencephalic audiometry* (EEA), and (2) *psychogalvanometry*—galvanic skin response (GSR), or *electrodermal audiometry* (EDA). Hogan provides an excellent account of attempts to utilize various autonomic responses as indices of auditory sensitivity.[124] In addition to GSR, he discusses cardiac, vascular, respiratory, and visual responses to auditory stimulation. EEG and GSR and other types of autonomic responses when used with auditory stimulation represent attempts to develop "objective" tests of hearing. The term *objective* implies a procedure that is scientifically precise and independent of errors of human judgment. Unfortunately, there has not yet been devised any method of measuring the hearing function that can be considered objective as we have just defined the word. And also unfortunately, the use of EEG and GSR testing methods with young children have not proved universally successful, and suitable techniques for utilizing other physiological indices of hearing with young children have not yet been evolved, although one method— Cardiac Evoked Response Audiometry (CERA)—shows promise on the basis of some preliminary experimental work at Columbia-Presbyterian Medical Center and the New York Foundling Hospital.[125]

[124] Donald D. Hogan, "Autonomic Responses as Supplementary Hearing Measures," in Robert T. Fulton and Lyle L. Lloyd, eds., *Audiometry for the Retarded* (Baltimore, Williams & Wilkins, 1969), pp. 238-262.
[125] "Cardiac Evoked Response Audiometry," Canberra Industries, Biomedical Systems Division, Meriden, Connecticut (undated).

The electroencephalograph measures the brain-wave activity of the subject. Neurologists and psychiatrists utilize the EEG for evidence of brain pathology or malfunctioning that would be represented by deviations from waves obtained with normal brains. It has been observed that brain-wave activity is subject to variability in the presence of external stimuli. In electroencephalography, the patient is kept as quiet and relaxed as possible, or even in a light sleep, which may require the use of some sedation. Even in this situation, the brain-wave pattern will show changes when sound stimuli are introduced at levels above the patient's threshold. Thus, attempts have been made to utilize reponses evoked in brain-wave activity as indicators of hearing sensitivity. Marcus was one of the first to report on the use of EEG in obtaining gross measures of hearing sensitivity in children.[126] Since he encountered technical difficulties in the use of an audiometer with the EEG equipment, his auditory stimuli were various noises. About half the children gave "appropriate" EEG responses to auditory stimulation but because of the lack of control over the intensity of the stimuli no information concerning threshold was obtained. Interpretation of the EEG record was on a subjective basis.

Later experimenters were able to utilize an audiometer as the source of auditory signals and could compare thresholds obtained through EEG methodology with those obtained with conventional audiometric procedures. Derbyshire and his colleagues established criteria for judging responses to auditory stimulation from reading the EEG record that contributed greatly to the objectification of the procedure.[127] Withrow and Goldstein described a procedure for obtaining simultaneous EEG and GSR tracings on subjects and combining the results of these two procedures in determining auditory thresholds.[128] They, too, employed special controls for objectifying the presentation of stimuli and interpreting the record. They reported that using the combined electrophysiological techniques they were successful in predicting thresholds within ± 10 dB of those obtained with conventional audiometry. Most investigators report that with EEG alone they can predict thresholds only within about ± 20 dB.

There are many difficulties at present in utilizing EEG for auditory measurements, particularly with children. One problem is the length of time required for an examination—about one and a half to two hours. Another problem is the establishment of the optimum degree of wakefulness on the part

[126] R. E. Marcus, "Hearing and Speech Problems in Children: Observations and Use of Electroencephalography," *A.M.A. Archives of Otolaryngology*, Vol. 53 (February, 1951), pp. 134-146.

[127] A. J. Derbyshire and J. C. Farley, "Sampling Auditory Responses at the Cortical Level—A Routine for EER Audiometric Testing," *Annals of Otology, Rhinology, and Laryngology*, Vol. 68 (September, 1959), pp. 675-697.

[128] F. B. Withrow, Jr. and R. Goldstein, "An Electrophysiological Procedure for Determination of Auditory Threshold in Children," *Laryngoscope*, Vol. 68 (September, 1958), pp. 1674-1699.

of the subject, and controlling the activity of the subject who is awake. The more active the subject, the more difficult it is to discriminate evoked responses from random brain-wave activity. The development of averaging or summing computers has greatly eased the problem of differentiating EEG responses to auditory stimuli from random brain-wave activity. The computer averages or algebraically sums the random activity so that it becomes essentially zero. The "unusual" brain-wave activity that is associated in time with the introduction of the auditory stimulus thus stands out in contrast to the relatively flat tracing that is the result of the averaging. Since the reports by Lowell *et al.* of the use of a special purpose analog computer with EEG auditory evaluations,[129] the literature has reflected the tremendous interest of laboratory and clinical investigators in Evoked Response Audiometry (ERA), or as Davis and Goldstein prefer to call it, Electric Response Audiometry, resulting in the same initials.[130] ERA refers to the use of EEG with an averaging or summing computer. It makes possible the evaluation of small changes in electrical activity of the brain that are present in the waking state and "except for children less than eighteen months of age and a few older ones who are unruly, electric response audiometry does not require putting the child to sleep," thus simplifying and shortening the procedure.[131]

McCandless and Best demonstrated that reliable summed evoked responses could be obtained with adults within 10 dB of voluntary threshold for clicks, and that evoked responses from children ranging in age from a few weeks to five years could be obtained at hearing levels of 30 dB.[132] Price *et al.* reported that the mean difference between the averaged evoked response and the voluntary threshold for eight adults was less than 5 dB.[133] The use of ERA in clinical evaluations of hearing in both children and adults was reported by McCandless. Children over age two could be tested satisfactorily with the technique, but younger children's test results were much more difficult to interpret.[134] McCandless sounds a note of caution regarding the interpretation of ERA data:

[129] Edgar L. Lowell, Carol I. Troffer, Edward A. Warburton, and Georgina M. Rushford, "Temporal Evannation: a New Approach in Diagnostic Audiology," *Journal of Speech and Hearing Disorders,* Vol. 25 (November, 1960), pp. 340-345.

Edgar L. Lowell, Carol Troffer Williams, Robert M. Ballinger, and Delphi Alvig, "Measurement of Auditory Threshold with a Special Purpose Analog Computer," *Journal of Speech and Hearing Research,* Vol. 4 (June, 1961), pp. 105-112.

[130] H. Davis and R. Goldstein, "Audiometry: Other Auditory Tests," in Hallowell Davis and S. Richard Silverman, eds., *Hearing and Deafness* (New York, Holt, Rinehart and Winston, 1970), p. 244.

[131] *Ibid.*

[132] Geary A. McCandless and LaVar Best, "Evoked Responses to Auditory Stimuli in Man Using a Summing Computer," *Journal of Speech and Hearing Research,* Vol. 7 (June, 1964), pp. 193-202.

[133] Lloyd L. Price, Benjamin Rosenblut, Robert Goldstein, and David C. Shepherd, "The Averaged Evoked Response to Auditory Stimulation," *Journal of Speech and Hearing Research,* Vol. 9 (September, 1966), pp. 361-370.

[134] Geary A. McCandless, "Clinical Application of Evoked Response Audiometry," *Journal of Speech and Hearing Research,* Vol. 10 (September, 1967), pp. 468-478.

It is safe to assume that appearance of an evoked potential indicates a sound has alerted the patient's cortex, but in no way does it imply that the patient can use auditory information meaningfully. The absence of a response, on the other hand, may not mean the child cannot hear, since some children with brain damage respond overtly to sound but give inconsistent and sometimes absent evoked responses. The interpretation of evoked response audiometry, therefore, must be undertaken with extreme caution.[135]

Davis *et al.* tested all the pupils at Central Institute for the Deaf whose thresholds for the speech frequencies were within the limits of the audiometer. Their conclusion was that ERA was feasible for school-age children. While the youngest age group (age four to ten) were more difficult to test, "adequate" ERA results were obtained with every child without the need for drugs, and excellent agreement was obtained between ERA and behavioral test results.[136]

Price reviewed the experimental and clinical work leading to the present state of ERA and cautioned against either placing too much reliance on the technique, or being too quick to discard it because of its limitations.[137] Later, in a journal article, Price again urged clinicians to proceed cautiously with the new technique and pointed to the need for further research to improve what already had been demonstrated to be a "clinically useful" tool. He made the point, however, that "evoked response audiometry at present is neither 'the answer' nor 'objective audiometry.' "[138]

Certainly ERA represents a "giant step" forward in the technique of evaluating hearing by EEG. Because of the expensive equipment required, its use will probably be confined to those clinics in medical centers, and certainly only clinicians who have received special training in EEG methodology and are fully aware of the limitations of the technique should attempt its use.

In the early years of conditioned GSR audiometry it appeared that this procedure would be feasible to employ with very young children and infants. It is a simpler method than EEG audiometry from the standpoint of instrumentation and test administration, but it, too, has drawbacks that severely limit its usefulness in the average audiology clinic. As we saw earlier in this chapter when we considered conditioned GSR audiometry in the context of functional hearing loss, the test results are adversely affected by muscular activity. Also we saw that there is an optimum degree of alertness required

---

135 *Ibid.,* p. 477.

136 Hallowell Davis, Shirley K. Hirsh, Joyce Shelnutt, and Clyde Bowers, "Further Validation of Evoked Response Audiometry," *Journal of Speech and Hearing Research,* Vol. 10 (December, 1967), pp. 717-732.

137 Lloyd L. Price, "Cortical-Evoked Response Audiometry," in Robert T. Fulton and Lyle L. Lloyd, eds., *Audiometry for the Retarded* (Baltimore, Williams & Wilkins, 1969), pp. 210-237.

138 Lloyd L. Price, "Evoked Response Audiometry: Some Considerations," *Journal of Speech and Hearing Disorders,* Vol. 34 (May, 1969), pp. 137-141.

from the patient before satisfactory responses can be elicited to auditory stimuli, especially those that are close to threshold. Children are usually so active that it is extremely difficult to differentiate responses to sound stimuli from random changes in skin resistance that occur as a result of the activity. There have been some attempts to quiet the physical activity of children with mild sedation, but unfortunately the sedation reduces the alertness of the child so that it is difficult to obtain adequate responses to the test stimuli. Another problem in using the GSR procedure with children is that the unconditioned stimulus, the electrical shock, has to be unpleasant before effective conditioning can be achieved. Many children react negatively to shock, or for that matter, to any unpleasant stimulus. We have seen that for an examiner to succeed in testing children he has to obtain the cooperation of his patients. The use of shock generally results in difficulty in maintaining the child's cooperation. Not infrequently the child in the GSR testing situation will cry. Crying causes such fluctuations in the GSR tracing that it is almost impossible to identify any changes associated with responses to tonal stimuli.

For GSR audiometry to result in valid and reliable measures of threshold, the method of administering the test and interpreting the record must be rigidly controlled. It is significant that the studies of the validity and reliability of conditioned GSR audiometry have been, almost without exception, performed with adult subjects. Techniques of GSR audiometry must be modified to some extent for young children, but it is still necessary to apply the "control" principles outlined for adults, such as adequate response criteria, use of control events, and so forth. The difficulties encountered in GSR testing of children are so great that many examiners prefer to rely on other techniques for assessing a child's hearing abilities. When it is used in the clinic, conditioned GSR audiometry should be interpreted with great caution, and it should be used as an adjunct to—not in place of—other methods of assessment.

Differentiating Deafness from Other Auditory Disorders

The audiologist is frequently confronted with the problem of making a differential diagnosis for children who apparently are not hearing but who may actually prove to have a normal peripheral hearing mechanism. There are other conditions that produce the behavioral symptom of apparent deafness. Myklebust has described the problem of differentiating the other disorders from genuine deafness and has suggested some techniques and procedures for making the differential diagnosis.[139] The child who is brain-injured, or aphasic, will frequently fail to attend to sound, so that he may be suspected of being deaf or hard-of-hearing. Other conditions that are confused with deafness are severe mental retardation, and psychological

[139] Helmer R. Myklebust, *Auditory Disorders in Children* (New York, Grune and Stratton, 1964).

disturbances, which may vary from emotional maladjustment resulting in a psychogenic hearing loss to a full-blown psychosis. Every person concerned with diagnosing language difficulties in children should be aware of the differentiating characteristics of the various disorders. A diagnosis of deafness in a particular child must be approached with caution, since the fact that a patient does not respond to sound in a testing situation is not incontrovertible evidence of an impairment of his hearing mechanism. The importance of a valid diagnosis is self-evident. A child who is mentally retarded and who has normal hearing does not belong in a school for the deaf. Likewise, a child who is severely emotionally disturbed requires entirely different handling from the child whose primary difficulty is an inability to hear normally. Differential diagnosis of auditory disorders is a subject in itself and is outside the scope of this book.

REFERENCES

Dale, D. M. C., *Applied Audiology for Children* (Springfield, Ill., Charles C Thomas, 1962).

Davis, Hallowell, and Silverman, S. Richard, eds., *Hearing and Deafness* (New York, Holt, Rinehart and Winston, 1970), Chap. 8.

Fulton, Robert T., and Lloyd, Lyle L., eds., *Audiometry for the Retarded* (Baltimore, Williams & Wilkins, 1969), Chaps. 3, 4, 6, 7, and 8.

Glorig, Aram, ed., *Audiometry: Principles and Practices* (Baltimore, Williams & Wilkins, 1965), Chaps. 9, 10, and 12.

Graham, A. Bruce, ed., *Sensorineural Hearing Processes and Disorders* (Boston, Little, Brown and Company, 1967), Chaps. 17, 18, 19, 20, 23, 24, and 27.

Jerger, James, ed., *Modern Developments in Audiology* (New York, Academic Press, 1963), Chaps. 3, 4, 5, and 9.

McConnell, Freeman, and Ward, Paul H., eds., *Deafness in Childhood* (Nashville, Vanderbilt University Press, 1967), Chaps. 2 and 5.

Miller, Maurice H., and Polisar, Ira A., *Audiological Evaluation of the Pediatric Patient* (Springfield, Ill., Charles C Thomas, 1964).

O'Neill, John J., and Oyer, Herbert J., *Applied Audiometry* (New York, Dodd, Mead & Co., 1966) ,Chaps. 7, 8, 9, 10, and 12.

Rose, Darrell E., ed., *Audiological Assessment* (Englewood Cliffs, N.J., Prentice-Hall, 1971). Chaps. 8, 10, and 12.

8

PUBLIC SCHOOL

HEARING CONSERVATION PROGRAMS

For many years the public schools have assumed responsibility for discovering cases of hearing impairment in school children. Hearing-conservation programs are now as much a part of school health examinations as measurements of height and weight and tests of visual acuity. In California, the legislature has made it mandatory for all school districts to test the hearing of all their pupils, although it was not specified how frequently the hearing of each pupil should be tested. Ideally, every pupil should be tested every year, but few districts can afford the personnel and equipment required to conduct annual examinations of all pupils. Some school systems plan to test each child every three years, scheduling tests each year, for example, for the first, fourth, seventh, and tenth grades. In addition, provision is made for testing children from any grade referred by teachers, school psychologists, or school speech specialists. Children transferring into the district would be tested at the time of their transfer.

Larger school districts operate their own hearing-conservation programs. Smaller schools may contract for hearing-testing services through the county superintendent's office. Some hearing-conservation programs have audiometrists whose sole responsibility it is to conduct hearing tests throughout the year. Other programs make use of school nurses, who of course have other responsibilities than the testing of hearing. Some larger school districts employ an audiologist, whose responsibility it is to supervise the hearing-conservation program, including the medical and educational follow-up of all children discovered to have impaired hearing.

The purposes of a school hearing-conservation program are to reduce to the absolute minimum the number of children with permanently impaired hearing, and to provide for the special educational needs of children whose hearing cannot be restored to normal limits through medical or surgical treatment. Since discovery of children with hearing losses is prerequisite to providing for their needs, the testing program is at the heart of hearing conservation. The success of a hearing-conservation program can be measured by the statistics developed in yearly testing. It is usually true that, in the first two or three years of a hearing-conservation program, testing may lead to the classification of as many as 10 per cent of a school population as having "medically significant" hearing losses, whereas, after the program has been in effect for a few years, this number may be reduced to a level of 3 to 5 per cent. In any school system, the greatest number of medically significant hearing losses will be discovered in the primary grades for the simple reason that very young children have a higher incidence of upper respiratory infections and of tonsil and adenoid problems. Because these conditions usually respond to proper medical treatment, it is important that they be discovered as soon as they become evident. In its early years, therefore, a hearing-conservation program should concentrate on the primary grades. The discovery and treatment of conditions producing hearing loss in the primary grades will have the result of reducing the number of hearing losses in the higher elementary grades and in junior and senior high school.

It is useless to discover cases of hearing impairment unless something is done to improve the situation for the children who have hearing problems. Therefore the medical and educational follow-up aspects of the hearing-conservation program are extremely important. This chapter will be concerned primarily with the various methods of discovering hearing impairments in school populations, but also, to some extent, with the requirements of medical and educational follow-up aspects of the hearing-conservation program.

TESTING ENVIRONMENT

It is often a problem to find a satisfactory room in which to give school audiometric examinations. In the past it has not been thought necessary to perform school tests in specially constructed rooms. Instead, it was felt that any room that was reasonably quiet would do. As a matter of fact, the screening level for individual sweep tests was traditionally set at 15 or 20 dB (re ASA–1951 calibration standards) because of the masking effect of room and outside noise in even "quiet" rooms. In 1960 a national conference on the subject of "identification audiometry" was held in Baltimore. The major findings of this conference have been reported in monograph form.[1] One of the strong recommendations that evolved from this conference was

[1] Frederic L. Darley, ed., "Identification Audiometry," *Journal of Speech and Hearing Disorders*, Monograph Supplement Number 9 (September, 1961).

that school testing must be performed in an adequate environment, so that a more stringent criterion for passing the screening test can be employed.

A good acoustic environment is necessary. It can safely be said that millions of dollars and thousands of man hours are now being spent on worthless programs simply because space has been utilized because of its convenience rather than because of its suitability for the purpose. If an examiner is screening at 15 dB above audiometric zero while the environment induces 20 dB of masking, spuriously large numbers of subjects will be identified as having hearing problems and will be referred on to successive stages of the program. Initial expenditure of money for a suitable testing environment results in substantial savings of money spent for the referral of children erroneously thought to have hearing impairment.[2]

Hopefully, school boards and school architects will plan for the inclusion of properly sound-isolated space for hearing testing in the construction of new school buildings. Since it is not economically feasible to remodel existing buildings to provide proper testing space, school authorities should consider the purchase of prefabricated booths that can be set up in existing space. Even though these booths are specially constructed to attenuate outside noise, care must be exercised to locate them in a quiet part of the building.

Assuming that specially constructed test rooms are not available, the school tests will have to be performed in the quietest space that can be found. Frequently the school nurse's office will be the most adequate space available. Regardless of which room is selected for the hearing tests, it is important that the ambient noise in and around the room be kept to a minimum. Since hearing testing involves only a few children of the total school population at a time, the rest are going about their regular activities. If there is much activity in the halls, or recess is in progress, the noise conditions in the testing room may become intolerable. Most principals will cooperate with the audiometrist by selecting a room for the testing which is on the opposite side of the building from the playground, and by restricting traffic in the hallway outside the testing room. Also, it is helpful if, during the days of testing, the bell system in the school is not operated. Rooms that are near lavatories should be avoided, if possible, since the noise of the plumbing may interfere with the testing. Since most schools do not have rooms to spare these days, finding a suitable place for conducting hearing tests may be a major undertaking.

Some school districts have solved the space problem by providing mobile testing units. These are buses or trailers, which are specially sound-treated and fitted out for the sole purpose of providing a suitable environment for hearing testing. Although some small mobile units are designed specifically for individual testing, most mobile units are equipped for group testing. Of course individual testing may also be done in these units. Since the size of the unit has practical limitations, the testing method must be restricted to groups of twenty or sometimes thirty children. The advantages of mobile units are

2 *Ibid.*, p. 27.

self-evident. Most important, they provide uniform testing conditions at every school. They can be driven to the quiet side of any school and be plugged in to the nearest electric outlet. When group equipment is decided upon, it can be permanently installed. An advantage not to be overlooked is that the fully equipped mobile unit is unquestionably a laboratory on wheels in which scientific work is accomplished, and impressionable children may be more inclined to cooperate with the audiometrist in such a setting than in the more familiar surroundings of a classroom.

GROUP TESTS VERSUS INDIVIDUAL TESTS

The first school hearing surveys were conducted in 1927 with a group test devised by Dr. Harvey Fletcher of the Bell Telephone Laboratories and produced commercially by the Western Electric Company.[3] This test, designated the Western Electric 4A test, consisted of a phonograph record of spoken numbers which "faded" from 30 to −3 dB. This test, popularly known as the "fading-numbers" or "group phonograph speech" test, was used extensively for over twenty years. It was succeeded by group forms of pure-tone tests. The primary advantage of a group test is that many more pupils can be tested in a hearing survey by a single audiometrist. Also, the administration of a group test sometimes is simplified so that an audiometrist with a minimum of training can successfully operate it. The disadvantage of a group test is that it may sacrifice accuracy of testing in order to cover a wider population. The primary purpose of any hearing test is to identify individuals with hearing impairments. If a group test does not perform this function satisfactorily, it is a poor instrument.

The advantage of an individual test is that it is the most accurate means known of assessing the hearing of each individual in a school population. The disadvantage of the individual test is that it is time-consuming, in comparison with the group test, and it requires an audiometrist who has skill in conducting individual tests of children. At the present time practically all school testing is performed on an individual basis. New group procedures are still being developed, however, and since the pendulum may swing again in the direction of group testing, the next section will include descriptions of the various group tests of the past and the present.

TYPES OF GROUP TESTS

The Fading-Numbers Test

The latest forms of this test consist of a phonograph recording of a woman saying paired one-digit numbers, such as five-three, four-two, one-seven, and

[3] Aram Glorig and Marion Downs, "Introduction to Audiometry," in Aram Glorig, ed., *Audiometry: Principles and Practices* (Baltimore, Williams & Wilkins, 1965), p. 11.

so forth. As many as forty individuals can be tested simultaneously, with each testee wearing a single earphone. The standard administration of the test calls for the testee to write the correct responses on a specially prepared test blank, such as that shown in Figure 8-1. The record is made so that the numbers

Santa Clara County Superintendent of Schools
Department of Pupil Personnel Services
GROUP SPEECH AUDIOMETER SCORE CARD

Name...Age...........Sex.............Date...........

Teacher...School...Grade...........

Hearing Loss (Decibels)	Left Ear				Right Ear				Hearing Loss (Decibels)
	1	2	3	4	5	6	7	8	
30									30
27									27
24									24
21									21
18									18
15									15
12									12
9									9
6									6
3									3
0									0
-3									-3

Hearing Score, Left Ear (Decibels):   Hearing Score, Right Ear (Decibels):

Figure 8-1.   Fading-numbers group test scoring sheet.

spoken at the top of each column are at a level of 30 dB above the normal threshold for one-digit numbers. As the test proceeds from the top to the bottom of a column, each number has been recorded at a level of 3 dB lower intensity than the preceding number, so that the last number in each series is at a level of −3 dB in relation to the normal threshold. There are four columns in which the complete series of 30 to −3 dB is run for each ear. The papers are scored by the tester, with a key to check the responses on each paper. Generally, it is required that a child pass this test at a level of 9 dB in at least one of the four columns before he is judged to have normal hearing in that ear. If he fails the test at the 9-dB level in either ear, he is required to repeat the group test with another group, with a different earphone to guard against the possibility that his first failure was due to a fault in the testing instrument.

In some school systems, all those who failed the group test were referred directly for a medical examination. In other places, it was standard practice to refer all who failed the second group test for an individual pure-tone hearing test. Medical referrals were then made on the basis of the pure-tone test results.

The fading-numbers test is easy to administer and score, which is the main reason why it remained in existence so long. Several studies demonstrated, however, that it is not an accurate means of assessing children's hearing. Since numbers serve as the test stimuli, it is possible for a subject who has good hearing at only the lower speech frequencies to guess which number is being said, even though he may not hear many consonants of speech. Thus, it has been demonstrated that children with losses as high as 30 to 50 dB at 1000 and 2000 Hz have been able to pass the fading-numbers test at the 9-dB level. Those who favor the fading-numbers test even today state that they are interested not in what a child's pure-tone loss may be but in how his hearing functions so far as speech is concerned. The criticism of this argument is that digits are not representative of running speech, and a child who passes the fading-numbers test may not be able to function adequately in a situation requiring his hearing and understanding running speech.

The Massachusetts Test

Dr. Philip Johnston of the Massachusetts State Department of Health devised a method of administering a pure-tone test on a group basis. It is referred to as the Massachusetts test.[4] With this method, it is possible to screen as many as forty children simultaneously, as with the fading-numbers test. In the Massachusetts test, three frequencies are utilized. Originally they were 500, 4000, and 8000 Hz. The three frequencies are presented at hearing levels of 20, 25, and 30 dB, respectively (re ASA–1951 calibration standards). The subjects are instructed to listen on signal from the audiometrist, and to circle a "yes" or "no" on the test paper, depending on whether they heard a burst of tone at the time they were to listen. Six trials are presented for each frequency, with the same hearing level on each trial. Following a prearranged plan, the audiometrist will occasionally not present a tone when the subjects are expecting one. Thus some "no" responses should appear on every paper. The papers are scored by counting the number of "no" responses. If the number of "no" responses at any frequency differs by more than two from the way in which the test was presented, the subject fails and must take another group test, with a different earphone. The test blank of the Massachusetts method is shown in Figure 8-2.

The Massachusetts test uses a pure-tone audiometer as the sound source and phones which must be matched in their frequency response at the three test frequencies. Because of the difficulty in matching phones at 8000 Hz,

4 Philip W. Johnston, "The Massachusetts Hearing Test," *Journal of the Acoustical Society of America*, Vol. 20 (September, 1948), pp. 697-703.

later instructions for the Massachusetts test have specified that the highest frequency tested should be 6000 Hz, as on the test blank shown in Figure 8-2.

Group Pure-Tone Hearing Test Record

Name_____ School_____ Grade_____
      Last   First

Date_____ Age_____ Teacher_____

I. Right Ear			Example			II. Left Ear		
500 Hz						**500 Hz**		
1	yes	no	1	yes	no	1	yes	no
2	yes	no	2	yes	no	2	yes	no
3	yes	no	3	yes	no	3	yes	no
4	yes	no	4	yes	no	4	yes	no
5	yes	no	5	yes	no	5	yes	no
6	yes	no	6	yes	no	6	yes	no
4000 Hz						**4000 Hz**		
1	**yes**	no				1	yes	no
2	yes	no				2	yes	no
3	yes	no				3	yes	no
4	yes	no				4	yes	no
5	yes	no				5	yes	no
6	**yes**	no				6	yes	no
6000 Hz						**6000 Hz**		
1	yes	no				1	yes	no
2	yes	no				2	yes	no
3	yes	no				3	yes	no
4	yes	no				4	yes	no
5	yes	no				5	yes	no
6	yes	no				6	yes	no

Figure 8-2.   The Massachusetts group test scoring blank.

In a comparison of the Massachusetts and the fading-numbers group tests, as measured against the standard of an individual sweep test (see section "The Individual Screening Test," in this chapter), Johnson discovered that the Massachusetts was far superior to the fading-numbers test in revealing cases of hearing impairment in a public school population.[5]

When multiple earphones are used with the pure-tone audiometer, a different calibration level must be used. Most audiometers used for screening

[5] Kenneth O. Johnson, "The Relative Efficiency of the Western Electric 4 CA Phonograph and Massachusetts Pure-Tone Group Hearing Tests," unpublished Ph.D. dissertation, Stanford University, 1952.

Kenneth O. Johnson and Hayes A. Newby, "Experimental Study of the Efficiency of Two Group Hearing Tests," *A.M.A. Archives of Otolaryngology*, Vol. 60 (December, 1954), pp. 702-710.

testing either already have jacks for use with multiple phones, or have provision for the installation of auxiliary jacks for this purpose so that the hearing-level dial readings reflect the changed calibration levels. If a school district wishes to utilize the Massachusetts type of group pure-tone test, or for that matter, any kind of group procedure employing an audiometer as the sound source, the manufacturer of the instrument should be consulted regarding any modifications that may be required to make the hearing-level dial readings accurate for multiple phones. The person who is responsible for the operation of the group test should then check the output of each of the phones to be used in the group test to make sure that the indicated hearing-level dial readings do represent the levels delivered to the earphones. It may be advisable to check some normal ears with the group equipment, comparing thresholds obtained at each frequency with the thresholds of the ears when tested individually. If necessary, corrections can be applied to bring the levels at the group phones in agreement with the levels delivered to a single phone in an individual test.

The Massachusetts method of group pure-tone testing may be modified to suit a specific school district's needs. Thus other frequencies may be selected, and different hearing levels adopted, provided only that the group test as modified is experimentally validated. A method of validation will be discussed later in this chapter.

The Pulse-Tone Group Test

A number of people have experimented with a group pure-tone test administered by the presentation of set numbers of pulses or spurts of tones, the subjects responding by writing on a test blank the number of pulses heard each time that the audiometrist signals the group to listen. Reger and Newby described a pulse-tone test that was designed to measure threshold hearing levels from 5 to 40 dB (re ASA–1951 calibration standards).[6]

In the Reger-Newby test, the first presentation of each frequency is at a hearing level of 40 dB. Successive presentations of that frequency are made at hearing levels of 30, 20, 15, 10, and 5 dB. A descending series is presented twice at each frequency. The subjects' responses are recorded on test blanks such as that shown in Figure 8-3. The audiometrist follows a predetermined pattern of tonal presentations, making adjustments of the frequency and hearing-level controls of the audiometer and the switch controlling the number of pulses presented. The test papers are scored by comparing them with the audiometrist's key. The point at which the subject was last able to give a correct response in one out of the two columns provided is determined to be his threshold for that frequency. Thresholds lower than 5 dB cannot be measured under the arrangement of tonal presentations described above.

6 Scott N. Reger and Hayes A. Newby, "A Group Pure-Tone Hearing Test," *Journal of Speech Disorders*, Vol. 12 (March, 1947), pp. 61-66.

GROUP HEARING TEST

DATE _____

NAME _____ AGE _____ SEX _____ EARPHONE NO. _____

LOCAL ADDRESS _____ TELEPHONE _____

RIGHT EAR

| 500 Hz | | 1000 Hz | | 2000 Hz | | 4000 Hz | | 6000 Hz | | HEARING LEVELS |
1	2	3	4	5	6	7	8	9	10	
										40
										30
										20
										15
										10
										5

LEFT EAR

| 500 Hz | | 1000 Hz | | 2000 Hz | | 4000 Hz | | 6000 Hz | | HEARING LEVELS |
1	2	3	4	5	6	7	8	9	10	
										40
										30
										20
										15
										1
										5

Figure 8-3. Group pulse-tone test form.

A loss of 20 dB at any of the test frequencies in either ear is considered to be a failure of the test. Newby found that in giving the test to university students it was possible to make medical referrals directly on the basis of the group test results, but when it was administered to school children he recommended that those failing the group test should be given an individual threshold test as a basis for medical referral.[7] The frequencies tested in the pulse-tone method depend upon the audiometrist's choice, the type of earphones available, and the time available for giving the group test. Reger and Newby recommended that five frequencies be used.

The equipment for the Reger-Newby pulse-tone test consists of a pure-tone audiometer, an interrupting device which controls the number of pulses of tone presented, an attention light which signals the group when to listen, and forty high-fidelity phones (such as TDH-39's) connected with the audiometer. Because forty phones change the intensity calibration of the audiometer, the audiometrist must make sure that the hearing-level dial readings of the audiometer do reflect accurately the levels delivered to the multiple phones, as described in the discussion of the Massachusetts test. Reger and Newby described an interrupter device which is mechanically operated. A commercial version of this test utilized a pulse automatically produced by a master tape. Gardner described a method of obtaining pulses by electronic means.[8]

The Reger-Newby pulse-tone group method is a useful test to secure accurate group test results that represent thresholds (within certain limits). It is a difficult test for the audiometrist to administer, however, since he must constantly be following a key and making split-second adjustments of the frequency and hearing-level controls of the audiometer and the pulse selector switch on the interrupter. Since experience has shown that with school children a follow-up individual test is indicated, rather than a direct medical referral on the basis of the group test results, the pulse-tone method can be modified to serve as a screening test of the Massachusetts type. In other words, in place of a series of decreasing intensities until near-threshold levels are reached, a number of tonal presentations at the same hearing level, for example, 25 dB at each frequency, can be substituted. This procedure simplifies the test administration considerably.

Hollien and Thompson developed a pulse-tone test modeled after the Reger-Newby test. An adult form of the test involved presentation of from zero to four pulses in a descending series of hearing levels from 45 to 15 dB (re ASA–1951 calibration standards) at four frequencies: 500, 1000, 4000, and 8000 Hz. For children the test was abbreviated. Presentations were made at hearing levels of 35, 25, 20, and 20 dB for three frequencies: 500,

[7] Hayes A. Newby, "Group Pure-Tone Hearing Testing in the Public Schools," *Journal of Speech Disorders,* Vol. 12 (December, 1947), pp. 357-362.

[8] Mark B. Gardner, "A Pulse-Tone Technique for Clinical Audiometric Measurements," *Journal of the Acoustical Society of America,* Vol. 19 (1947), pp. 592-599.

1000, and 4000 Hz. Forty phones were connected to a Beltone 10-A audiometer. The pulses were presented manually. A mock-up chart of the answer sheet at the front of the room helped subjects keep their place. On the answer sheet for each presentation there appeared five digits—01234. The subject responded by crossing out the number corresponding to the pulses he heard. This test was used successfully with children as young as third graders.[9]

A later version of the Hollien-Thompson test was used successfully with first graders. Except for changing from 0–4 pulses to 0–3 pulses, the test was the same as that used with the older children, although some modifications in technique were made. Instead of the mock-up chart of the answer sheet, an electrically lighted box duplicating the answer sheet was placed in the front of the room. For each presentation of the stimulus, the row corresponding to the one on the answer sheet to be marked was lighted up. The answer sheet itself was printed in larger type than that used in the earlier version of the test. In an alternate form of the test, a filmstrip of the answer sheet was projected on a screen with the correct row indicated by a colored overlay.[10]

The Johnston Group Pure-Tone Screening Test

All the group tests described above require some form of written response on the part of the test subjects. This limits the usefulness of the tests in public school work to the age levels at which reasonably accurate written responses can be expected. The instructions for the fading-numbers test, the Massachusetts test, and the Reger-Newby version of the pulse-tone group test specify that results cannot be expected with children younger than third graders. Johnston, the originator of the Massachusetts technique, devised a group pure-tone procedure which could be utilized with children as young as kindergarteners.[11] This test is now referred to as the Johnston group pure-tone test.

The procedure for the Johnston test calls for ten children to be seated in a semicircle around a table. The audiometrist instructs them to keep their eyes closed, and when they hear a tone through their earphone to raise their hands. He informs them that some of the time certain earphones will be disconnected and therefore cautions them to pay no attention to anyone else's responses but to listen and respond only if they hear the tone.

The test utilizes a pure-tone audiometer which has a jack for use with ten earphones. While Johnston suggested that the test could be performed at all

9 Harry Hollien and Carl L. Thompson, "A Group Screening Test of Hearing," *Journal of Auditory Research*, Vol. 7 (January, 1967), pp. 85-92.

10 Harry Hollien and Carl L. Thompson, "Forms C and D of the Hollien-Thompson Group Screening Test of Hearing," *Journal of Auditory Research*, Vol. 8 (April, 1968), pp. 143-150.

11 Philip W. Johnston, "An Efficient Group Screening Test," *Journal of Speech and Hearing Disorders*, Vol. 17 (March, 1952), pp. 8-12.

frequencies from 125 through 6000 Hz at a hearing level of 15 dB (re ASA-1951) at each frequency, it is advisable to eliminate 125 and 250 Hz, since these frequencies are easily masked by room noise. Magnetic earphones which are adequate through 6000 Hz are chosen for the test. A push button is wired into the tray of phones, so that when the button is depressed two phones are cut out of the circuit. This is the audiometrist's means of assuring "honest" responses from the test subjects. The tester follows much the same procedure as that used in individual sweep frequency testing but succeeds in screening ten children simultaneously.

Other Group Tests

Meyerson has described a group speech audiometric test which has simple words containing various English sounds as the test stimuli.[12] He describes a technique of administering this speech test in recorded form to ten children simultaneously. The children indicate that they have heard a word by pointing to the appropriate mimeographed picture out of a group on a sheet in front of them. Meyerson claims that the test succeeds in locating the children who have losses through the speech frequencies as measured by the pure-tone audiometer and also locates children whose hearing sensitivity may be normal, but who are unable to respond to spoken stimuli. His test, therefore, measures both sensitivity of hearing and what some writers have referred to as "auding," the ability to comprehend the spoken word.

Recently a test similar to Meyerson's has been developed for use with pre-school children. This test, described by Griffing, Simonton, and Hedgecock, is called VASC, for "Verbal Auditory Screening for Children."[13] The test, administered to two children simultaneously, consists of tape-recorded spondee words divided into four lists. Each list contains twelve words, spanning a range of speech hearing levels from 51 to 15 dB in 4-dB steps of attenuation. The last three words in a list are all delivered at the 15-dB hearing level. The child responds to the test by pointing to a picture that represents the test word. To pass the test, he must correctly identify two of the three words presented at the 15-dB level. This test has received considerable publicity in the popular press because it can be administered by volunteers who observe each child's responses and score them as "right," "wrong," or "no response." Using a commercially available form of the VASC test, Mencher and McCulloch compared this test with individual pure-tone screening on a group of kindergarten children. They reported that the VASC test failed to identify children with losses from 30 to 40 dB (re ANSI–1969 calibration standards) in the speech range, and those with losses of 30 to 50 dB in the 4000

[12] Lee Meyerson, "Hearing for Speech in Children: A Verbal Audiometric Test," unpublished Ph.D. dissertation, Stanford University, 1951.

[13] T. S. Griffing, K. M. Simonton, and L. D. Hedgecock, "Verbal Auditory Screening for Preschool Children," *Transactions of the American Academy of Ophthalmology and Otolaryngology*, Vol. 71 (1967), pp. 105-110.

to 6000 Hz range.[14] They suggest that considerable experimentation with the VASC test is indicated before it can be considered to be an adequate screening instrument.

DETERMINING THE EFFICIENCY OF GROUP TESTS

As stated previously, the purpose of a school hearing test is to discover cases of hearing impairment; therefore, the primary requisite of any group test is that it must be capable of identifying the children in a school population who have hearing losses. There is another aspect of group test efficiency, however, which must be considered. The efficient group test not only discovers cases of hearing impairment; it also correctly identifies children whose hearing is normal. If a group test fails many children who on individual re-examination are discovered to have normal hearing, it causes the audiometrist to waste his time in needless retesting. Efficiency of a group test, then, is determined both by how well it correctly identifies children with hearing losses and by how well it correctly identifies those with normal hearing. No group test is perfect in both respects. With any group test, it is necessary to make a compromise between these two aspects of efficiency.

By adjusting the criterion of test failure, most group tests may be made close to 100 per cent efficient in discovering cases of hearing impairment but only at the expense of failing some individuals with normal hearing. There will always be some children who will fail the group test because of their inability to follow instructions. Also, the stricter the criterion is for passing the group test, the more children with normal hearing there will be who will fail the test. Nevertheless, so long as the number of children needlessly retested is not exorbitantly great, it is better to be strict in setting the criterion for passing or failing the group test, because the efficiency of the test should be judged primarily on how well it discovers cases of actual hearing loss.

In order to check the efficiency of a group test, it is advisable to test a minimum of 100 children with both the group test and an individual pure-tone threshold test. The efficiency of the group test will then be judged according to how well it identifies children with hearing losses and those with normal hearing in comparison with the individual test, which must be assumed to be completely accurate. As the efficiency of the group test will be most critical for children in the lower grades, where the greatest number of hearing losses is found, the experimental subjects for the efficiency check should be drawn from the third and fourth grades. In any group of 100 third and fourth graders, there will probably be from three to five who will fail to pass the criteria for normal hearing on an individual test. These are the

14 George T. Mencher and Barbara F. McCulloch, "Auditory Screening of Kindergarten Children Using the VASC," *Journal of Speech and Hearing Disorders*, Vol. 35 (August, 1970), pp. 241-247.

children who should fail the group test. As we have said previously, however, some children with normal hearing will also fail the group test because they were not paying attention or because they did not follow the instructions properly.

In the next section of this chapter, reference is made to the criteria of a "medically significant" hearing loss as based on complete individual pure-tone audiometry. Since these criteria may be definitely stated, it is a simple matter to determine which of the 100 children have failed the individual test. The rest, by definition, have "normal" hearing. The audiometrist is interested in knowing how the group test classifies the 100 children, and he wants to adjust the criterion for failure of the group test so that it will properly classify the maximum number. One way of accomplishing this task is by drawing up a graphic representation of data in the form of a tetrachoric table.[15] This is a method by which statisticians compute correlations, but for our purpose it is simply a convenient way of comparing and contrasting the group and individual test results. Table 8-1 shows a tetrachoric table arranged for comparing the results of individual and group testing.

Table 8-1. The Tetrachoric Table

| | | Individual Test | |
		% showing significant loss	% showing no significant loss
Group Test	% showing significant loss	a	b
	% showing no significant loss	c	d

The tetrachoric table contains four "cells," which are labeled a, b, c, and d. Agreement between the group and the individual tests is represented by percentages which appear in cells a and d, whereas disagreement is indicated by the percentages recorded in cells b and c. If it were possible to design a group test which operated with perfect efficiency, the percentage values in cells b and c would each be zero. No group test is perfect, however, and we must settle for the best efficiency that can reasonably be achieved. Cell c is the most important one in the table, for our purposes, for percentages recorded there represent children who pass the group test but are shown on the individual test to have "medically significant" hearing losses. Every effort must be made to keep the percentages in cell c as close to zero as possible. The percentages recorded in cell b represented "wasted effort" on the part of the audiometrists. These are children who failed the group test, but who do not meet the individual test criteria for "medically significant" hearing losses.

15 Hayes A. Newby, "Evaluating the Efficiency of Group Screening Tests of Hearing," *Journal of Speech and Hearing Disorders,* Vol. 13 (September, 1948), pp. 236-240.

If the percentage in cell *b* becomes too high, the audiometrist is having to spend so much time in individually testing "normal" ears that the group test has lost its time-saving advantage over the individual method of screening school children.

If an analysis with the tetrachoric table reveals that a group test is passing too many children who should fail, it is possible that the criterion for passing or failing the group test is at the wrong level. To test this hypothesis, see what effect a change in the group test criterion would have on the tetrachoric analysis. If making the criterion for passing the test more rigorous results in lowering the percentage in cell *c* to an acceptable level without increasing the percentage in cell *b* by an unreasonable amount, the criterion for passing the group test should be altered. If reducing the percentage in cell *c* can be accomplished only at the cost of greatly increasing the percentage in cell *b*, then the group test is unacceptably inefficient and should not be used. As stated earlier, the efficiency of a group test is dependent upon its success both in identifying individuals with hearing loss and in correctly identifying individuals whose hearing is normal. The criterion of failure of the group test which is finally selected must be a compromise which gives a reasonable performance in both aspects of efficiency. A good group test is one which has good efficiency in identifying the hearing losses and reasonably good efficiency in identifying the normals. A group test is inadequate if (1) it has poor efficiency in selecting those with hearing losses, or (2) it fails such a high percentage of the population who actually have normal hearing that it results in little or no saving of time. It is possible to analyze the efficiency of any group test by the method suggested above. Moreover, by this method, the best criterion of failure for the group test can be selected.

THE INDIVIDUAL SCREENING TEST

Most school districts prefer the individual type of screening examination because of its admittedly greater accuracy in discovering cases of hearing impairment. As was pointed out earlier, the disadvantage of the individual method is the time that it consumes; however, some people have speculated that because of the inadequacies of certain group tests in discovering cases of hearing impairment the expense to the school district in the long run is greater with the group test than it would be to hire additional audiometrists to screen everyone individually.

A technique referred to as the "sweep" test has been devised to enable individual screening at a rapid rate. In the sweep test the audiometrist sets the hearing-level dial of the audiometer at a fixed level, usually 20 or 25 dB (re ANSI–1969 calibration standards), and then "sweeps" from low through high frequencies, checking to see if the subject is responding at each frequency.

The frequencies tested are usually 500, 1000, 2000, 4000, and 6000 Hz. 250 Hz is not included because it is easily masked by room noise. The highest frequency tested is 6000 Hz instead of 8000 Hz because of the possibility of standing waves interfering with accurate measurement at 8000 Hz. As was mentioned earlier in this chapter, one of the recommendations of the 1960 conference on identification audiometry was that adequate testing environments be provided in schools so that more stringent criteria for passing tests may be employed. Assuming a proper testing environment, the conference recommended that a hearing level of 10 dB be employed for all frequencies except 4000 Hz. The recommended screening level for 4000 Hz was 20 dB, in recognition of the common occurrence of 4000 Hz "dips" considered to be insignificant.[16] Of course these hearing levels were in reference to the ASA–1951 calibration standards. The corresponding hearing levels in reference to the ANSI–1969 calibration standards (for the Western Electric 705-A earphone) would be 20 dB at 1000, 2000, and 6000 Hz, and 25 dB at 500 and 4000 Hz. In other words, the new standard shifted audiometric zero by 10 dB at 1000, 2000, and 6000 Hz, by 15 dB at 500 Hz, but only by 5 dB at 4000 Hz. All of these differences are approximations of the actual values, rounded to the nearest 5-dB step. The actual values are given in Table 5-2 in Chapter 5. The choice of a 20-dB screening level for the speech frequencies was rationalized on the basis that in some situations individuals with hearing levels of 25 dB experience difficulty in understanding speech. If screening is performed at a hearing level of 25 dB, a child with a 25-dB hearing level is passed. A 20-dB hearing level passing criterion would screen out children with 25-dB hearing levels for additional testing.

The audiometrist should take precautions to see that the subject is responding accurately. If he uses the interrupter switch at each frequency he can check the validity of the subject's responses. The audiometrist should instruct the child to raise a finger when he hears a tone and lower it when the tone goes away, or he may ask the child to respond orally if he prefers. Then he places the earphones over the child's ears. While the prescribed hearing levels for 500 and 4000 Hz are at 25 dB, the audiometrist can save time by checking all five frequencies at the 20-dB hearing level. Then, only if the child does not respond at 20 dB at 500 and/or 4000 Hz will it be necessary to check him at 25 dB. In beginning the test, the frequency control is set at 500 Hz and the hearing-level control at 30 dB (so that the initial stimulus will be more clearly audible). The ear-selector switch is on "right ear." A tone is presented and left on until the child responds. If he does not respond immediately the hearing level should be increased to 40 dB and the tone be presented again. As soon as the child responds that he hears the tone by raising his finger, the examiner releases the interrupter switch, and the child's finger should lower. The hearing-level control is then set at 20 dB and the tone is presented again. The child's finger should be raised. Leaving the tone on, the examiner

16 Darley, ed., *op. cit.*, p. 31.

switches to 1000 Hz. The child's finger should remain raised. Now the interrupter is released and the finger should lower. The examiner switches to 2000 Hz and depresses the interrupter. The finger should be raised. Leaving the tone on, the examiner switches to 4000 Hz, and the finger should stay up. The examiner releases the interrupter, and the child should lower his finger. The frequency control is switched to 6000 Hz and the interrupter is depressed. The child's finger should be raised. Leaving the tone on, the examiner switches to the left ear, with the frequency control still at 6000 Hz and the hearing-level control at 20 dB. The finger should remain up. The examiner then follows the same sequence of events as he covers all the test frequencies in descending order in the left ear. The test ends with the frequency control back at 500 Hz, and the examiner is ready for the next child. This time he can start the test with the left ear, so all he needs to do to start the test is to set the hearing-level control at 30 dB. Every other child will receive the stimulus first in his left ear. Some examiners might feel more comfortable with a procedure that always tests a child's right ear first, in which case it is a simple matter to reset the ear-selector switch at the conclusion of each screening test.

If a child should not respond at the 20-dB level for 500 or 4000 Hz, he must be checked at 25 dB at these frequencies, which of course slows down the test somewhat. Even so, using the technique just described, a competent examiner should be able to screen from twenty to thirty children an hour. In the interest of most efficient use of time, three children should be standing by watching the testing procedure. Then as soon as one child is finished, another can take his place, and an additional child is admitted to the room to wait his turn. Besides providing a steady flow of testees, this procedure minimizes the instructions required, since each child observes the tests of three children before his turn arrives.

In the sweep test the audiometrist is interested in knowing only whether or not a given pupil can hear at the screening level. If the pupil does not respond at the appropriate hearing level at any one of the frequencies screened, he fails the sweep test and must be retested later with an individual threshold test, as described in Chapter 5. Some audiometrists prefer to do the threshold test immediately upon discovering a pupil who fails the sweep test. This procedure interrupts the steady flow of subjects to the test room, however, and thus decreases the efficiency of the procedure.

In 1957 a "limited frequency" screening procedure was suggested by Doctors House and Glorig.[17] From analyzing a sizable sample of audio-

---

[17] Howard P. House, "A New Instrument and Concept for the Rapid Detection of a Possible Hearing Impairment," *Transactions of the American Academy of Opthalmology and Otolaryngology,* Vol. 61 (March-April, 1957), pp. 228-230.

Howard P. House and Aram Glorig, "A New Concept of Auditory Screening," *Laryngoscope,* Vol. 67 (July, 1957), pp. 661-668.

Aram Glorig and Howard P. House, "A New Concept of Auditory Screening," *A.M.A. Archives of Otolaryngology,* Vol. 66 (August, 1957), pp. 228-232.

grams, House and Glorig concluded that practically every hearing problem, regardless of its etiology, was characterized by some hearing loss at 4000 Hz. It occurred to them, then, that a test at only 4000 Hz should be a quick means of screening a large population. If an individual could hear a 4000-Hz tone at a standard screening level, the presumption was that he had no significant hearing loss at any other frequency. Originally, House and Glorig were interested in developing a quick procedure for use in "monitoring" the hearing of workers in industry, so significant changes in an individual worker's hearing, presumably as a result of his exposure to noise, could be detected early. Based on their recommendations, Ambco Electronics in Los Angeles designed and built a battery-powered, transitorized screening audiometer which they designated "Oto-Chek." This instrument produced a single frequency, 4000 Hz, at three hearing levels: 20, 35, and 50 dB (re ASA–1951).

House and Glorig suggested the single-frequency Oto-Chek would also be useful in school screening testing programs, and they reported some data on the efficiency of such a test in school programs. They indicated, however, that a two-frequency test would be even more efficient and suggested that these frequencies should be 4000 and 2000 Hz. Ambco Electronics built a second model of their Oto-Chek primarily for use in school screening testing programs. This instrument produced 4000- and 2000-Hz tones at two hearing levels: 15 and 35 dB (re ASA–1951). House and Glorig recommended that a school test begin at 4000 Hz with a presentation of the tone at the 35-dB hearing level, so the subject would have a strong stimulus to which to respond. If he responds, the 4000-Hz tone is then presented at the 15-dB level. If he responds again, he passes the screening test in that ear. If he does not respond to the 15-dB signal at 4000 Hz, the frequency is switched to 2000 Hz. If he can respond to the 2000-Hz tone at the 15-dB hearing level he passes the test, and the assumption is made that he has an "insignificant" dip at 4000 Hz (somewhere between 15 and 35 dB). If he does not hear the 2000-Hz tone at the 15-dB level, he fails the test. The same procedure is, of course, followed with each ear. The current model of the Oto-Chek is shown in Figure 8-4. On the current model the two hearing levels available at each frequency are 25 and 45 dB (re ISO–1964 or ANSI–1969 calibration standards). The single-frequency model of the Oto-Chek is no longer in production.

One advantage for the two-frequency screening procedure with the Oto-Chek cited by House and Glorig is that the test can be performed satisfactorily in the average school room; that is, no specially sound-treated room is necessary, since high frequencies are resistant to masking by room noise. Other advantages cited were the speed of the test and the simplicity of the equipment and the procedure. It was assumed that screen-testing with the Oto-Chek would require no special training in audiometry. Of course, children failing the Oto-Chek test would be referred to a qualified audiometrist for a complete threshold test.

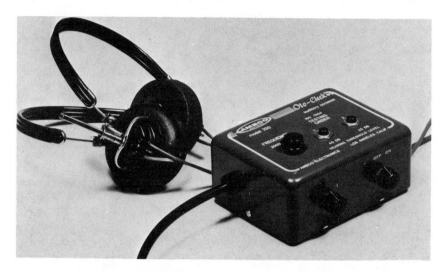

Figure 8-4. The two-frequency Oto-Chek. (Reproduced by permission of Ambco Electronics, Los Angeles, California.)

The appearance of the articles by House and Glorig advocating the use of limited-frequency screening testing in the schools provoked a rash of articles reporting on experimentation with the procedure, most of which concluded that limited-frequency screening was not an acceptable substitute for a complete sweep-frequency screening test, although some suggested that a two-frequency test would be adequate if some frequency other than 2000 Hz were combined with 4000 Hz.[18] The most frequent suggestion was that either 500 Hz or 1000 Hz should be combined with 4000 Hz. Farrant, for example, advocated a two-frequency screen test consisting of 500 and 4000 Hz presented at a hearing level of 15 dB (re ASA–1951).[19] He states that such a test has been used in Australian schools since 1951. Some investigators report that the limited-frequency concept of screening is based on valid

[18] Clifton F. Lawrence and Wallace Rubin, "The Efficiency of Limited Frequency Audiometric Screening in a School Hearing Conservation Program," *A.M.A. Archives of Otolaryngology*, Vol. 69 (May, 1959), pp. 606-611.

Charles Lightfoot, Richard A. Buckingham, and Mary Neville Kelly, "A Check on Oto-Chek," *A.M.A. Archives of Otolaryngology*, Vol. 70 (July, 1959), pp. 103-113.

Douglas Ann Stevens and G. Don Davidson, "Screening Tests of Hearing," *Journal of Speech and Hearing Disorders*, Vol. 24 (August, 1959), pp. 258-261.

Bruce M. Siegenthaler and Ronald K. Sommers, "Abbreviated Sweep-Check Procedures for School Hearing Testing," *Journal of Speech and Hearing Disorders*, Vol. 24 (August, 1959), pp. 249-257.

Maurice H. Miller and Jeanne L. Bella, "Limitations of Selected Frequency Audiometry in the Public Schools," *Journal of Speech and Hearing Disorders*, Vol. 24 (November, 1959), pp. 402-407.

W. Ruth Maxwell and G. Don Davidson, "Limited-Frequency Screening and Ear Pathology," *Journal of Speech and Hearing Disorders*, Vol. 26 (May, 1961), pp. 122-125.

[19] R. H. Farrant, "The Audiometric Testing of Children in Schools and Kindergartens," *Journal of Auditory Research*, Vol. 1 (September, 1960), p. 8.

principles and believe that the method of one- or two-frequency screening has merit for use in the schools.[20] At the present writing, one can only say that the question of whether or not limited-frequency screening testing is an appropriate procedure to apply in the schools has not been finally answered. Since five frequencies can be screened in a matter of a minute or so for each ear, the time saved by checking only two frequencies would be minimal, so most audiometrists prefer not to take the chance of missing any child with impaired hearing by using limited-frequency screening.

While the screening levels of 20 dB at 1000, 2000, and 6000 Hz and 25 dB at 500 and 4000 Hz were recommended by the conference on identification audiometry only if an adequate testing environment were available, these screening levels have been generally adopted regardless of the adequacy of the test space. The reports on the experience of school testing programs employing these levels have been good by and large.[21] Some suggestions have been made for revising the criteria for passing the screening test. Lloyd suggested that in the interest of saving time during the screening procedure a uniform screening hearing level of 20 dB be employed.[22] Melnick et al., who discovered that many of their screening failures occurred at the frequency of 6000 Hz, suggested that the screening hearing level should be the same at 6000 Hz as at 4000 Hz.[23]

Following the screening test, each child who has failed to hear one or more frequencies in either ear at the prescribed hearing level should receive a threshold hearing test. Some hearing conservation programs prefer to administer a second screening test before referring children for threshold testing. In other words, those children who failed the first screening test would be screened again on another day, and only those who failed both screening tests would be given threshold tests. Melnick et al. report data indicating that about one-fourth of those children who failed a single screening test passed a second screening test.[24] There are various reasons why a child might pass the second test after having failed the first: he might have been fright-

---

[20] Ira M. Ventry and Hayes A. Newby, "Validity of the One-Frequency Screening Principle for Public School Children," *Journal of Speech and Hearing Research*, Vol. 2 (June, 1959), pp. 147-151.

Max C. Norton and Elizabeth Lux, "Double Frequency Auditory Screening in Public Schools," *Journal of Speech and Hearing Disorders*, Vol. 25 (August, 1960), pp. 293-299.

Clair N. Hanley and Barbara G. Gaddie, "The Use of Single-Frequency Audiometry in the Screening of School Children," *Journal of Speech and Hearing Disorders*, Vol. 27 (August, 1962), pp. 258-264.

[21] Marion P. Downs, Mildred E. Doster, and Marlin Weaver, "Dilemmas in Identification Audiometry," *Journal of Speech and Hearing Disorders*, Vol. 30 (November, 1965), pp. 360-364.

Harold J. Weber, Frank J. McGovern, and David Zink, "An Evaluation of 1000 Children with Hearing Loss," *Journal of Speech and Hearing Disorders*, Vol. 32 (November, 1967), pp. 343-354.

[22] Lyle L. Lloyd, "Comments on 'Dilemmas in Identification Audiometry,'" *Journal of Speech and Hearing Disorders*, Vol. 31 (May, 1966), pp. 161-165.

[23] William Melnick, Eldon L. Eagles, and Herbert S. Levine, "Evaluation of a Recommended Program of Identification Audiometry with School-Age Children," *Journal of Speech and Hearing Disorders*, Vol. 29 (February, 1964), pp. 3-13.

[24] *Ibid.*, pp. 6-7.

ened or he might have misunderstood the instructions during the first test; he could have had a cold or other upper respiratory condition that reduced his hearing sensitivity on the initial screening; or his hearing sensitivity actually might be on the borderline of normal, so that a very slight shift of threshold for whatever reason—perhaps just a matter of concentration or attention—could move him from the "fail" group to the "pass" group.

FOLLOW-UP OF THE SCHOOL TESTS

The success of a hearing-conservation program depends on the adequacy of medical and educational follow-up of pupils discovered to have "medically significant" hearing impairments. What is meant by a medically significant hearing impairment? The term was used in a classic monograph by Newhart and Reger that for many years was the "Bible" of school hearing-conservation programs. Newhart and Reger said that a "hearing loss probably is of medical significance" if the impairment in either ear was at least 20 dB (re ASA–1951) for two or more frequencies. If the testing was performed in "an exceedingly quiet location," an impairment of 15 dB at two frequencies would constitute a medically significant loss.[25]

The 1960 conference on identification audiometry recommended that the same criteria should be applied for referring a child for an otological examination that are recommended for failure of a screening test. It will be recalled that to pass a screening test a pupil must hear 1000, 2000, and 6000 Hz at a hearing level of 20 dB, and 500 and 4000 Hz at a hearing level of 25 dB. These are the screening levels recommended by the conference corrected to ANSI–1969 calibration standards (for the Western Electric 705-A earphone). Thus a "medically significant" loss today consists of a threshold hearing level of 25 dB or more at 1000, 2000, or 6000 Hz, or 30 dB or more at 500 or 4000 Hz. If a pupil is found on a follow-up threshold test to have a "significant" loss at any frequency in either ear, he should be referred for an otological examination. Since presumably threshold testing is conducted in a suitable acoustic environment, it can be expected that some of the children who failed the screening test—or perhaps two screening tests—will prove to have hearing within acceptable limits on the threshold test. Not infrequently children will fail the screening test(s) at only the frequency of 500 Hz but will be found on threshold testing not to have a significant loss at that frequency. What this tells us is that the screening test was performed in an "unsuitable" acoustic environment, so that the "failure" at 500 Hz was really the result of the masking effect of room noise. It was the recognition of the susceptibility of 500 Hz to masking by room noise that prompted the

[25] Horace Newhart and Scott N. Reger, "Syllabus of Audiometric Procedures in the Administration of a Program for the Conservation of Hearing of School Children," Supplement to the *Transactions of the American Academy of Ophthalmology and Otolaryngology* (April, 1945), pp. 17 and 18.

conference on identification audiometry to recommend that otological referrals should be based on threshold hearing levels for the frequencies of 1000 Hz and above unless the follow-up tests were performed in an acceptable acoustic environment.[26]

If possible, bone-conduction tests with masking when appropriate should be given to all those pupils who have medically significant losses by air conduction. The comparison of air- and bone-conduction hearing levels on the school audiogram will assist the otologist to a diagnosis of a given pupil's hearing impairment. It is recognized that not all school districts will be equipped or have adequately trained personnel available to perform bone-conduction testing, in which case the audiogram will contain air-conduction threshold hearing levels only.

Experience has demonstrated that many school children have losses of 30 dB or more at only 4000 or 6000 Hz. Almost invariably an otologist who examines children with this type of high-frequency loss finds no demonstrable pathology and nothing in the child's history of significance. Many otologists feel that such high-frequency losses are congenital and static (not progressive). Since the success of a hearing-conservation program depends upon securing the cooperation of the examining otologist, it is important that he feel that his time is well spent. It may be advisable, therefore, for the school audiometrist to assign priorities to the pupils identified as having "significant" hearing impairments. Those with losses only at 4000 or 6000 Hz would be given the lowest priority. Thus the otologist can make the decision as to whether or not he should give individual examinations to each of the pupils in the low-priority group. Highest priority would be assigned to those who have a significant loss at any of the speech frequencies. And the next priority would include those children who have losses at *both* 4000 and 6000 Hz. Regardless of the priority of their hearing losses, all children who are found to have a medically significant loss should be retested in the schools at intervals of no greater than a year. Only by comparing the results of successive tests can it be determined whether a given loss is static or changing.

The purpose of identification audiometry is to discover cases of medically significant hearing impairment so that appropriate medical and/or educational follow-up procedures can be instituted. It would be nice if identification audiometry could also identify all those children who have otologically abnormal ears, but unfortunately that is not the case. School hearing tests alone identify very few of the otologically abnormal ears in a school population, as has been demonstrated by Eagles and by Eagles and Wishik, reporting on a study of hearing in children in Pittsburgh under the sponsorship of the American Academy of Ophthalmology and Otolaryngology and the Graduate School of Public Health at the University of Pittsburgh. All children in the study were given an otological examination in addition to a hearing test. It was found that the median hearing levels of the otologically abnormal

26 Darley, ed., *op. cit.,* p. 31.

group varied by only 2 to 4 dB from the median hearing levels of the normal group. If only the speech frequencies are considered, 90 per cent of the children in the otologically abnormal group could pass a screening test at the 15 dB level (re ASA–1951)—about 25 dB (re ANSI–1969).[27] Since so many of the otologically abnormal children have hearing levels within the range of normal, they could not be screened out by any hearing test. They can be identified only by an otological examination. The purpose of a school hearing-conservation program has to be confined, therefore, to identifying children whose hearing is sufficiently impaired that they might experience some difficulty in certain listening situations.

Medical Follow-up

All pupils found to have medically significant losses on the basis of the threshold test following the screening procedure should be referred for a medical follow-up. Many school systems, in cooperation with the crippled children services of the state department of health, conduct periodic otological clinics for the purpose of giving medical examinations to children who have failed the school hearing test. As was stated above, maximum otological cooperation can be achieved by grouping pupils who have failed the hearing test in terms of the priority of their hearing losses. The otologist can thus give his attention first to pupils who have losses that might interfere with their ability to communicate. The duty of the examining otologist is to determine whether there is any condition of the ear or any significant information in the medical history of the child which could account for his hearing loss. The examining otologist thus makes a diagnosis and recommends treatment if he feels that the hearing loss is one which could be helped through medical or surgical care.

In one follow-up of 1000 pupils who were found to have medically significant hearing losses, 43 per cent were diagnosed as conductive losses, 23 per cent as sensori-neural losses exclusive of 4000 Hz "drop-off," and 34 per cent were individuals whose only significant loss was at 4000 Hz. Through age eleven, the greatest number of impairments were conductive, with the highest incidence in the age group of six to seven. Beginning at age twelve, the 4000 Hz drop-off constituted the greatest number of cases, with the highest incidence at the oldest age group—sixteen and older. In the group of medically significant losses as a whole, 62 per cent were male and 38 per cent were female.[28]

[27] Eldon L. Eagles, "Hearing Levels in Children and Implications for Identification Audiometry," *Ibid.*, Appendix B, pp. 52-62.

Eldon L. Eagles and Samuel M. Wishik, "A Study of Hearing in Children. I. Objectives and Preliminary Findings," *Transactions of the American Academy of Ophthalmology and Otolaryngology* (May-June, 1961), pp. 261-282.

[28] Weber *et al.*, *op. cit.*, pp. 344-346.

The findings of the examining otologist are recorded on the pupil's health record. These findings and recommendations are transmitted by the school to the pupil's parents. The parents are urged to take their child to their own family physician for the fulfillment of the recommendations that the examining otologist has made. If the parents are financially unable to provide the medical or surgical care that has been recommended, the crippled children services can assume this responsibility also.

The medical follow-up of a child discovered to have hearing impairment should include examinations by the examining otologist after the child has received medical or surgical care, so that the otologist can determine the effectiveness of the treatment. Audiometric tests should be administered before re-examination by the otologist, as the effectiveness of the treatment may be demonstrated by an improvement in the child's hearing. The value of the medical follow-up of children discovered to have significant hearing losses is demonstrated in a report, which indicates that 34 per cent of the children who received treatment after their failure of the school tests demonstrated on subsequent tests a return to normal levels of hearing.[29] "Treatment" was defined as having included at least one known visit to a physician. Many children taken to a physician by their parents were found to have permanent and irreversible hearing losses. If these children are not considered in the statistics, 57 per cent of those who received medical "treatment" demonstrated a return to normal levels of hearing. By contrast, only 18 per cent of the children who did not receive medical "treatment" showed an improvement in hearing to normal levels on subsequent tests.

Educational Follow-Up

As stated above, the effectiveness of a school hearing-conservation program is directly related to the thoroughness with which the follow-up program is conducted. In the otological examination, pupils whose hearing might be improved through medical or surgical care are identified, and provision is made to have the child given appropriate treatment. Many children with discovered hearing impairment are found to have a loss that is irreversible even with medical care. In other words, these children will have congenital losses of a sensori-neural type, sensori-neural losses through adventitious causes, or static impairments due to previous middle ear pathology. Then the otologist can make no medical recommendations. He can state only that the child has a permanent and irremediable type of impairment. This pupil then becomes the concern of the schools, which must provide whatever help of an educational character is required to assist him in overcoming or minimizing his hearing handicap.

[29] Robert M. Cameron, Summary of Hearing Conservation Program for 1955-1956 School Year, unpublished report submitted to the Palo Alto, California, Unified School District, 1956.

Naturally the type of educational program planned will depend upon the nature and degree of hearing impairment that an individual child demonstrates. His need for amplification should be considered. Perhaps in certain classroom situations he should be provided with a desk-type hearing aid which many schools make available during school hours to hearing-handicapped pupils. It may be that he would benefit from having his own, wearable hearing aid. Even though he does not need amplification, he may benefit from some instruction in speechreading. Children with permanent hearing impairments may also have speech problems, and so they may need to be enrolled in a speech correction program. Even though a particular child may not have a speech problem at the time his hearing loss is discovered, it is possible that with the passage of time his speech will deteriorate unless he is given "preventive speech therapy."

It is doubtful that children will be discovered in the public school system with such profound hearing impairments as would necessitate placement in a class for the deaf. Such children would be so obviously handicapped that they would be known without a hearing-conservation program. It is possible, however, that a child may be discovered in the school hearing tests to have a mild hearing impairment of a progressive nature, and in a few years' time become so profoundly impaired that he has to be placed in a special class for the deaf. The educational follow-up program in the schools, therefore, should include periodic audiometric examinations for all pupils who have been found to have a hearing loss. It is only through the follow-up tests that the progressive type of hearing impairment can be discovered.

In addition to providing special educational services for the child who is hard-of-hearing, the schools have the responsibility of informing parents of the extent of handicap that their child has and helping parents to assist their child. Some parents are completely upset at the discovery that they have a child with a hearing impariment. The schools and the physician must interpret the meaning of a specific hearing loss and counsel the parents on what can and cannot be done to help the child. The subject of parental counseling, as well as other aspects of the training of hearing-impaired children, will be discussed further in Chapter 11.

FUNCTIONAL HEARING PROBLEMS IN CHILDREN

Recently considerable attention has been focused on a very interesting clinical finding: the child who manifests a functional or nonorganic hearing problem. Juers was one of the first clinicians to make reference to the existence of this problem.[30] More recently articles on the subject have

[30] Arthur L. Juers, "Pure Tone Threshold and Hearing for Speech—Diagnostic Significance of Inconsistencies," *Laryngoscope,* Vol. 66 (April, 1956), pp. 402-409.

appeared by audiologists working in clinical settings to which many children who fail school audiometric tests are referred for further evaluation.[31]

In a typical case of a child found to have a functional hearing problem, he will not have been suspected by parents or teachers of having a hearing impairment until he fails a school hearing test. Usually he will be seen by a physician after the parents have been notified by the school that their child has a hearing impairment, and if a hearing test is performed in the physician's office, generally the child will exhibit a bilateral hearing "loss" with air- and bone-conduction hearing levels of from 40 to 60 dB. The physician may or may not suspect the authenticity of the audiogram. In any event the otological examination is negative in its findings, although there may be a history suggesting previous disease of the middle ear, and the physician refers the child to a hearing center or clinic for a complete hearing evaluation. Not infrequently, the referral will be for the purpose of selecting a hearing aid.

When the child is interviewed by the examining audiologist, it will usually be noted that he readily follows normal conversation. This observation is, of course, inconsistent with the degree of loss the child has shown on previous tests and should immediately alert the examiner to the possibility of a functional hearing problem. If the examiner were to start his evaluation with a pure-tone test, in all probability he would obtain an audiogram that would agree substantially with the ones obtained at school and in the physician's office. When he suspects the presence of a functional hearing problem, the examiner would be well-advised to commence his evaluation with the speech audiometer, monaurally with live voice. Best results will ordinarily be obtained with an ascending technique, that is, starting with the hearing-level control at minimum intensity and increasing intensity until the child responds.

[31] Robert L. Berk and Alan S. Feldman, "Functional Hearing Loss in Children," *New England Journal of Medicine*, Vol. 259 (July, 1958), pp. 214-216.

Richard F. Dixon and Hayes A. Newby, "Children with Nonorganic Hearing Problems," *A.M.A. Archives of Otolaryngology*, Vol. 70 (November, 1959), pp. 619-623.

Bengt Barr, "Nonorganic Hearing Problems in School-Children," *Acta Otolaryngologica*, Vol. 52 (1960), pp. 337-346.

Seymour J. Brockman and Gloria H. Holversten, "Pseudo Neural Hypacusis in Children," *Laryngoscope*, Vol. 70 (June, 1960), pp. 825-839.

George J. Leshin, "Childhood Nonorganic Hearing Loss," *Journal of Speech and Hearing Disorders*, Vol. 25 (August, 1960), pp. 290-292.

Donald R. Calvert, John P. Moncur, D. Wayne Smith, and Jack Snyder, "Nonorganic Hearing Loss in School-Age Children," *The Voice* (The Journal of the California Speech and Hearing Association), Vol. 10 (November, 1961), pp. 6-11.

William Rintelmann and Earl Harford, "The Detection and Assessment of Pseudo-hypoacusis Among School-Age Children," *Journal of Speech and Hearing Disorders*, Vol. 28 (May, 1963), pp. 141-152.

John L. Peterson, "Nonorganic Hearing Loss in Children and Békésy Audiometry," *Journal of Speech and Hearing Disorders*, Vol. 28 (May, 1963), pp. 153-158.

Peter A. Campanelli, "Simulated Hearing Losses in School Children Following Identification Audiometry," *Journal of Audiotry Research*, Vol. 3 (1963), pp. 91-108.

The examiner may start his evaluation by asking the child casual questions about himself or his family, or conversing on a subject that he thinks will be of interest to the child, for example, pets, sports, or television programs. If the child responds to the examiner's questions in each ear at zero or near-zero dB hearing level, then a more formal speech-reception threshold can be obtained, using spondee words. If the child does not respond to the spondee words immediately, the examiner should "coax" a response from him. It may be necessary to urge the child to respond on almost every word. On rare occasions, the examiner may have to employ delayed auditory feedback to verify the presence of a functional hearing problem. Usually, however, SRT's within the range of normal can be established by using a combination of informal conversation and spondee words. Once an SRT has been established in each ear, the examiner should perform discrimination tests with PB word lists in each ear. Typically, the child will exhibit excellent discrimination at suprathreshold levels with no urging from the examiner.

Once the examiner has established SRT and obtained a discrimination score in each ear, he begins a pure-tone evaluation. It is best for the examiner to remain outside the test room, assuming that his equipment permits remote pure-tone testing. Before commencing the pure-tone test, the examiner should make sure that the child understands what it is he is to listen for and how he is to respond on the pure-tone test. It is probably best to make no mention to the child of the results of earlier tests he has had at school or elsewhere. The examiner then proceeds to establish pure-tone thresholds in the conventional way. If the child fails to respond at levels consistent with his performance in speech audiometry, the examiner should stop the test, inform the child that he apparently misunderstood the directions, and emphasize the necessity of the child's responding just as soon as he is aware of the presence of the tone. The examiner may decide to present the tone in pulses and have the child report the number of pulses he hears in each presentation. Perhaps because this is a new kind of task, the child may respond at appropriate hearing levels. Ross cautions that the emphasis should be on the counting task rather than on hearing, and he suggests alternating intensities above and below the child's admitted thresholds. Of course any responses "below" threshold establish new threshold hearing levels.[32] Incidentally, the technique of having the child report the number of pulses he hears may be successful even if he does not report them correctly. Sometimes a child will consistently respond with the incorrect number after a series of pulses has been presented, but he will always respond at the appropriate time. Sometimes a child will respond "no" or "none" each time a series of tones is presented, and it is possible to obtain reliable threshold measurements based on his negative responses.

In most cases, by utilizing unusual techniques when necessary, the exami-

[32] Mark Ross, "The Variable Intensity Pulse Count Method (VIPCM) for the Detection and Measurement of the Pure-Tone Thresholds of Children with Functional Hearing Losses," *Journal of Speech and Hearing Disorders*, Vol. 29 (November, 1964), pp. 477-482.

ner can obtain pure-tone threshold measurements that agree well with the previously-established speech thresholds. Only rarely is it necessary to employ neurophysiological techniques to establish thresholds. It is important that the examiner always treat the child with dignity and respect and give the child an opportunity to perform in a manner consistent with his actual hearing levels without suffering "loss of face." In other words, the examiner must avoid giving the child any impression that he is being accused of attempting to deceive the examiner.

While occasionally it is obvious that a particular child who manifests a functional hearing problem is emotionally disturbed, in most instances there is no apparent reason for the child to exhibit atypical auditory behavior, and indeed it is only in a test situation that there is any indication of abnormal hearing. Reporting on their experiences with forty children found to have functional hearing problems, Dixon and Newby said:

> Most of the children seemed to be performing well academically, to be intellectually normal, and were without noticeable emotional disturbances. Nine children displayed symptoms which might be related to their "hearing problem." These symptoms included functional articulatory speech disorders, and–according to parent reports–strong sibling rivalry, persistent enuresis, anxiety reactions, possible nonorganic visual difficulties, and lack of satisfactory academic progress. It should be reemphasized, however, that children with any symptoms or history of psychological significance were definitely in the minority–less than 25 per cent of the total group. On the basis of our own observations, we cannot state why these children performed as they did on hearing tests.[33]

As stated earlier, the first clue an examiner obtains that a child may be exhibiting a functional hearing problem is that his ability to follow ordinary conversation is inconsistent with the degree of impairment he has demonstrated in tests. School audiometrists should be aware of discrepancies between a child's auditory behavior and his test results. Too frequently, however, there is a tendency for those associated with the child to assume the validity of an audiometric test and to ignore the evidence of their own observation. It is not unusual to find that educational decisions of considerable importance to a child's future may be based on erroneous audiometric results. In the group of forty children studied by Dixon and Newby, fourteen were receiving instruction in speechreading, receiving auditory training, or had been given preferential seating in the classroom; two were in special classes for the hard of hearing; one was in a class for the deaf; and one had been furnished with a hearing aid. All of these children were found to have normal hearing.[34] The lesson to be learned from such experiences is that audiometrists, and others concerned with planning a child's educational program, must not place blind dependence on the results of an audiometric test when a child's behavior belies the evidence of the audiogram.

[33] Dixon and Newby, *op. cit.*, p. 620.
[34] *Ibid.*

9

INDUSTRIAL AUDIOLOGY

As we saw in Chapter 3, one of the causes of a sensori-neural hearing impairment is exposure to noise. In our modern industrialized civilization, hardly anyone can escape some exposure to noise. Even the farmer, who traditionally is associated with the quiet environment of the wide open spaces, employs mechanized labor-saving devices that are noise producing and thus potentially damaging to his hearing. The term "presbycusis" refers to the gradually increasing loss of hearing acuity associated with increasing age. It is quite possible that our daily exposure to just ordinary environmental noises contributes substantially to the "aging" of our hearing mechanism. There is evidence to suggest that primitive tribesmen in Africa who are completely removed from the noises of our modern civilization do not show any appreciable decrease in hearing acuity with advancing age.[1] Glorig has suggested that a better word to describe the progressive loss of hearing associated with increasing age would be "sociocusis"—the loss of hearing acuity due to all of the hazards of living in our modern society, disease and noise exposure as well as aging.[2] As noise becomes an increasingly important problem in our modern civilization, the control of noise and protection of the individual from damage as the result of exposure to noise become increasingly important. A variety of professional skills is required to deal with all of the facets of noise control and hearing conservation. Included among the specialists whose skills are brought to bear on these problems are

[1] Samuel Rosen, Moe Bergman, Dietrich Plester, Aly El-Mofty, and Mohamed Hamad Satti, "Presbycusis Study of a Relatively Noise-Free Population in the Sudan," *Annals of Otology, Rhinology, and Laryngology,* Vol. 71 (September, 1962), pp. 727-743.
[2] Aram Glorig, Jr., *Noise and Your Ear* (New York, Grune & Stratton, 1958), p. 141.

the expert in acoustics, the industrial engineer, the architect, the industrial hygienist, the safety engineer, the industrial physician, the otologist, and the audiologist. This chapter will deal with the complexities of the problems created by noise, particularly in the context of industry, and the means of control of these problems.

NOISE-INDUCED HEARING LOSS

Noise may cause a sudden hearing loss, as in the case of a blast or explosion that may rupture the tympanic membrane and also "jar loose" some of the hair cells of the organ of Corti in the cochlea, or noise may exert an insidious long-term effect on the hair cells that produces a gradually-increasing hearing loss. The sudden loss of hearing from noise is called "acoustic trauma," while the gradual diminution of hearing acuity associated with noise exposure is referred to as "noise-induced hearing loss." The amount of hearing impairment incurred from noise exposure is proportional to the intensity of the stimulus and the length of the exposure. Also there is the matter of individual susceptibility to noise to consider. People differ considerably in their ability to withstand noise.

From animal experiments it has been determined that the sensori-neural loss associated with noise exposure is cochlear in origin. Confirmation of this conclusion comes from recruitment studies of humans who have incurred noise-induced hearing impairment. Typically, such individuals will demonstrate recruitment at the affected frequencies in loudness balance tests, or will yield SISI scores that are characteristic of cochlear involvement. Usually the individual exposed to noise will manifest initially a "dip" or "notch" centered around 4000 Hz on the pure-tone audiogram. In its beginning stages, noise-induced hearing loss is reversible; that is, if the individual is removed from the noisy environment, his hearing will gradually improve until it reaches the pre-exposure level. For example, a worker tested on Friday evening after five days of on-the-job exposure to industrial noise may evidence a notch of 10 dB at 3000 Hz, 20 dB at 4000 Hz, and 10 dB at 6000 Hz, with all other frequencies at the zero-dB hearing level. After a week end away from the noisy environment, this same worker may yield an audiogram on Monday morning that shows zero-dB hearing level at all of the audiometric frequencies. The presumed explanation for this finding is that certain of the hair cells responsible for the reception of the frequencies from 3000 through 6000 Hz have not been destroyed or irreparably damaged by the noise exposure but have been "fatigued," and with rest they can recover their normal function. The results of fatigue we refer to as "temporary threshold shift," abbreviated TTS. TTS can be demonstrated in the laboratory by presenting an ear with a fatiguing stimulus for as short a period as ten to fifteen minutes.

Now let us return to the example cited above of the worker who demonstrated TTS at the end of a week of exposure to industrial noise. On a

Monday morning his hearing is back to its normal level. But then he spends another week in his noisy work and again on Friday night his audiogram shows a notch. Perhaps by the following Monday morning his hearing will be back to its normal level. If, however, this procedure is repeated for many weeks and months, there will come a time when even after a week end of rest the worker's hearing at the affected frequencies will not quite return to its former level of acuity. With succeeding months of continued noise exposure on the job, the worker will demonstrate on his Friday evening audiograms a deepening and widening notch. Perhaps his audiogram will show levels of 10 dB at 2000 Hz, 20 dB at 3000 Hz, 40 dB at 4000 Hz, 20 dB at 6000 Hz, and 10 dB at 8000 Hz. On Monday morning it may be found that instead of returning to zero dB at all frequencies, his hearing levels are 10 dB at 3000 Hz, 20 dB at 4000 Hz, and 10 dB at 6000 Hz. In other words, this worker is now demonstrating some "permanent" noise-induced hearing loss in addition to a TTS. The word "permanent" is enclosed in quotation marks, because it is possible that if this worker were removed from his noisy work environment for a period of several weeks or months his hearing might gradually return to its former levels. On the other hand, it might not. One thing is sure: if this hypothetical worker remains in his noisy job for a period of several years, the degree of his permanent hearing loss will increase both in the depth and width of the notch until the speech frequencies are affected and the worker realizes that he is in fact hard of hearing. Figure 9-1 demonstrates a typical progression in hearing loss due to noise exposure with the passage of time.

What is particularly insidious about noise-induced hearing loss is that it can occur without the affected individual's being aware that his hearing is being damaged. As we saw in Chapter 2, sound does not become uncomfortably loud for most people until it reaches a sound pressure level of 120 dB, and it does not produce pain until the sound pressure level reaches at least 140 dB. Unfortunately, sound pressure levels of considerably less than 120 dB can produce permanent damage to the ear in time. No one would endure sound pressure levels in excess of 120 dB for long because of the discomfort, but we might be willing to work indefinitely in noise levels of 95 to 100 dB without suspecting that the noise was damaging us in any way.

Another way in which noise-induced hearing loss is insidious is that almost invariably the first evidence of damage to the ears is found in the frequencies above the speech range. One can incur a substantial loss at frequencies above 2000 Hz without being aware of any difficulty in communication under good listening conditions. Only when the notch widens to include 2000 Hz is there any noticeable effect on our hearing for speech. Most people would not complain of being hard of hearing until there is some noticeable effect on their understanding of speech. By the time 2000 Hz is involved, there may be a considerable degree of permanent noise-induced hearing loss in the higher frequencies.

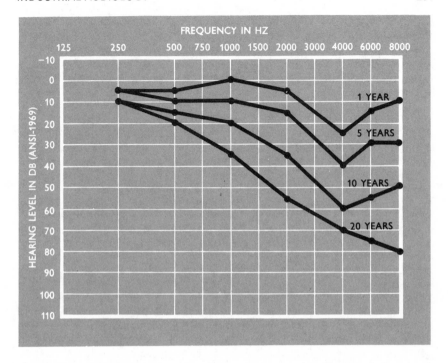

Figure 9-1.   Typical progression in hearing loss as a function of years of exposure to industrial noise of high intensity. Both ears would be affected similarly.

In advanced stages, noise-induced hearing loss may produce a sharply sloping audiogram curve for frequencies above 500 Hz. While initially there is a notch effect, with the greatest loss somewhere between 3000 and 6000 Hz, in time the notch tends to become obliterated, so that the audiogram of the individual with noise-induced hearing loss becomes indistinguishable from other sensori-neural losses. Thus the individual with noise-induced hearing loss that extends into the speech frequencies has problems in communication that are characteristic of those with typical sensori-neural impairment— primarily problems of speech discrimination. Because the hearing at 500 Hz and below is usually not affected, a hearing aid may not be of much help.

THE MEDICOLEGAL PROBLEM

History

Following the lead of several European countries, the United States in 1908 enacted the first workmen's compensation law under which civilian employees of the federal government were protected against economic loss arising out of accidental injuries incurred on the job. By 1915 some thirty states had formulated workmen's compensation laws, and by 1949 all of the states had enacted compensation legislation.[3] Originally, compensation laws covered only accidental injuries, but subsequently the laws of most states were expanded to include occupational disease. In some states occupational diseases covered under the compensation laws were specified in "schedules," while in other states the coverage was expanded to include any occupational disease which the claimant could prove was caused by his employment. In order to qualify for benefits under either the accidental injury or occupational disease provision of workmen's compensation, a claimant had to establish a loss of earnings.

When a loss of hearing is associated with a blast or single traumatic incident, it is clearly covered under the accidental injury provision of workmen's compensation. In cases involving the gradual onset of hearing impairment associated with one's occupation, the occupational disease provision of workmen's compensation would be applicable in those states where the definition of occupational disease is sufficiently broad to include noise-induced hearing impairment. In some states, a ruling has been made that a gradual hearing impairment associated with one's occupation is actually a series of separate "accidents" the effect of which is cumulative, so that such a noise-induced hearing impairment is held to be an accidental injury.

In 1948, a new principle in workmen's compensation was established through a ruling of the New York Court of Appeals by which compensation for a noise-induced hearing loss was awarded to a claimant who had not lost any time from his job and had thus demonstrated no loss of his earnings. This decision resulted in the filing of many claims in New York State for noise-induced hearing impairment.[4] In the early 1950's a similar decision was rendered in Wisconsin. In both New York and Wisconsin, special legislation was enacted to establish a basis for compensating employees for occupational loss of hearing, rather than depending on the broad coverage provided by the laws relating to occupational diseases in general. In 1959 the state of Missouri followed the lead of New York and Wisconsin in writing special legislation to cover the problem of occupational hearing loss. Now in all but fifteen states there are legislative provisions for compensation for occupational hearing loss, and in two of the fifteen under certain circumstances a worker can receive compensation for noise-induced hearing impairment.[5] In general, the legislation that has been

[3] Harry A. Nelson, "Legal Liability for Loss of Hearing," Cyril M. Harris, ed., *Handbook of Noise Control* (New York, McGraw-Hill, 1957), Chap. 38, p. 4.

[4] Charles R. Williams, "Medicolegal Aspects," in Joseph Sataloff, *Industrial Deafness* (New York, McGraw-Hill, 1957), Chap. 5, p. 53.

[5] Meyer S. Fox, "Hearing Loss Statutes in the United States and Canada," in Appendix to *Guide for the Conservation of Hearing in Noise*, Supplement to the *Transactions of the American Academy of Ophthalmology and Otolaryngology*, 1969.

enacted by other states recognizes the principles of compensation established in New York, Wisconsin, and Missouri. Let us, therefore, examine briefly the provisions of the laws of these three states.

Provisions of the Law in New York, Wisconsin, and Missouri[6]

In all three states, noise-induced hearing loss was considered to be an occupational disease, and a schedule of benefits was outlined. The principle that compensation is dependent on demonstrated wage loss was abandoned. In Wisconsin and Missouri the new schedules reduced the amount of compensation payable for complete or partial loss of hearing in comparison to what the law provides in cases of traumatic hearing loss, but in New York no differentiation was made between the amount payable for occupational hearing loss and for traumatic hearing loss. In Wisconsin and Missouri, the "date of disablement" is considered to be the last day of a six months' period of separation from the noisy work that caused the hearing impairment, while in New York it is the last day of a six months' period following separation from the employment in which the noise exposure was received. In New York, in other words, there is no date of disability until the employee terminates his relation with the employer. In Wisconsin and Missouri, the purpose of the six months' waiting period is to allow for any recovery of hearing once the claimant has been removed from his noisy work environment. In New York, in addition to serving this purpose, the six months' waiting period following cessation of employment in which the exposure was incurred permits the employer to spread out the payment of awards over a period of time and helps to solve the problem of "accrued liability" by providing more time to meet financial obligations for which no provision had been made by employers or insurance companies during the years while liability was accruing. According to Symons, there is an additional advantage in the New York system, since employers are encouraged to institute noise control procedures without facing the danger that such procedures will focus workers' attention on noise problems and produce a flood of claims for noise-induced hearing loss.[7]

The laws hold the last employer liable for all of a claimant's noise-induced hearing impairment, unless that employer can present evidence that the employee had some hearing impairment at the time he commenced employment with him. If it can be demonstrated that the claimant incurred some of his hearing impairment in previous work situations, then those employers are held responsible for their "share" of the claimant's hearing impairment. This provision of the laws points up the importance of employers' instituting hearing testing as part of the physical examination

[6] *Background for Loss of Hearing Claims* (Chicago, American Mutual Insurance Alliance, 1964), pp. 1-7.

[7] Noel S. Symons, "Workmen's Compensation Benefits for Occupational Hearing Loss," *Noise Control*, Vol. 4 (September, 1958), pp. 29 and 30.

procedure for all new employees. A given employer can then be held responsible for only that amount of hearing impairment an employee incurs after
he commences work for that employer.

The states of New York, Wisconsin, and Missouri have all adopted
the so-called AAOO method of computing percentage of hearing loss for
purposes of determining degree of disability. It will be recalled from
Chapter 5 that this method utilizes the average dB loss through the frequencies of 500, 1000, and 2000 Hz. As illustrated in Figure 5-12, the
percentage loss in each ear is determined by subtracting 26 dB from the
average dB loss through these three frequencies and then multiplying the
remainder by $1\frac{1}{2}$ per cent. Binaural percentage hearing loss is computed by
weighting the better ear five times the poorer ear.

A question that confronted the legislatures of the three states with which we
are concerned was whether or not to make an allowance for presbycusis in
determining an employer's liability for an employee's hearing impairment.
In New York no allowance is made for presbycusis. In Wisconsin, the practice for a number of years was to deduct from the percentage of compensable
hearing loss $\frac{1}{2}$ per cent for each year of age over fifty. Wisconsin then changed
its procedure and ceased to make any allowance for presbycusis. The Missouri
law provides that before the percentage of hearing loss is determined, $\frac{1}{2}$ dB
for each year of age over forty shall be subtracted from the total average dB
loss. The calculation is made on the basis of the employee's age at the time of
his last exposure to industrial noise. At the present time (1970) seventeen
states make corrections for presbycusis, either on a formula basis as in
Missouri, or on the basis of medical evidence.[8] As more research information
is accumulated concerning the effect of the aging process on human hearing,
it can be anticipated that the laws of the various states will become uniform
on the matter of making allowances for prebycusis in determining compensable hearing impairment.

In arriving at the amount of money an employee should receive as compensation for occupational hearing loss, reference must be made to the
schedule of compensation payments established for complete loss of hearing.
The amount of compensation due to a particular claimant then depends on
the percentage of hearing impairment he demonstrates. Thus, in Missouri,
for example, the schedule calls for the payment of one hundred weeks of
compensation for total occupational deafness of both ears. A claimant who
has a binaural percentage compensable hearing loss of 50 per cent would be
entitled to fifty weeks of compensation. The weighting factor of five for the
better ear utilized in the AAOO formula is demonstrated by the provision
in the Missouri law for only seventeen weeks of compensation payments for
total occupational deafness of one ear, or in other words, about one-fifth of
the allowable compensation for total deafness of both ears.[9]

8 Fox, *op. cit.*
9 *Ibid.*

The States of New York, Wisconsin, and Missouri led the way in legislation to provide compensation for occupational hearing loss. In all three of these states, the legislation enacted was the result of the cooperative efforts of labor, management, and medical and allied medical specialty groups, who joined to produce laws that were fair to both labor and industry and that were predicated on the best scientific information concerning the effect of noise on hearing. It is probably just a matter of time until all fifty states have developed legislation to deal with the economic problem of noise-induced hearing impairment.

NOISE MEASUREMENTS

In order to determine whether or not an employer has a noise hazard problem, it is necessary to obtain accurate measurements of the noise levels at various locations within a factory. In addition to measurements of the overall sound level in a given location, it is necessary to have information concerning the spectral composition of the noise, since the danger of noise depends upon both its intensity and frequency components. Noise measurements are made with an instrument called a sound-level meter, and spectral analyses are made with various kinds of analyzers.

The Sound-Level Meter

"A sound-level meter is an instrument including a microphone, an amplifier, an output meter, and frequency weighting networks for the measurement of noise and sound levels in a specified manner." [10] Measurements obtained with a sound-level meter are referred to as "sound levels," which are weighted sound pressure levels. The weighting networks provide three frequency response characteristics, referred to as A, B, and C, the values of which are specified by the American National Standards Institute.[11] The purpose of the weighting networks is to approximate the loudness function of the human ear at three different intensity levels. The A and B networks resemble equal loudness contours of the normal ear made at loudness levels of 40 and 70 phons, respectively. Network C provides a "flat" frequency response approximating the equal loudness contour at 100 phons. Readings obtained when the C network is employed and the meter is used with a flat response microphone are sound pressure levels. Network A discriminates against low frequencies, and network B is intermediate in low frequency weighting between A and C. Readings obtained with networks A and B are

[10] "American Standard Acoustical Terminology (Including Mechanical Shock and Vibration)," *American Standards Association Bulletin* (S1.1-1960, New York, American Standards Association—now American National Standards Institute).

[11] "General Purpose Sound Level Meters," *American Standards Association Bulletin* (S1.4-1961, New York, American Standards Association—now American National Standards Institute).

"sound levels" rather than sound pressure levels. The weighting network employed in a particular sound-level measurement should always be specified. For example, if a reading of 50 dB were obtained when the A network was used, it should be reported as a sound level of 50 dB(A), or, as seems to be the trend today, simply 50 dBA. Some manufacturers recommend that all three networks be used in measuring every noise. In the past it was customary to use A weighting for levels below 55 dB, B weighting for levels between 55 and 85 dB, and C weighting for levels above 85 dB. Now, however, A weightings are most commonly used regardless of level.[12] Gross information as to the frequency characteristics of the noise being measured may be secured by comparing the sound levels obtained by all three networks. If the readings are essentially the same, the noise is predominantly high frequency in spectrum; that is, its most prominent characteristics lie above 600 Hz. If lower sound-level readings are obtained with the A and B networks than with C, the noise is predominantly of low frequency. The greater the difference between the readings obtained with A and C networks, the more heavily weighted the noise is in the lower frequencies (below 600 Hz).[13] A typical sound-level meter is shown in Figure 9-2.

A sound-level meter is useful for measuring overall sound levels of continuing, or steady-state noises. For measuring the levels of impulsive noises, such as a gun shot, it is necessary to use an impact-noise analyzer in conjunction with a sound-level meter. The meter response of the sound-level meter is too slow to give an accurate reading on an impulsive noise.

Noise Analyzers

The hazard of a particular noise usually cannot be determined without analyzing its frequency components. If a noise survey indicates that the overall sound levels obtained in a particular location are potentially hazardous, then an analysis of the frequency components of the noise is in order. The most commonly used instrument for this purpose is an octave-band analyzer, which, as its name implies, measures the sound levels in various bands, each of which is one octave in width. When this instrument is used with the sound-level meter, the sound levels obtained in these bands are called octave-band levels. The "preferred" octave bands have center frequencies of 31.5, 63, 125, 250, 500, 1000, 2000, 4000, 8000, and 16000 Hz. Older octave-band analyzers included the following bands: 18.75–37.5, 37.5–75, 75–150, 150–300, 300–600, 600–1200, 1200–2400, 2400–4800, 4800–9600, and 9600–19200 Hz. Many test codes specify band levels in terms of the older bands, and considerable data have been reported based on the older series. Octave-band levels reported in the older series can be

[12] Arnold P. G. Peterson and Ervin E. Gross, Jr., *Handbook of Noise Measurement* (West Concord, Mass., General Radio Company, 1967), pp. 8-10, 46.

[13] Charles R. Williams, "Principles of Noise Measurement," in Sataloff, *op. cit.*, Chap. 7, p. 85.

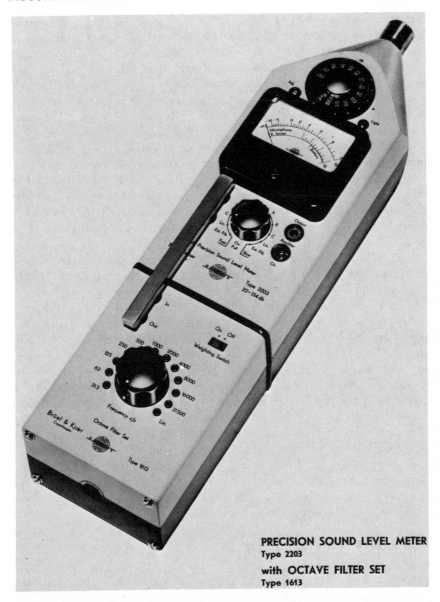

PRECISION SOUND LEVEL METER
Type 2203

with **OCTAVE FILTER SET**
Type 1613

Figure 9-2. A sound-level meter with attached octave filter set—octave-band analyzer. (Reproduced by permission of B & K Instruments, Inc., Cleveland, Ohio.)

converted to octave-band levels based on the preferred center frequencies by referring to a table in the ANSI standard.[14] In Figure 9-2 the octave-band analyzer is attached to the sound-level meter.

In addition to the octave-band analyzer, other types of analyzers are available: half-octave and third-octave analyzers, and continuously tunable narrow-band analyzers that accept a band of only 1/30 octave in width. As the band width of an analyzer becomes narrower, the more precise is the information yielded about the frequency components of a noise. In general, however, the octave-band analyzer yields sufficiently precise information to make judgments concerning the hazard of a particular industrial noise and it is rarely necessary to obtain more detailed information than the octave-band analyzer provides. Figure 9-3 illustrates the difference in the shape of the curves obtained when the same noise is analyzed with both an octave-band analyzer and a half-octave band analyzer.

For industrial noise surveys, generally an octave-band analyzer is used in conjunction with a sound-level meter for analyses in the field. On occasion, however, it is desirable to make a more thorough study of certain industrial noises than can easily be accomplished in the field. In such cases, tape recordings may be made of the noises for later analysis in the laboratory. Such recordings should be made with tape recorders of broadcast quality. If the noise to be analyzed is of relatively short duration, or if only a brief recording has been made, a tape loop can be constructed so that the signal is continually passed over the playback head of the recorder. A take-up reel is suspended in the loop to maintain sufficient pressure of the tape on the playback head. Figure 9-4 illustrates the use of a tape loop. The output of the recorder is fed to the particular analyzer being used. The readings obtained from the analyzer can be recorded as the energy in each band is measured, and the results can then be plotted on graph paper in the manner indicated in Figure 9-3. If a graphic level recorder is available, the energy in each band can be graphed automatically to produce the type of record shown in Figure 9-5.

Conducting a Noise Survey

Noise surveys are conducted usually for two basic reasons: to evaluate the hazard of noise for employees so that suitable protective measures may be taken to conserve hearing, and to obtain information concerning the noisiness of various pieces of machinery or manufacturing processes for the purpose of improving design or improving the method of installation of equipment. In addition to constituting a hazard to hearing, noise may interfere with communication and have other annoying effects. Techniques

[14] "USA Standard Specification for Octave, Half-Octave, and Third-Octave Band Filter Sets," *United States of America Standards Institute Bulletin* (S1.11-1966, New York, United States of America Standards Institute—now American National Standards Institute), Appendix A.

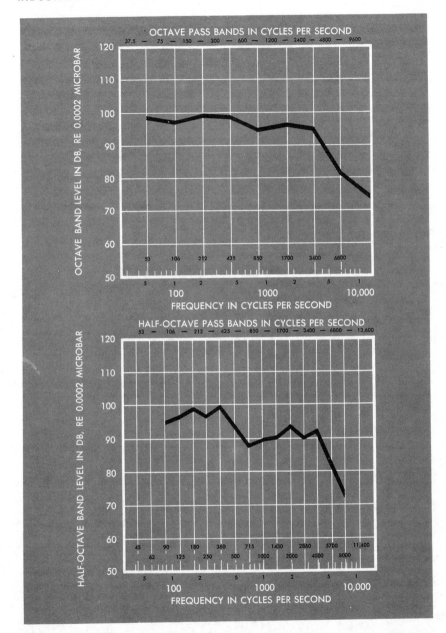

Figure 9-3.   Comparison of octave-band analysis and half-octave band analysis of an industrial noise. (From Lewis S. Goodfriend, "Measurement of Noise," *Noise Control,* Vol. 7 [March-April, 1961]. Used by permission.)

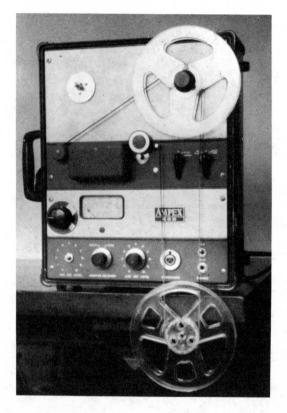

Figure 9-4.   Tape recorder with tape loop. (From Lewis S. Goodfriend, "Measurement of Noise," *Noise Control,* Vol. 7 [March-April, 1961]. Used by permission.)

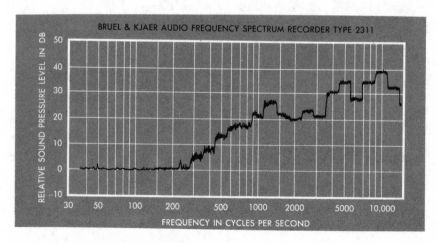

Figure 9-5.   Graphic record of one-third octave analysis of a stream of air. (Reproduced by permission of B & K Instruments, Inc., Cleveland, Ohio.)

have been evolved for translating the results of noise measurements into the subjective effects of the noise on exposed personnel, as we shall see later. In any event, a thorough study of the physical properties of noise is an essential first step to the development of a hearing conservation program, or to the development of noise control procedures.

As Williams has said, noise measurement is an art, requiring not only technical proficiency in the handling of equipment but a considerable amount of judgment in determining where measurements should be made and what kinds of analyses of noises are indicated.[15] Noise measurements should be attempted only by individuals who are thoroughly acquainted with the uses and limitations of the equipment employed and who have an adequate background in the physical principles involved in noise measurement. The instructions contained in various technical manuals in regard to such matters as combining sound intensities, assessing the effect of background noise, choosing the right microphone and knowing what corrections must be made for the particular microphone used, and correcting measurements for cable length, the angle of incidence, and the effects of reflected sound are most bewildering to the novice. The validity of the measurements obtained is in direct proportion to the degree of knowledge on the part of the individual conducting a survey. It is not the purpose of this section to give detailed information concerning the use of measuring equipment, but rather to give the reader some appreciation of what is involved in conducting a noise survey.

The first step is to make sure that all equipment is calibrated and in proper working order. This determination in itself is no simple matter and requires an understanding not only of the particular instruments to be used, but also of the physical principles involved in sound measurement. Once the equipment is found to be performing satisfactorily, then the next step is to select the locations where measurements will be taken. This step is accomplished by obtaining rough measurements of the overall intensity at various positions around the noise source to be evaluated. If the primary purpose of the survey is to assess the hazard to the hearing of the employees who work in the environment, then the microphone placement should approximate the location of employees who work around the sound source. If the purpose of the survey is to derive the total acoustic power output and the directional characteristics of the noise source, the measurements should be made in systematic geometric patterns around the noise source regardless of the location of the employees. In either event, the initial rough measurements of overall intensity may be made with the sound-level meter.

When the locations at which measurements are to be made have been selected, accurate readings of the overall levels at each location are taken with the sound-level meter. The locations at which readings are made

15 Charles R. Williams, "Principles of Noise Measurement," in Sataloff, *op. cit.*, Chap. 7, p. 77.

should be plotted on a floor plan and clearly labeled, so that at some later time the measurements can be duplicated in the same locations. Once the overall sound levels have been recorded at each of the selected locations, the octave-band measurements should be made, or, if the spectral analysis is to be accomplished later in the laboratory, tape recordings should be made at each location. The overall levels of the noise should be checked with the sound-level meter after the octave-band readings are obtained in order to make sure that the noise has not fluctuated appreciably since the time of the initial readings, and also as a check on the accuracy of the first readings. The accuracy of the octave-band analysis should be checked by adding the intensities in each band and comparing the total with the overall sound level obtained at a particular location. The procedure for adding octave-band levels to compare with overall level involves the use of a table that can be found in any manual dealing with the technical aspects of sound measurement.

The recording of the data obtained is most important, since it should be possible for someone else subsequently to duplicate the conditions of any noise survey from the information supplied on a report. The specific items of equipment utilized in the survey should be described by name, model, and even serial number. The settings of the equipment, for example, the weighting network employed and the meter speed utilized in making sound-level measurements, should be specified. The time of day and the duration of the measurements, and any corrections applied for microphone, cable, etc., should be recorded. The environment in which the noise source is located should be completely described, and the location of employees in relation to the noise source and the length of time of their daily exposure to the noise should be recorded. In other words, a complete description of the noise being measured, the way in which the measurements were obtained, and any extraneous factors that may have exerted any influence on the measurements obtained should be included in any report of the results of a noise survey. Williams gives an excellent description of the procedures for conducting a noise survey and recording the results of the survey.[16]

DAMAGE-RISK CRITERIA

For many years experts have sought an answer to the question as to the levels of noise to which the average individual may be exposed during his working lifetime without incurring noise-induced hearing impairment. Those acquainted with the problem of noise-induced hearing impairment realize that there are many factors that must be considered in evaluating the hazard of noise. These include: the overall level of the noise, the frequency composition of the noise, the duration and distribution of exposure to the noise during the work day, and the number of years of exposure

[16] *Ibid.*, Chaps. 7 and 8, pp. 77-112.

during one's lifetime. Another factor to be considered is the range of individual susceptibility to noise-induced hearing loss.[17]

In order to set the stage for the current (1970) thinking on how best to specify noise exposures that are "safe" for one's working lifetime, it will be helpful to review the principal efforts in this direction of the past twenty years. Kryter, in 1950, suggested that an overall measurement of noise level was insufficient to yield information concerning the hazard to hearing presented by a given noise. He underlined the importance of making spectral analyses of noises in estimating their potential danger, and he suggested that the critical bands concept derived from masking experiments might profitably be employed in predicting the degree of hearing impairment from noise exposure. A "critical band" is the narrowest band that just masks out the pure tone that is the central frequency of the band when both the band and the central frequency contain equal sound power. In what he admitted might be a conservative "guess," Kryter suggested that the maximum safe sound pressure level at any critical band for "long and intermittent exposures" was 85 dB.[18]

According to Yaffe and Jones,[19] Parrack introduced the concept of a "damage-risk criterion" about a year after the Kryter monograph appeared, and this concept was elaborated by Rosenblith and Stevens,[20] who proposed allowable safe limits for lifetime exposures for both wide-band and narrow-band noise in terms of octave-band levels. The Rosenblith and Stevens damage-risk criterion has been widely quoted and incorporated into various noise regulations and safety orders. It is reproduced in Figure 9-6.

Rosenblith and Stevens admit that their damage-risk criterion is based on incomplete data, and they anticipate that new curves will be derived from additional laboratory and field data. They do not hold any brief for the exact values plotted in the two curves of Figure 9-6 but feel that they are accurate within ±10 dB. In the Rosenblith and Stevens criterion the assumption is made that the risk of damage is greater for pure-tone stimuli, or noise in which the major portion of the energy is concentrated in a very narrow band of frequencies, than for wide-band noise.

In 1954 there appeared a report by a subcommittee of the American Standards Association that attempted to relate hearing loss to noise exposure based on an analysis of data obtained from workers in industry.[21]

[17] *Guide for the Conservation of Hearing in Noise, op. cit.,* p. 9.

[18] Karl D. Kryter, "The Effects of Noise on Man," *Journal of Speech and Hearing Disorders,* Monograph Supplement 1 (September, 1950), pp. 36 and 37.

[19] Charles D. Yaffe and Herbert H. Jones, *Noise and Hearing* (Washington, D. C., Public Health Service Publication No. 850, U. S. Government Printing Office, 1961), p. 43.

[20] Walter A. Rosenblith and Kenneth N. Stevens, *Handbook of Acoustic Noise Control, Vol. II, Noise and Man* (Wright-Patterson Air Force Base, Ohio, Wright Air Development Center Technical Report 52-204, 1953).

[21] *The Relations of Hearing Loss to Noise Exposure,* Report of the Z24-X-2 Exploratory Subcommittee of the American Standards Association Z24 Sectional Committee on Acoustics, Vibration, and Mechanical Shock (New York, American Standards Association—now American National Standards Institute—1954).

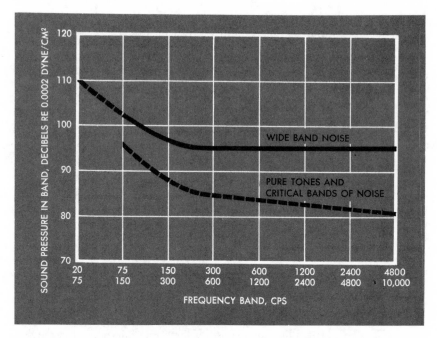

Figure 9-6. Damage-risk criterion for steady noise and for lifetime exposures. (From Walter A. Rosenblith and Kenneth M. Stevens, *Handbook of Acoustic Noise Control,* Vol. II, Technical Report 52-204, Wright Air Development Center, June, 1953. Used by permission.)

"Trend" curves were developed that provided a means of estimating the degree of hearing loss at 1000, 2000, and 4000 Hz to be expected on the average for certain specified years of exposure of workers to steady noise. The hearing levels at 1000 and 2000 Hz were shown to be more closely related to the octave-band level at 300–600 Hz than to any other octave-band level, whereas the hearing level at 4000 Hz was most closely related to the octave-band level at 1200–2400 Hz. The authors reported that they did not attempt to set damage-risk criteria or even to imply that it was possible to specify the limit of safe exposure at that time. Among other questions that the authors of this report raised was the following: "What percentage of the people exposed to industrial noise should a standard be designed to protect? In view of the large individual differences in susceptibility to noise exposure, should a noise standard be aimed at preventing hearing losses in 50 per cent, 90 per cent, or even 99 per cent of the population?"[22] An answer to this question must, of course, be forthcoming before allowable limits of noise exposure can be defined.

[22] *Ibid.,* p. 55.

In 1956 the Air Force issued a regulation defining the limits of allowable noise exposure for Air Force personnel.[23] The allowable lifetime (25 years) limit for an eight-hour day exposure to broad-band noise with ears unprotected was defined as a maximum band-pressure level of 85 dB at each of four octave bands: 300–600, 600–1200, 1200–2400, and 2400–4800 Hz. The Air Force recommends that when the band-pressure level in any of these bands exceeds 85 dB, personnel should wear ear protectors. When the band-pressure level in any of these bands reaches 95 dB the use of ear protectors is mandatory. Based on the assumption that a short exposure to a noise of high intensity is equal in its injurious effect to a long exposure to a noise of lesser intensity, the Air Force regulation presents a method for calculating the allowable exposure time limits without ear protection for various band-pressure levels in excess of 85 dB by converting them to values equivalent to an eight-hour day of exposure to band-pressure levels of 85 dB. The same thing is done for allowable exposure time limits with ear protection for various band-pressure levels in excess of 95 dB. By using a nomogram reproduced in the Air Force regulation, one can determine the allowable or "safe" time limit with or without ear protection for exposure to any given noise whose spectrum is known. The time limits are expressed in terms of the number of minutes a day to which personnel can be exposed to given noise intensities. Different allowances are made for different kinds of ear protectors, and an allowance is made also when the noise is found to be of the narrow-band type. The Air Force regulation employed the "equal energy hypothesis" that trades duration of exposure with intensity level of the stimulus. In other words, according to this hypothesis, the hazard to the hearing is the same for a stimulus of I intensity and D duration as it would be for a stimulus of 2I intensity and D/2 duration. By referring to Table 2-2 in Chapter 2, it can be seen that doubling intensity (power ratio) produces an increase of 3 dB. Thus, if a damage-risk criterion specifies that an exposure to an octave-band level of 85 dB for eight hours a day is allowable, the following exposures would also be allowable: 88 dB for four hours, 91 dB for two hours, 94 dB for one hour, 97 dB for thirty minutes, 100 dB for fifteen minutes, etc.

The Subcommittee on Noise in Industry in 1957 stated that because of the limited information regarding the relations between noise exposure and hearing impairment it was not possible to specify "safe" levels of exposure. The Subcommittee took cognizance of the findings that workers exposed to noise tended to develop hearing impairments at frequencies higher than the dominant frequency of the noise stimulus. On the premise that it was most important to protect workers' hearing at the speech frequencies (500, 1000, and 2000 Hz), the Subcommittee suggested that the octave-band levels at the two bands of 300–600 and 600–1200 Hz were the most important to consider

23 *Hazardous Noise Exposure*, Air Force Regulation No. 160-3 (Washington, D.C., Department of the Air Force, 29 October 1956).

in the development of damage-risk criteria.ⁱThe Subcommittee then proposed the following "tentative hearing conservation level," to be applied
only in the case of long term exposure to broad-band steady noises that have
comparatively flat spectra: [24]

> If the sound energy of the noise is distributed more or less evenly throughout the
> eight octave bands, and if a person is to be exposed to this noise regularly for many
> hours a day, five days a week for many years, then: if the noise level in either the
> 300–600 cycle band or the 600–1200 cycle band is 85 dB, the initiation of noise-
> exposure control and tests of hearing is advisable. The more the octave band levels
> exceed 85 dB the more urgent is the need for hearing conservation.

The Subcommittee points out that the 85 dB level it specifies applies only to
the octave-band levels in two bands; that the over-all sound pressure level
of a noise may be as much as 20 dB higher than the level in a particular
octave band.

Rudmose, in 1957, reviewed the report of the Z24-X-2 Exploratory Subcommittee of the American Standards Association (now the American
National Standards Association), referred to previously in this section, and
suggested a method for determining "safe" exposure limits.[25] His method is
based on the "trend curves" for estimating hearing loss developed by the
ASA Subcommittee, on data derived from hearing studies conducted at the
Wisconsin State Fair, and on the principles of relating hearing impairment
to compensation that were established by the Advisory Medical Committee
to the State of Wisconsin at the time when that state was developing regulations for adjudicating claims for noise-induced hearing impairment. Rudmose
assumes that industry should aim to protect 80 per cent of the workers, or in
other words that efforts should be made to control noise to the point where
no more than 20 per cent of the workers would incur compensable hearing
impairment. Since the Wisconsin regulations related compensation to impairment only through the frequencies of 500, 1000, and 2000 Hz, the
Rudmose method concentrates on the 300–600 Hz octave band which Subcommittee Z24-X-2 had found to be most closely related to hearing impairment for frequencies below 4000 Hz. Based on a number of assumptions,
some of which would be untenable in certain circumstances, Rudmose
developed a series of charts showing the percentage of compensable hearing
loss (by the Wisconsin standards of that time) that would be equalled or
exceeded by 20 per cent of a group of workers as related to the band-pressure
level in the 300–600 Hz octave band and the number of years of exposure.
Separate charts were constructed for different age groups, thus reflecting the

---

[24] *Guide for the Conservation of Hearing in Noise* (Los Angeles, Subcommittee on Noise in
Industry of the Committee on Conservation of Hearing, and Research Center, Subcommittee
on Noise in Industry, 1957), pp. 14 and 15.

[25] Wayne Rudmose, "Hearing Loss Resulting from Noise Exposure," in Harris, *op. cit.*,
Chap. 7.

effect of presbycusis.[26] While from these charts it is possible to derive damage-risk criteria (for the 300–600 Hz octave band only), Rudmose is more interested in proposing a method for industry, or actually society, to employ in arriving at damage-risk criteria than he is in suggesting a specific criterion. He says,

It is hoped that Fig. 7-9 [the charts referred to above] will form the foundation for industry to set its own criteria for noise exposure. It is obvious that no single number can be chosen as an undeniable criterion. Whether the matter is one of fully protecting 80 or 90 per cent of the workers or just 50 per cent is a policy decision industry must make. Certainly it seems reasonable that industry will try to protect as high a percentage of its employees as possible.[27]

Rosenwinkel and Stewart conducted a study of some 270 workers in a large machine shop, relating their audiograms to the length of time on the job and using a group of 290 office workers with the same distribution of ages as controls. The spectrum of the noise to which the experimental group was exposed was relatively flat through eight octave bands, with the highest octave-band level at 80 dB (300–600 Hz octave band). The authors asked the question: "Does a continuous occupational exposure to a steady state noise of 80 dB per octave band cause a measurable change in pure tone hearing sensitivity during man's normal working life span?" Their data showed that while the differences between the experimental and control groups were minimal up to a mean exposure time of 16 years, comparisons between the groups indicate increasingly greater differences as the time of exposure increases beyond 16 years. The groups differ significantly, however, only for the frequencies higher than 2000 Hz. The group that had a mean exposure time of 34 years demonstrated hearing levels at 4000 Hz that exceeded the control group's hearing levels at that frequency by an average of 25 dB. The authors concluded that while the experimental group's average hearing loss did not fall within the compensable range even for the longest exposure times, the difference between the hearing levels of the experimental and control groups at 4000 Hz demonstrated that exposure to steady-state noise that does not exceed a level of 80 dB in any octave band can produce measurable reduction in hearing sensitivity over a normal working life span.[28]

In 1961, Yaffe and Jones reported on a study of the hearing acuity of prisoners who were exposed to various kinds of noisy work environments in federal prisons. The study was conducted over a period of seven years. The authors relate their data on shift in hearing level in prisoners in various working environments to various published damage-risk criteria and

[26] *Ibid.*, p. 12.

[27] *Ibid.*, p. 13.

[28] N. E. Rosenwinkel and K. C. Stewart, "The Relationship of Hearing Loss to Steady State Noise Exposure," *American Industrial Hygiene Association Quarterly*, Vol. 18 (September, 1957), pp. 227-230.

reach the conclusion that their data lend considerable support to the criterion for exposure to wide-band noise that had been proposed in 1953 by Rosenblith and Stevens (see Figure 9-6). Their findings did not justify a lowering of the criterion for narrow-band noise, however, as Rosenblith and Stevens had proposed. Yaffe and Jones also agree with the recommendations of the Subcommittee on Noise in Industry that hearing conservation measures should be instituted when steady-state broad-band noise is characterized by octave-band levels as high as 85 dB.[29]

As can be seen by a comparison of the sources cited in this section, there is not yet agreement on the levels of noise to which workers may be exposed over long periods of time without incurring hearing impairment. If one is concerned only with compensable hearing impairment, then it would appear from the Rosenwinkel and Stewart study that octave-band levels of 80 dB and less are "safe," at least for the average worker over a lifetime of work exposure. One can only speculate as to what Rosenwinkel and Stewart would have concluded if they had applied Rudmose's principle of protecting 80 per cent of the workers. It is possible that 20 per cent of their experimental group might have incurred sufficient hearing impairment to warrant compensation from noise exposure that did not exceed 80 dB in any octave band. The Rosenblith and Stevens criterion has been widely quoted, and as we have just seen, the Yaffe and Jones study lends it considerable support. Yet even Yaffe and Jones favor the adoption of the more conservative practice advocated by the Subcommittee on Noise in Industry of becoming concerned when octave-band levels reach 85 dB. Air Force Regulation 160-3 represents a reasonable compromise between the Rosenblith and Stevens criterion and the recommendations of the Subcommittee on Noise in Industry in recommending the use of ear protectors when octave-band levels exceed 85 dB, and requiring the use of ear protectors when octave-band levels reach 95 dB.

In 1961, Glorig, Ward, and Nixon proposed damage-risk criteria for continuous steady-noise exposures for five hours a day, five days a week for many years; continuous steady-noise exposures for less than five hours a day, five days a week for many years; and steady-noise that is intermittently on during the day, five days a week for many years.[30] Their recommendations are based on extensive research relating TTS to PTS (permanent threshold shift) and set the pattern for later thinking in regard to industrial hearing conservation.

Glorig, Ward, and Nixon's damage-risk criteria are based on research findings that if a worker demonstrates no "significant" TTS at the end of a day's exposure to noise, he will not develop a PTS for "habitual"

---

[29] Yaffe and Jones, *op. cit.*

[30] Aram Glorig, W. Dixon Ward, and James Nixon, "Damage Risk Criteria and Noise-Induced Hearing Loss," *A.M.A. Archives of Otolaryngology,* Vol. 74 (October, 1961), pp. 413-423.

exposure to that noise over a period of years. While most TTS studies have been concerned with 4000 Hz, the frequency that generally shows the greatest loss from noise exposure, Glorig, Ward, and Nixon propose using the TTS at 2000 Hz for predicting PTS at 2000 Hz, and their criteria are based on avoiding PTS at 2000 Hz resulting from a lifetime noise exposure for 85 to 90 per cent of the exposed population. Their reasoning for employing 2000 Hz instead of 4000 Hz for TTS and PTS studies is twofold: (1) PTS for 4000 Hz reaches a maximum after 10 to 12 years, regardless of the level of the exposure noise; beyond this time further increases in hearing level at 4000 Hz seem to be a function of aging. (2) 2000 Hz is the highest of the "speech frequencies," and hearing conservation measures should be aimed at protecting the worker's ability to hear and understand speech; generally, the frequencies above 2000 Hz are "expendable," in the sense that they are not important in communication by speech.

The criterion for steady (not impulsive) noise that is on for more than five hours a day is the International Organization for Standardization Noise Rating Number 85 (N-85). This refers to curves of octave-band levels covering a range from N-0 to N-130 in steps of 5 numbers. The numbers coincide with the sound pressure level in dB re 0.0002 dyne/cm^2 for the octave band centered on the frequency of 1000 Hz. The curves of noise rating, which bear a resemblance to the sound pressure level graphs of phon curves, were based on various studies and "educated opinions" of acoustical consultants from several countries and unanimously accepted by the group of consultants meeting in Stuttgart in 1959 under the aegis of the International Organization for Standardization. A noise having a rating of N-85 would have the following maximum levels at each octave band:[31]

Octave Mid-Frequency, Hz	Sound Pressure Level, dB	Octave Mid-Frequency, Hz	Sound Pressure Level, dB
63	102	1000	85
125	95	2000	82
250	91	4000	80
500	87	8000	79

The noise exposure criterion applicable to steady noise that is on less than five hours a day is determined from data relating noise rating numbers and exposure time in minutes (up to 300 minutes) with the amount of TTS at 2000 Hz. After the "acceptable" amount of TTS at 2000 Hz has been decided, one can determine from the data how many minutes' exposure to a noise of a given rating is allowable to avoid PTS at 2000 Hz over a period of years of such exposure. Glorig, Ward, and Nixon suggest that 12 dB should be the maximum allowable TTS at 2000 Hz as measured at the end of a working day. According to studies relating TTS

31 *Ibid.*, p. 421.

and PTS, this criterion of allowable TTS will not result in any significant PTS at 2000 Hz for habitual exposure.

Additional data enable one to determine the relations between the "on-time," "off-time," and number of exposure cycles (combinations of on-time and off-time) allowable for exposure to intermittent steady-noise of particular noise ratings. Glorig, Ward, and Nixon's criteria are based on recommendations of the International Organization for Standardization, which has also proposed methods of utilizing the noise rating numbers for determining the effect of noise on communication, and the annoyance effect of noise.

In 1966, Kryter *et al.* published the recommendations of a working group of the National Academy of Science–National Research Council Committee on Hearing, Bioacoustics, and Biomechanics (NAS–NRS CHABA, usually identified simply as CHABA).[32] The working group was established as the result of a request to CHABA by the Office of the Surgeon General of the U.S. Army to "reevaluate, on the basis of new knowledge in this field, the question of damage-risk criteria for exposure to sound." The working group adopted as its basic criterion the acceptability of noise exposures that would result in noise-induced permanent threshold shifts (NIPTS) after ten years of near-daily exposure of no more than 10 dB at 1000 Hz or lower frequencies, 15 dB at 2000 Hz, or 20 dB at 3000 Hz or higher frequencies. The working group believed that if the median NIPTS could be held at these levels, only 20 per cent of workers exposed to levels of noise producing this median amount of NIPTS would incur compensable hearing impairments in a lifetime of work. The assumption was made that NIPTS from a particular noise environment over a period of years would be no greater than TTS measured two minutes after a full working day's exposure to that environment. In other words, it was assumed that essentially $TTS_2 = NIPTS_{10yr}$, so that a given noise environment would be safe if it resulted in median TTS_2's of no more than 10 dB at 1000 Hz and lower, 15 dB at 2000 Hz, and 20 dB at 3000 Hz and higher. Based on field studies of NIPTS of workers in industries and laboratory studies of TTS, the working group then developed a series of damage risk contours for various conditions of steady-state and intermittent noise exposures. With spectral information on the noise, one can determine from the contours the maximum allowable time per day for exposure to steady-state or intermittent noise, or the maximum allowable level for short bursts of noise (two minutes or less in duration), or the amount of intervening quiet required between long bursts of noise (more than two minutes).

Botsford combined and consolidated the CHABA contours into fewer graphs. As a further simplification he suggested the use of A-weighted

[32] K. D. Kryter, W. Dixon Ward, James D. Miller, and Donald H. Eldredge, "Hazardous Exposure to Intermittent and Steady-State Noise," *Journal of the Acoustical Society of America,* Vol. 39 (March, 1966), pp. 451-464.

sound levels, instead of octave- or third-octave-band levels, which makes possible the combining of the CHABA contours into a single graph specifying the total allowable on-time per day and the allowable number of exposure cycles per day for manufacturing noises of various dBA levels.[33] While casting some doubt on the usefulness of TTS_2 as a predictor of NIPTS, Eldredge and Miller support the notion of utilizing equinoxious contours based on TTS data which "allow us to chart our way through the complexities introduced by brief exposures, rest periods away from noise, etc., and provide the best guides to safety that we have." [34]

More research is needed before we can state with any great certainty that a specific proportion of workers will develop compensable hearing impairments when exposed for a certain period of time to noise that has certain characteristics. More research is particularly needed to understand the relationships between hearing impairment and intermittent exposure to wide-band noise (as contrasted with continuous exposure), exposure to narrow-band continuous and intermittent noise, and exposure to impulsive or impact noises. In the meantime, the problem of compensation for noise-induced hearing impairment is with us, and the federal and state governments and industries are having to make arbitrary decisions based on what data are available.

In May, 1969, the federal government put into effect an addition to the Walsh-Healey Public Contracts Act that places limitations on noise levels permissible in plants that have federal contracts in excess of $10,000.[35] Noise exposures are expressed in dBA with meter on slow response. Contours are provided for translating octave-band levels into dBA values. Table 9-1 gives the allowable noise exposures under the Walsh-Healey Act.

Table 9-1. Permissible daily noise exposures according to the Walsh-Healey Act.

Duration per day, hours	Sound level, dBA
8	90
6	92
4	95
3	97
2	100
$1\frac{1}{2}$	102
1	105
$\frac{1}{2}$	110
$\frac{1}{4}$ or less	115

[33] James H. Botsford, "Simple Method for Identifying Acceptable Noise Exposures," *Journal of the Acoustical Society of America*, Vol. 42 (October, 1967), pp. 810-819.

[34] Donald H. Eldredge and James D. Miller, "Acceptable Noise Exposures—Damage Risk Criteria," in W. Dixon Ward and James E. Fricke, eds., *Noise as a Public Health Hazard*, *ASHA Reports 4* (Washington, The American Speech and Hearing Association, 1969), pp. 110-120.

[35] *Federal Register*, Vol. 34, No. 96, 7891-7954, May 20, 1969. Rules and Regulations 50-204.10.

Note that the Walsh-Healey Act criteria depart from the equal energy principle, or what has come to be known as the 3-dB rule. The equal energy principle has been considered by many to be overly conservative, since it does not take into account the recovery from fatigue that occurs during periods of relative quiet or harmless noise between bursts of intense noise. According to the equal energy theory, the hazard is the same from an eight-hour continuous exposure to 90 dBA of noise as it is for four one-hour exposures to 93 dBA of noise distributed over an eight-hour day. The Walsh-Healey Act adopts a 5-dB rule that presumably compensates for the decreased hazard of an intermittent noise. Thus, according to the Walsh-Healey Act, 90 dBA of continuous exposure for eight hours is equivalent to four hours of 95 dBA exposure in an eight-hour day, whether that exposure is continuous or intermittent. In the 1969 revision of the *Guide for the Conservation of Hearing in Noise,* tables for determining acceptable noise exposures for less than eight hours a day based on dBA sound levels are given according to both the 3-dB rule and the 5-dB rule.[36]

The Walsh-Healey Act specifies a method for evaluating the cumulative effect of a series of exposures of different dBA levels and durations in terms of the criterion measure of a continuous eight-hour exposure to 90 dBA of noise. The method assumes a continuous monitoring of plant noise with a sound-level meter and keeping a record of the duration of each exposure in excess of 90 dBA. The ratio of actual exposure time to allowable exposure time for each dBA level is computed. These ratios are then summed for the day. If the sum does not exceed unity (1.0), the Walsh-Healey criterion has been met.[37] For example, assume that during an eight-hour day workers were exposed to the following dBA levels for the indicated times: 95 dBA for $1\frac{1}{2}$ hours, 97 dBA for 1 hour, and 105 dBA for 15 minutes ($\frac{1}{4}$ hour). The following ratios of actual to allowable exposure times in hours would then be as follows (the allowable time taken from Table 9-1): 1.5/4, 1/3, and .25/1. These ratios reduce to .375, .333, and .250, respectively, and their sum is .958. Since this sum is less than 1.0, the Walsh-Healey criterion has not been exceeded. While the kind of monitoring required to evaluate plant noise in terms of the Walsh-Healey provisions can be done with a sound-level meter and a watch, a much more convenient method is to utilize a graphic recorder in conjunction with a sound-level meter. Presumably, the microphone of the meter would be placed in a location representing the average position of workers exposed to the noise, since it would not be feasible to conduct measurements at the ear level of every worker. The Walsh-Healey Act states that where noise levels are found in excess of those permissible, "feasible administrative or engineering controls shall be utilized." If these fail to reduce the noise levels to acceptable values, then

---

[36] *Guide for the Conservation of Hearing in Noise,* 1969, *op. cit.,* pp. 17-20.
[37] *Federal Register, op. cit.*

"personal protective equipment shall be provided and used." [38] Incidentally, the Walsh-Healey Act specifies that exposure to impulsive noise should not exceed 140 dB peak sound pressure level.

Following the lead of the federal government, the state of California in 1970 rewrote its standards for occupational noise exposure to specify the same allowable exposures to intermittent or continuous noise that were incorporated in the addition to the Walsh-Healey Act and reproduced in Table 9-1.[39] The 1970 revision replaced the standards for occupational noise exposure that had been in effect in California since November, 1962. The exposure levels specified in the 1962 orders had been exactly those proposed in 1953 by Rosenblith and Stevens and reproduced in Figure 9-6. Also, the 1962 standards had incorporated the equal energy concept (halving exposure time increases the permissible exposure level by 3 dB). Thus the 1970 revision lowers the allowable exposure level for an eight-hour day from band levels of 95 dB to sound levels of 90 dBA and substitutes the 5-dB rule for the 3-dB rule.

It is likely that at some future date the Walsh-Healey Act will reduce the allowable exposure level for an eight-hour day from 90 dBA to 85 dBA. On December 29, 1970, the President of the United States signed into law an Occupational Safety and Health Act that extends to all manufacturing plants engaging in interstate commerce the safety and health standards now required of U.S. Government contractors through the Walsh-Healey Act. Thus some 55 million workers will now receive the protection to their hearing afforded by the provisions of the Walsh-Healey Act.

Ward reported on a series of experiments in which TTS and recovery time were studied with a group of twelve normal-hearing young adults. The purpose of the experiments was to validate the damage-risk contours for steady and intermittent noise exposures that had been developed by the CHABA working group.[40] Specifically, Ward wished to see if the various CHABA contours were in fact accurate in predicting median TTS_2's of 10 dB at 1000 Hz and below, 15 dB at 2000 Hz, or 20 dB at 3000 Hz and above. He found that the CHABA contours are appropriate for eight hours of steady continuous noise. The contours for eight-hour exposures to intermittent noise consisting of short bursts are apparently accurate in terms of predicted TTS_2's, but when the stimulus is a band of high frequencies (1400–2000 Hz) and the band level exceeds 100 dB, the recovery time to pre-exposure hearing levels may exceed sixteen hours, meaning that workers would begin a workday with some residual TTS. It was for intermittent noises consisting of longer bursts that the CHABA contours were most in error, since even for

[38] *Ibid.*, 50-204.10(b).

[39] Revision of "Noise Control Safety Orders," Group 6.1, "General Industry Safety Orders" (Division of Industrial Safety, State of California Human Relations Agency, Department of Industrial Relations), effective September 19, 1970.

[40] Kryter *et al.*, *op. cit.*

exposures of relatively low intensity the recovery time for TTS_2 was significantly longer than had been assumed in the formulation of the contours. Ward suggests that the CHABA contours for longer bursts—and Botsford's derived single set of curves[41]—should be revised, since Ward's findings indicate that the longer the duration of the bursts, the shorter should be the allowable cumulative daily exposure time. Ward concluded that TTS_2 was not a satisfactory measure to employ in evaluating the hazard of noise exposure. Because of the delayed recovery time from longer noise bursts and from shorter bursts of high frequency and high intensity, he suggests that TTS measured at some longer interval than two minutes following a day's exposure should be employed. While ideally TTS_{1000}—sixteen hours later—should be the measure used to assure that workers would not begin a day with some residual TTS, Ward reports that TTS_{30} would have been adequate to rank-order the TTS's of the subjects in his experiment. From inspecting the recovery curves of his subjects, Ward concluded that the CHABA contours should be constructed so that a particular allowable exposure would produce no more than median TTS_{30}'s of 5 dB at 1000 Hz and lower, 7.5 dB at 2000 Hz, or 10 dB at 3000 Hz and higher. In passing, Ward observed that the 5-dB rule utilized in the Walsh-Healey Act is as erroneous in underprotecting for steady noise as the 3-dB rule is in overprotecting for intermittent noises. He believes that the CHABA method of presenting damage-risk criteria—with suitable modifications based on his and others' research—is at present superior to other methods of predicting the hazard of intermittent noise exposure that ignore the temporal distribution of energy, that is, the length of noise bursts, and the intervals between noise bursts.[42]

Thus concludes our review of the development of damage-risk criteria for the past twenty years. In some respects we have made little progress in defining the "safe" limits of noise exposure from the time that Kryter suggested that the maximum allowable critical-band level for continuous steady-state noise should be 85 dB, or Rosenblith and Stevens placed the safe limit for wide-band noise at 95 dB for the octave band 300–600 Hz and higher octave bands. As Ward said at the 1968 Conference on Noise as a Public Health Hazard, ". . . when the worker's noise environment is below 80 dBA, the probability is zero that the noise caused his hearing loss; when the level has been 95 dBA, the probability is about 50 per cent. At 105 dBA, steady, continuous exposure produces losses in nearly all men who are habitually exposed."[43] The earlier attempts to specify damage-risk criteria largely ignored intermittent noise. We now know that the temporal distribution of energy in intermittent noise is important, and that we cannot

41 Botsford, *op. cit.*

42 W. Dixon Ward, "Temporary Threshold Shift and Damage-Risk Criteria for Intermittent Noise Exposures," *Journal of the Acoustical Society of America*, Vol. 48 (August, 1970), pp. 561-574.

43 W. Dixon Ward, "Effects of Noise on Hearing Thresholds," in Ward and Fricke, eds., *op. cit.*, p. 44.

assume that any fixed rule for equating intermittent to continuous noise (such as the 3-dB or 5-dB rules) will be suitable. Probably the answer to predicting the hazard of intermittent noise will lie in the development of damage-risk contours of the type proposed by CHABA, or perhaps simplified as Botsford has suggested. But, as Ward in his 1970 article points out, the present contours need revision based on further research relating TTS and NIPTS. We can anticipate revisions in present federal and state regulations regarding noise exposures as new information becomes available.

INTERFERENCE OF NOISE WITH COMMUNICATION

Quite apart from the potentially damaging effects of noise exposure to the hearing, noise can create problems that require noise-control procedures. One of these problems concerns interference with speech. Because of the obvious importance of maintaining adequate communication in military activities, a great deal of research on the interference effects of noise on speech has been sponsored by the Army, Navy, and Air Force. Naturally, the importance of maintaining speech communication in the presence of various kinds of noise has been recognized by industries also, and particularly by the American Telephone and Telegraph Company, whose Bell Laboratories have contributed a great deal of our present knowledge of the characteristics of speech and the effects of distortion and masking on speech intelligibility.

In order to make an accurate assessment of the effect of noise on speech communication, it is necessary to conduct speech intelligibility tests with actual talkers and listeners in the presence of the interfering noise. The test materials utilized may be sentences, digits, bisyllabic words, monosyllabic words, or nonsense syllables. The listeners are scored as to the percentage of the speech materials heard correctly, in the manner of scoring discrimination tests in speech audiometry as explained in Chapter 6. Since it is not practical to conduct this kind of testing in the presence of the actual noise with which one is concerned, in practice the noise is recorded and the speech intelligibility testing is performed in the laboratory in the presence of the recorded noise. From such experiments it is known that speech intelligibility is affected by both the intensity and the frequency characteristics of an interfering noise. The relationship between the intensity of the speech and the intensity of the noise is known as the "signal-to-noise ratio," abbreviated S/N. According to Licklider and Miller, "For most noises encountered in practical situations, S/N should exceed 6 dB for satisfactory communication, although the presence of speech is detectable for S/N as low as —18 dB." [44]

[44] J. C. R. Licklider and George A. Miller, "The Perception of Speech," S. S. Stevens, ed., *Handbook of Experimental Psychology* (New York, John Wiley & Sons, 1951), Chap. 26, p. 1049.

Figure 9-7 from Licklider and Miller, adapted from Hawkins and Stevens,[45] shows the effect of white noise on thresholds of detectability and intelligibility of running speech. It will be noted from Figure 9-7 that the threshold of intelligibility is not seriously affected until the sound pressure level of the noise exceeds the sound pressure level of the speech by about 10 dB (S/N of —10 dB). As the sound pressure level of the noise is increased above 30 to 40 dB, the threshold of intelligibility is proportionally increased, so that the S/N of —10 dB remains constant over a wide range of intensities in the case of this experiment involving running speech and white noise. For other kinds of speech materials and different kinds of noise, the relationships between the threshold of intelligibility and the level of the interfering noise would not necessarily be the same.

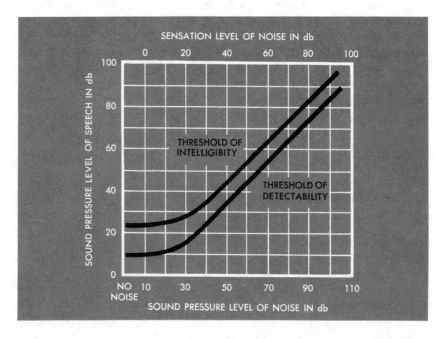

Figure 9-7. The effect of white noise on thresholds of detectability and intelligibility of running speech. (Reproduced from *Handbook of Experimental Psycology* by permission of the publishers.)

Because of the expense and time involved in measuring the effects of noise on the intelligibility of speech in this manner, engineers have sought simpler ways of arriving at interference effects of noise on speech communication. A widely accepted method is to compute what has been termed the "articulation index" by analyzing the intensity and frequency components

[45] J. E. Hawkins, Jr. and S. S. Stevens, "The Masking of Pure Tones and of Speech by White Noise," *Journal of the Acoustical Society of America*, Vol. 22 (January, 1950), p. 12.

of both the speech signal and the noise and working out their interactions mathematically on the basis of data available from laboratory experiments in psychoacoustics. French and Steinberg [46] of the Bell Laboratories developed a method for arriving at the articulation index based on the following assumptions: (1) the range of important speech frequencies is from 200 to 6100 Hz; (2) this range can be divided into 20 frequency bands, each of which contributes equally to the intelligibility of speech provided the signal-to-noise ratios are equal in each band; (3) a 30 dB change in signal-to-noise ratio will span the entire range of word intelligibility scores from zero to almost 100 per cent; (4) each of the 20 frequency bands will contribute 0.05 (5 per cent) to the articulation index, and each decibel of the signal-to-noise ratio in the band will contribute 1/30 of this 0.05 of the articulation index. [47] Thus to calculate the articulation index in a given situation, one needs to determine the signal-to-noise ratio (at the ear of the listener) in each of 20 frequency bands of specified width to arrive at the proportion of the 0.05 that band contributes to the total articulation index. The sum of the contributions of each band then is the articulation index. Figure 9-8 from Hawley and Kryter plots typical intelligibility curves in relation to articulation index. According to Beranek, speech communication is probably satisfactory if the articulation index exceeds 0.6 (60 per cent), unsatisfactory if it is less than 0.3 (30 per cent), and in between these two values more study is required before decisions can be made regarding the adequacy of communication. [48]

Calculation of the articulation index is not a simple matter, since it is necessary to determine the signal-to-noise ratio for 20 frequency bands, a process that requires special laboratory equipment. A simpler means of estimating the effect of noise on speech communication has been devised, making use of octave-band levels as measured in a typical noise survey. What is called the "speech interference level," abbreviated SIL, can be obtained by computing the arithmetic average of the octave-band levels in the three octave bands of 600–1200, 1200–2400, and 2400–4800 Hz. It has been determined that reliable speech communication can exist when the over-all rms (root-mean-square) level of undistorted speech is 12 dB above the speech interference level at the ear of the listener. This relationship between speech level and noise level is equivalent to an articulation index of 0.4. [49] Beranek suggests that if the band level in the 300–600 Hz band exceeds the band level in the 600–1200 Hz band, the speech interference level should be computed by including the level in the 300–600 Hz band in the average. [50]

[46] N. R. French and J. C. Steinberg, "Factors Governing the Intelligibility of Speech Sounds," *Journal of the Acoustical Society of America*, Vol. 19 (January, 1947), pp. 90-119.

[47] Mones E. Hawley and Karl D. Kryter, "Effects of Noise on Speech," in Harris, *op. cit.*, Chap. 9, p. 6.

[48] Leo L. Beranek, *Acoustics* (New York, McGraw-Hill, 1954), p. 415.

[49] Hawley and Kryter, *op. cit.*, p. 10.

[50] Beranek, *op. cit.*, p. 419.

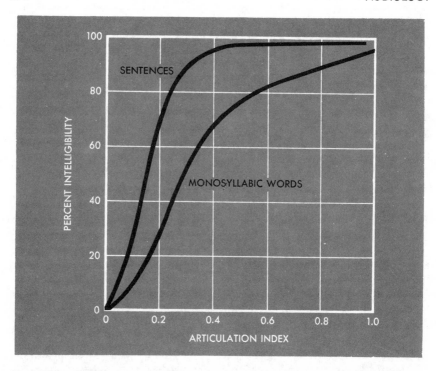

Figure 9-8. The relation of intelligibility to articulation index. (From Mones E. Hawley and Karl D. Kryter, "Effects of Noise on Speech," in Cyril M. Harris, ed., *Handbook of Noise Control.* Copyright 1957. New York, McGraw-Hill Book Co., Inc. Used by permission.)

Beranek has worked out a table that represents the speech interference levels that "barely permit reliable word intelligibility" at various distances between speaker and listener, and at various voice levels, assuming that no reflecting surfaces are present. This information is presented in Table 9-2.

Table 9-2. Speech interference levels (in dB re 0.0002 dyne/cm²) that barely permit reliable word intelligibility at the distances and voice levels indicated. (After L. L. Beranek, "Airplane Quieting II—Specification of Acceptable Noise Levels," *Transactions American Society Mechanical Engineers*, Vol. 67 (1947), pp. 97–100, in Beranek's *Acoustics*, 1954, McGraw-Hill.)

Distance, feet	Normal	Voice Level Raised	(average male) Very Loud	Shouting
0.5	71	77	83	89
1	65	71	77	83
2	59	65	71	77
3	55	61	67	73
4	53	59	65	71
5	51	57	63	69
6	49	55	61	67
12	43	49	55	61

If women's voices are involved, the speech interference levels should be decreased by 5 dB from those values shown in Table 9-2.

Webster has related SIL's based on the average of band levels in the three octaves with the preferred center frequencies of 500, 1000, and 2000 Hz to those shown in Table 9-2. The correction from the data reported in Table 9-2 which were based on the octave bands 600–1200, 1200–2400, and 2400–4800 Hz to data based on octave bands with center frequencies of 500, 1000, and 2000 Hz involves simply adding 5 dB to each of the values in Table 9-2.[51] Later, Webster refers to this SIL based on the preferred center frequencies for octave-band analyzers as PSIL, the "P" standing for "preferred."[52] Table 9-4 in Burns's book transposes Beranek's table reproduced here as Table 9-2 to PSIL values by adding 5 dB to each SIL.[53] The speech-interfering effect of various noises can also be rated by A-weighted sound-level meter readings, or by modifying dBA readings by the difference between C-weighted and A-weighted levels as suggested by Botsford.[54]

OTHER EFFECTS OF NOISE

Physiological Effects

The literature on the physiological effects of exposure to noise of high intensity is rather sparse. Kryter[55] cites a study performed by Parrack, Eldredge, and Koster for the Engineering Division of the Air Materiel Command in 1948 of the effects of exposure to noise from turbo-jet engines and from sirens at sound pressure levels of around 150 dB. In addition to producing severe temporary threshold shifts, the noise was reported to produce some heating of the skin, a sensation of vibration in the bones of the cranium and movement of air in the sinuses and nasal passages, some blurring of the vision, and some difficulty in maintaining posture thought to be associated with the proprioceptive reflex mechanism.

Broadbent also refers to the Parrack, Eldredge, and Koster study, and in addition he mentions some biological effects noted in response to sudden, unexpected sound, such as a shot.[56] He notes that in such situations there will be observed a rise in blood pressure, an increase in pressure inside the

[51] J. C. Webster, "Speech Communications as Limited by Ambient Noise," *Journal of the Acoustical Society of America*, Vol. 37 (April, 1965), p. 694.

[52] John C. Webster, "Effects of Noise on Speech Intelligibility," in Ward and Fricke, eds., *op. cit.*, p. 68.

[53] William Burns, *Noise and Man* (Philadelphia, J. B. Lippincott Company, 1969), p. 132.

[54] Webster, in Ward and Fricke, eds., *op. cit.*, pp. 60-63.

James A. Botsford, "Predicting Speech Interference and Annoyance from A-Weighted Sound Levels," *Journal of the Acoustical Society of America*, Vol. 42 (November, 1967), p. 1151 (abstract).

[55] Kryter, *op. cit.*, p. 21.

[56] Donald E. Broadbent, "Effects of Noise on Behavior," in Harris, *op cit.*, Chap. 10, pp. 8-10.

head, increased perspiration, increase in heart rate, changes in breathing, and perhaps general muscular contractions. The significance of these reactions is that, if they are repeated frequently, they may cause harmful effects to the health, for example, digestive disorders, since one of the byproducts of such startle responses is a decrease in peristalsis and in the flow of saliva and gastric juices. Broadbent also mentions the possibility of harm resulting from increased activity of the adrenal glands in response to sudden, unexpected noise. Apparently, however, there are no long term effects from repeated exposures to "unexpected" noises, since with repetition a noise no longer serves to produce a startle effect. Broadbent also refers to a study that indicated such biological effects as increased blood pressure, heart rate, and respiration rate tended to disappear or adapt over long periods of exposure to intense noise.

Glorig, while recognizing that there may be some effects on respiration, circulation, and balance from exposure to noises that are of very low frequency and very high intensity concludes that noise exposures encountered in industry are not likely to produce biologically harmful effects. He says, "We cannot make a categorical statement that noise exposure has no ill effects on human behavior, but I feel that we can safely say that the behavioral effects of noise are not now a general health problem. The complaints of noise-induced annoyance and fatigue are probably more closely related to motivation or the lack thereof than to actual mental or organic pathology."[57]

Davis dispels the notion that there are any mysterious biological effects from exposure to certain sounds or combinations of sounds, or from exposure to ultrasonic frequencies. He says, "There is no magic in any strange disharmony or in any high-frequency 'ultrasonic death ray' at any practical intensity." [58]

In engineering contexts, noise and vibration are considered to be problems of equal concern to the acoustical engineer. "Vibration is an oscillation wherein the quantity is a parameter that defines the motion of a mechanical system."[59] "A mechanical system is an aggregate of matter comprising a defined configuration of mass, mechanical stiffness, and mechanical resistance."[60] The human body comes under this definition of a mechanical system and is affected by vibration. The body as a whole is subjected to vibration while in a rough-riding vehicle, and harmful effects may result from such abuse. One of the receptors for mechanical stimulation is the auditory system, and another is the vestibular system. Frequently these interact, so that high-intensity sound stimulation can produce reflexive head

---

[57] Glorig, *op. cit.*, p. 107.

[58] Hallowell Davis, "Abnormal Hearing and Deafness," in Hallowell Davis and S. Richard Silverman, eds., *Hearing and Deafness* (New York, Holt, Rinehart and Winston, 1970), Chap. 4, p. 118.

[59] "American Standard Acoustical Terminology," *op. cit.*, p. 9.

[60] *Ibid.*, p. 16.

motions and displacement of the visual field. It is not the purpose of this section to discuss the biological effects of vibration but only to mention that high-intensity noise stimulation sufficient to produce vibratory effects can cause other physiological effects than have been discussed.[61]

Psychological Effects

Many studies have been conducted on the psychological effects of exposure to noise. These have included studies of the ability of subjects to perform various kinds of tasks in the presence of noise, and studies of the annoyance of noise. Miller[62] has summarized the results of a number of these studies:

1. Noise does not appear to affect significantly the mental or motor skills of individuals. In the performance of simple tasks, action becomes automatic and is not adversely influenced by noise. In the performance of difficult tasks, action is concentrated on the task and the noise is ignored.

2. With prolonged exposure to noise, individuals become adapted to the noise environment. Short-term changes in the noise environment require short periods of readjustment and frequently produce short-time improvements in performance because of the break in an otherwise monotonous environment.

3. High noise levels give rise to feelings of annoyance and irritability, and possibly fatigue.

Miller points out that higher noise levels are more disturbing than lower levels; a noise having most of its energy in a narrow band, thus producing a whine or hum, is more annoying than a noise with a broad spectrum; an impact, or intermittent type of noise, is more annoying than a steady-state noise; and (excluding impact noises) longer noises are more disturbing than shorter ones.[63]

Broadbent observes that a high-pitched noise (above 1500 Hz) is more annoying than a low-pitched noise of the same loudness, and he suggests that the reduction of high-frequency components in a noise will yield greater benefits than reduction of low frequencies.[64] Another factor that is involved in assessing annoyance is the localization of the noise. Apparently a noise that cannot be localized is more annoying than one that can be. Other parameters contributing to annoyance are the degree to which a given noise is "necessary" or "unnecessary," and the degree to which a noise is inappropriate to one's own activities. The unnecessary noise evokes more complaints, and a noise that is manifestly inappropriate to a situation—such as a laugh at a funeral—is most annoying.[65]

61 David E. Goldman, "Effects of Vibration on Man," in Harris, *op. cit.*, Chap. 11, p. 3.

62 Laymon N. Miller, "Does Noise Affect You and Your Work?" *Safety Maintenance* (June, 1956), p. 44.

63 *Ibid.*, p. 45.

64 Broadbent, *op. cit.*, p. 5.

65 *Ibid.*, pp. 7-8.

THE CONTROL OF INDUSTRIAL NOISE

The control of noise may be desirable in order to reduce the hazard of noise-induced hearing impairment, to improve communication, or to reduce annoyance. The reduction of noise can be accomplished through improved engineering design of machinery, through the proper mounting of machinery, through alterations in the path of sound emanating from the machinery, and finally through the use of ear protectors that reduce the level of sound reaching the hearing mechanism.

Improved Engineering Design

If designers of machinery had in mind the desirability of minimizing noise, many of the noise control measures now needed in factories would become unnecessary. Frequently parts for machines can be designed of materials that are relatively noiseless at no sacrifice of efficiency, durability, or expense. Sometimes the design of machinery to minimize noise production may create additional expense, but when the costs of instituting noise control procedures in factories and the possible economic effects of workmen's compensation claims are compared with the cost of machinery, the additional initial investment for "quiet" machines may appear to be well worthwhile. Manufacturers of machinery are responsive to consumers' demands, so if the consumers insist on quieter machinery and are willing to pay the price, the manufacturers of machinery will produce quieter products.

Peterson and Gross refer to some ways in which the control of noise at its source can be achieved:[66]

(1) Decrease the energy available for driving the vibrating system.
(2) Change the coupling between this energy and the acoustical radiating system.
(3) Change the structure that radiates the sound so that less is radiated.

While the suggestions of Peterson and Gross refer to the modification of existing machinery, they could apply as well to the original design of the machinery. The energy that drives the vibrating system can be decreased by keeping the speed of moving parts as slow as possible, by keeping air streams at low velocity, and by using structural materials that inherently are less noisy. Noise resulting from the coupling system can be reduced by providing special mounts for the machinery that absorb vibration, and by installing mufflers on intake and exhaust systems. Changing the radiating structure may involve only reducing the external surface areas of vibrating parts, or it may involve special treatment of the radiating surfaces to reduce the efficiency of radiation.

66 Peterson and Gross, *op. cit.*, p. 164.

Alterations in the Pathway of Sound

Peterson and Gross suggest three ways in which noise control can be achieved through altering the pathway of sound:[67]

(1)   Change in relative position of source and listener.
(2)   Change in acoustic environment.
(3)   Introduction of attenuating structures between source and listener.

If most of the noise is directly radiated from the source, rather than being bounced off reflecting surfaces, it may be sufficient simply to move employees further away from the noise source—at least those employees who do not have to be close to the source. If the source is directional, then rotating it to achieve minimum exposure of the workers around the source may be helpful. The acoustic environment can be changed by adding acoustical absorbing material to the room in which the machinery is located. Acoustical tiles and other absorbing materials are useful primarily in reducing noise levels at some distance from the source, and in reducing the sound energy that is reflected from walls and ceiling. Such acoustical treatment does not substantially reduce the noise that emanates directly from the source, and so such treatment will not be very effective in protecting workers who are in the vicinity of the noise source.

Usually the most effective way of altering the pathway of sound to achieve noise control is through the use of attenuating structures of various types. These may consist of walls, standing or hanging barriers, or even total enclosures of the sound source. By using one or more enclosures around a machine, it is possible to reduce the noise level by almost any desired amount. It must be kept in mind, however, that the isolating integrity of an enclosure can be nullified if sound can be transmitted through ventilating ducts, or doors and windows in the enclosure. Ducts should be lined with absorbing materials and built with interior baffles like a muffler, and doors and windows should be designed for maximum acoustical attenuating characteristics in the same manner that openings into audiometric "sound-proof" rooms are designed. It goes without saying that as the complexity of the enclosure increases, the expense of the noise control measure increases. Thus, as we stated earlier, it may be more economical in the long run to pay an increased price for a machine that is designed to minimize noise, than to go to the expense of isolating the machine in an enclosure. Figure 9-9 from Peterson and Gross [68] shows a hypothetical example of what typically can be anticipated in the way of noise reduction by various noise control measures. First

[67] *Ibid.*, pp. 164-165.
[68] *Ibid.*, pp. 167-168.

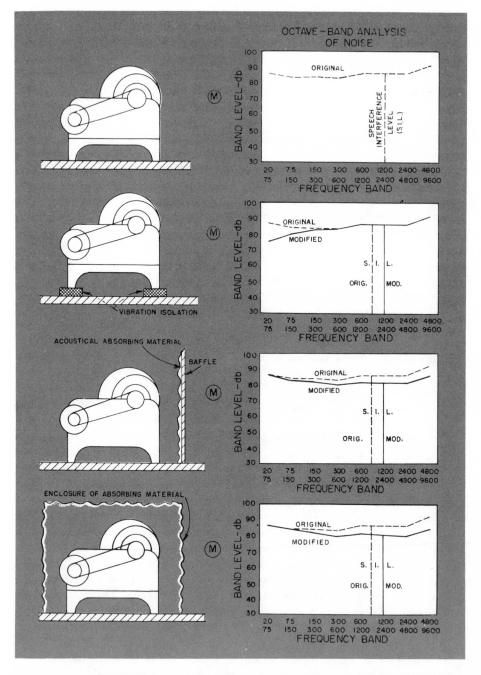

Figure 9-9.   Noise reduction by various noise control measures. (Reproduced by permission of General Radio Company from Arnold P. G. Peterson and Ervin E. Gross, Jr., *Handbook of Noise Measurement*, 1967.)

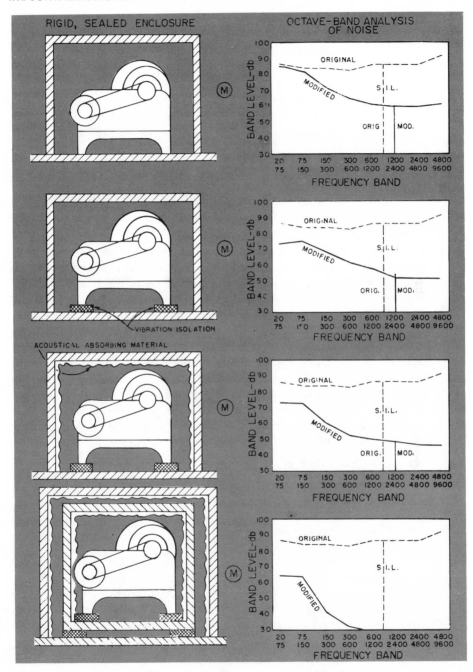

Figure 9-9 *continued*

this figure shows the octave-band levels measured at the position "M" of the noise produced by a machine that is simply sitting on the floor of a factory. The machine produces a wide-band noise that is relatively flat through all of the eight octave bands. The band levels range from about 83 to 92 dB. The next seven parts of the figure show the decrease in band levels that would typically occur with various kinds of noise control measures, from the use of vibration mounts to the employment of a double enclosure of rigid, sealed type and vibration mounts on both the machine and the inner enclosure. It should be noted that enclosing the machine with sound-absorbing material alone is an ineffective means of reducing noise; a massive, rigid, sealed enclosure is much more effective. Lining the interior of a rigid structure with sound-absorbing material, however, increases its effectiveness.

Ear Protectors

If it is impossible or for some reason not feasible to control noise at its source, or to create barriers to the radiation of noise from its source, so that the resulting sound level is potentially hazardous to the hearing, the individuals exposed to the noise may be protected by using "ear protectors." These are of two types: those that are inserted in the external canal, and those that fit over the entire auricle. Insert-type protectors may be of the disposable variety, such as wax-impregnated cotton, or they may be of rubber or neoprene. The latter types are made in from three to five sizes for different size ear canals. To be effective, an insert must fit the canal snugly, so that there is no leakage around the insert. The same individual may require one size in one ear, and a different size in the other ear. Initially, inserts should be fitted by a trained person to insure that the proper size is selected. Maas gives the following instructions for fitting ear protectors:[69]

> In fitting, it helps to pull up and back on the ear lobe slightly. This enlarges and tends to straighten the entrance to the ear canal, making it easier to insert a proper-sized device. When the lobe is released, the tissues of the canal will then hold the protector firmly in the ear. If properly fitted and inserted, the device will seem to *stay put* when an attempt is made to withdraw it.

Ear muffs are becoming increasingly popular as ear protectors. They have the advantage of not requiring special fitting, as do the inserts, and they may be more comfortable for long-time wear. Also they are somewhat more efficient in attenuating sound than inserts. The disadvantage to the ear muffs is that there may be a problem in getting an adequate seal when they are worn with glasses, and they are uncomfortable to wear in hot rooms. Initially the cost of the ear muffs is higher, but over a period of time they may not prove to be any more expensive than the insert types, which are easily lost and may have to be replaced several times. An additional advantage of the muff is that a supervisor can see at a glance whether or not a worker is

[69] Roger Maas, "Ear Protection—Why? . . . How?" *Supervision* (February, 1960), p. 19.

utilizing his ear protectors. Ear muffs may have liquid-filled seals that further increase their attenuating characteristics. Muffs may be fitted into a helmet that protects the whole head. Muffs may also be used as cushions for earphones, thus serving a dual purpose. Typical muffs are shown in Figure 9-10.

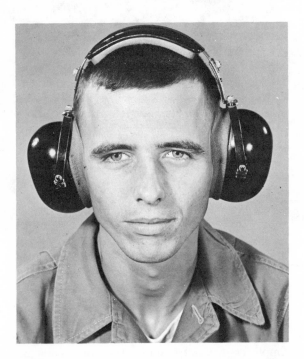

Figure 9-10.   Typical ear muffs. (From Elizabeth Guild, "Ears Can Be Protected," *Noise Control*, Vol. 4 [September, 1958]. Used by permission.)

In conditions of extreme noise, it may be necessary to wear both the insert-type protectors and ear muffs. The two types of protectors used together result in better attenuation than that provided by either one alone. Figure 9-11 shows the attenuating characteristics of muffs, plugs (inserts), and a combination of the two protectors as reported in an Air Force study by Guild.[70] More recently Webster and Rubin [71] have reported the results of comparative studies of various ear protectors for the Navy. Generally, their results agree within 5 dB with those shown in Figure 9-11, except at 4000 Hz, where they found the maximum attenuation achieved by combining inserts with muffs was about 45 dB instead of the 51 dB reported by Guild.

[70] Elizabeth Guild, "Ears Can Be Protected," *Noise Control*, Vol. 4 (September, 1958), p. 35.
[71] J. C. Webster and E. R. Rubin, "Noise Attenuation of Ear-Protective Devices," *Sound*, Vol. 1 (September-October, 1962), pp. 34-46.

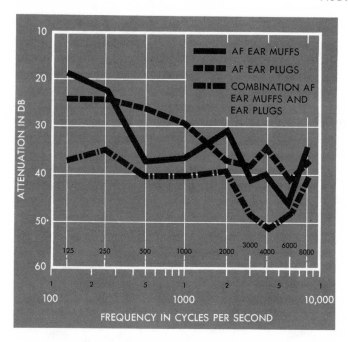

Figure 9-11. Attenuating characteristics of ear protectors. (From Elizabeth Guild, "Ears Can Be Protected," *Noise Control*, Vol. 4 [September, 1958]. Used by permission.)

It is of concern to supervisory personnel that while good protective devices are available, it is not easy to persuade workers to use them. Maas reports a study by the Employers Mutual Liability Insurance Company of Wausau, Wisconsin indicating that only 22.5 per cent of 1148 plants polled reported having had much success with getting workers to accept ear protectors for a period of six months or more.[72] Maas lists some of the following reasons given by workers for not utilizing ear protection: the protectors "hurt" and are uncomfortable, they are too much bother, they get lost, they cause headaches and nervousness, with the protectors in place one cannot hear sounds he wants to hear, and one gets used to the noise so it does not bother him.[73] If ear protectors are properly selected and fitted, they need not be uncomfortable. With ear protectors it is actually easier to carry on conversation in a noisy environment than without them. The hardest argument to overcome is that the noise really does not bother one when he gets used to it. Many men seem to feel that they are being "sissy" if they use ear protectors. They like to think that their ears are "tougher" than other people's, and they believe it would be an admission of weakness to use ear protectors. As we

[72] Roger A. Maas, "Hearing Protection in Industry," *Nursing Outlook*, Vol. 9 (May, 1961), p. 281.

[73] *Ibid.*

said at the beginning of this chapter, noise is insidious in its effect on the hearing, since noise levels below those required to produce the sensation of discomfort may cause permanent damage, and in the absence of regular audiometric tests a worker may incur a serious hearing loss in the higher frequencies without being aware of it. The experience of insurance companies and factory management has been that it is necessary to carry on continuing employee education programs as to the need for and advantage of ear protection, and even to insist on threat of discharge from employment that employees in certain very noisy operations wear ear protection at all times. At the same time, management has the responsibility for seeing that ear protection is available to every employee in noisy areas, and that the protectors issued are of proper size and fit for maximum comfort.

Incidentally, a word should be said about the ineffectiveness of dry cotton as ear protection. Because for many years there were no specially-designed ear protectors manufactured, cotton was used by individuals who were exposed to gunfire in the armed services. In comparison with the attenuation provided by even a relatively inefficient ear plug of rubber or neoprene, however, dry cotton is almost useless.

Fletcher has described an ingenious method for making use of the ear's own protective device, the intra-aural muscle reflex, for protection from impulsive sounds, such as bursts of gunfire.[74] When the tensor tympani and stapedius muscles contract, the amount of sound transmitted to the inner ear is reduced. In a burst of machine-gun fire, the muscles will contract after the first shot, but that first shot may cause damage to the hair cells of the cochlea. It takes 9 msec for the ear reflex to occur, whereas the rise time of a gun shot is less than 2 msec. Fletcher devised a system for presenting a subject a 1000-Hz tone through a loudspeaker at a sound pressure level of 98 dB some 200 msec before a burst from a machine gun was fired. Thus the ear reflex was activated prior to the initial shot of the burst. Fletcher then compared the amount of TTS obtained from two groups of subjects firing machine guns: one in which the acoustic reflex was activated in the manner described, and the other (control group) in which there was no activation of the acoustic reflex prior to the first shot. His results indicated that the experimental group showed an average of 10 dB less TTS than the control group for frequencies of 1000 Hz and higher. He states that for certain "highly sensitive" individuals, the protection afforded by the acoustic reflex may be as great as 50 dB at some frequencies.[75] Fletcher then compared the protective effect of the ear reflex with that of an ear insert protector. He found that the ear reflex produced slightly better protection for frequencies of 1000 Hz and lower, but that the insert provided superior protection for frequencies higher than 1000 Hz.[76] While Fletcher's work is interesting, it is doubtful if a method of

---

[74] John L. Fletcher, "Reflex Response of Middle-Ear Muscles: Protection of the Ear from Noise," *Sound,* Vol. 1 (March-April, 1962), pp. 17-23.

[75] *Ibid.,* p. 20.

[76] *Ibid.*

activating the ear reflex will prove feasible for industrial use, especially since readily available ear protectors provide almost as good protection for the lower frequencies as does the ear reflex, and better protection for the higher frequencies.

INDUSTRIAL HEARING CONSERVATION PROGRAMS

Since noise-induced hearing impairment has become a compensable disability, the area of hearing conservation has assumed an economic importance to industry and to the insurance companies that write industrial compensation insurance. The principle of apportionment of liability, referred to earlier in this chapter, holds an employer liable for only that portion of a claimant's hearing loss that was incurred during his period of work for that employer, provided the employer can prove that the claimant had some hearing loss at the time he started his employment. It follows, then, that to protect himself against being held liable for all of a claimant's hearing loss, an employer must perform a hearing test on each new employee. This initial audiogram then becomes a "reference" with which future audiograms will be compared to determine what changes if any have occurred in an employee's hearing levels during his period of employment. Since the decision as to where to place a new employee may hinge to some extent upon the degree of "toughness" or "tenderness" of his ears, the initial audiogram is frequently called a "pre-placement audiogram." If in his initial audiogram a new employee shows evidence that he has incurred some noise-induced hearing impairment, the employer is warned that placing this employee in a noisy work environment may be inviting a future claim, because the employee has already demonstrated a susceptibility to noise.

Another purpose of the reference audiogram is to identify individuals who have hearing problems whether or not they are related to noise exposure. Such individuals should have careful diagnostic audiometry performed to determine whether their hearing impairments are conductive, sensori-neural, or mixed in type, and, insofar as it can be determined, the site of the lesion and its etiology. Naturally, an otological examination is required to establish the medical diagnosis of any hearing impairments identified by reference audiograms. Individuals who are found to have hearing impairments that are treatable by medical or surgical means should be advised to seek treatment in the interest of conserving their hearing. The primary interest in discovering hearing impairments that are not related to noise exposure, however, so far as the employer is concerned, is his protection from future claims that noise exposure on the job has been the primary agent in producing an employee's hearing impairment when in fact there may have been an entirely different etiology.

Establishing a system through which the hearing of all new employees is routinely tested is certainly desirable, for the reasons that have been cited.

It may not, however, be economically feasible for an employer to provide hearing tests for all new employees. If this is the case, then there should be provision for obtaining reference audiograms for all new employees who will be working in environments that the employer considers to be at least potentially hazardous to the hearing.

For those employees who are working in noisy environments, there should be provision for periodic retesting to determine whether or not there has been a change in hearing level. Since exposure to noise is known to produce a temporary threshold shift, the periodic retests, referred to frequently as "monitoring audiometry," should be performed on Monday mornings after the employee has had the week end to recover. After 48 hours, any change in hearing levels from the reference audiogram should be regarded as "persistent" if not permanent threshold shift. The detection of a persistent threshold shift should alert management to the need for taking action to prevent further deterioration of an employee's hearing. This action may be in the form of insisting that he use available ear protection, in attempting to reduce excessive noise levels at their source through improved engineering, in limiting the employee's exposure time if this is possible, or in extreme cases removing the employee entirely from the noisy environment in which he has been working.

As in the case of reference audiograms, monitoring audiometry also serves the purpose of discovering changes in hearing levels that may be due to an etiology other than noise exposure. Whenever monitoring audiometry reveals significant differences from the reference audiogram, there should be an audiological and otological evaluation of the employee whose hearing has been affected to determine wherever possible the cause for the change in hearing levels that has occurred. Glorig suggests that the first monitoring audiogram should be scheduled for a period of about 90 days after the employee commences work, unless the employee himself complains of hearing impairment or tinnitus, in which case the first monitoring audiogram should be obtained earlier. If the first retest following the reference audiogram shows that there has been no change at any frequency of more than 10 dB, then future monitoring audiograms can be scheduled at yearly intervals.[77]

The Reference Audiogram

The reference audiogram should be obtained under conditions of testing that assure good validity. The room in which the testing is performed should be properly sound treated for excluding outside interference. A normal-hearing listener wearing the usual binaural earphones with MX41/AR cushions should be able to hear all test tones from 500 through 6000 Hz at zero-dB hearing level re ANSI-1969 calibration standards provided the octave-band levels for the octave bands with preferred center frequencies do not exceed the following values within the test room: [78]

[77] Glorig, *op. cit.*, p. 129.
[78] *Guide for Conservation of Hearing in Noise, op. cit.*, p. 37.

500 Hz	30 dB
1000 Hz	30 dB
2000 Hz	37 dB
4000 Hz	47 dB
8000 Hz	52 dB

Of course the amount of attenuation required to achieve the necessary levels within the room will depend on the amount of noise in the environment in which the test room is placed.

The reference audiogram should include thresholds by air conduction for the following frequencies: 250, 500, 1000, 2000, 3000, 4000, and 6000 Hz. The frequency of 3000 Hz is included because some states utilize this frequency in computing percentage of hearing loss for purposes of compensation, and also because a loss at 3000 Hz is known to affect discrimination of speech materials under conditions of difficult listening.[79] The highest frequency tested is 6000 Hz rather than 8000 Hz, because of the comparative unreliability of test results at 8000 Hz.[80] Some authorities prefer to include 250 Hz as a test frequency, but most favor its elimination. Whether or not it is included will depend upon local preferences and legal requirements.

The reference audiogram is usually obtained by a nurse or audiometric technician operating a pure-tone audiometer in the standard method for individual threshold testing. Automatic audiometry, however, on either an individual or a group basis, is becoming more popular, especially in those industrial situations in which there is a large turn-over of the labor force, so that it is not feasible to administer individual tests in the customary manner because of the sheer numbers to be tested. A number of automatic audiometers have been developed experimentally, and several have been used in practical testing situations. Rudmose describes the various kinds of automatic audiometers that have been devised.[81] We shall be concerned here with a brief description of only the Rudmose Model ARJ recording audiometer, which has had extensive use in both military and industrial settings. The development of this audiometer was described by McMurray and Rudmose in 1956.[82]

The Rudmose ARJ audiometer is a discrete frequency Békésy-type instrument (see Chapter 7) that measures hearing levels from zero to 100 dB at the frequencies of 500, 1000, 2000, 3000, 4000, and 6000 Hz. The subject wears a headset containing two earphones, and he controls the intensity of the signal by pushing a button when he hears and releasing the button when

[79] J. Donald Harris, H. L. Haines, and C. K. Myers, "The Importance of Hearing at 3 KC for Understanding Speeded Speech," *Laryngoscope,* Vol. 70 (February, 1960), pp. 131-146.

[80] Hallowell Davis, Gordon Hoople, and Horace O. Parrack, "The Medical Principles of Monitoring Audiometry," *A.M.A. Archives of Industrial Health,* Vol. 17 (January, 1958), p. 18.

[81] Wayne Rudmose, "Automatic Audiometry," in James F. Jerger, ed., *Modern Developments in Audiology* (New York, Academic Press, 1963), Chap. 2, pp. 30-75.

[82] R. F. McMurray and Wayne Rudmose, "An Automatic Audiometer for Industrial Medicine," *Noise Control,* Vol. 2 (January, 1956), pp. 33-36.

he does not hear. The pushbutton controls an attenuator motor that increases or decreases the intensity of the test tone. The left ear is tested first, and the order of frequency presentation is from lowest to highest. Each frequency is presented for about thirty seconds. At the operator's choice the tone may be either continuous or pulsed. The attenuator position is constantly recorded by a stylus tapping a typewriter ribbon, thus making a series of dots on an audiogram card. The attenuator movements for the frequency under test are confined to the space between the vertical lines on the card. The frequency changes as a vertical line passes under the printer. At the conclusion of the threshold determination at 6000 Hz, the signal is automatically switched to the right earphone, and the test of the right ear is begun at the frequency of 500 Hz. The Rudmose audiometer is pictured in Figure 9-12, and the audiogram obtained with this instrument is shown in Figure 9-13.

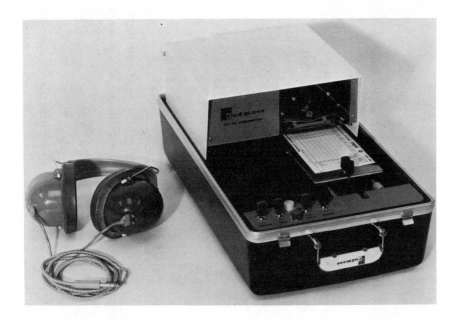

Figure 9-12.   The Rudmose automatic audiometer with earphones in Otocup enclosures (Reproduced by permission of Tracor, Inc., The Medical Instruments Division, Austin, Texas.)

The Rudmose audiometer was originally designed for individual testing, but it has been adapted for use as a group audiometer by combining several attenuators with their recording devices with a master oscillator. As many as ten individuals can be tested simultaneously with this equipment. Rudmose suggests that with the use of earphone enclosures, which he calls "Otocups,"

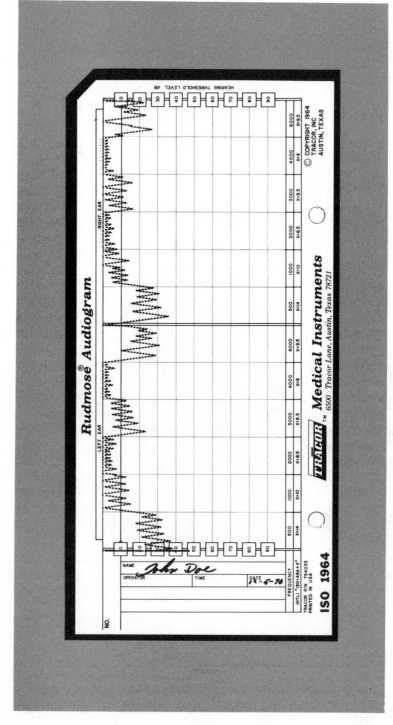

Figure 9-13. Audiogram obtained with Rudmose automatic audiometer. (Reproduced by permission of Tracor, Inc., The Medical Instrument: Division, Austin, Texas.)

an attenuation of ambient noise comparable to that provided by a single-wall test booth can be achieved.

Other automatic audiometers have been designed with "programers" that present single pulses of tone to a listener who responds by pushing a button if he hears. The machine then attenuates the tone by 10 dB and presents another stimulus. As long as the subject responds correctly, the tone is attenuated in 10-dB steps. When the subject does not respond, the next presentation is at a level 5 dB higher in intensity. When the subject again responds, the intensity of the tone is decreased in 5-dB steps. Several threshold crossings are provided and the machine then makes a "decision" as to threshold at that frequency, which is printed out automatically in numbers by an electric typewriter. Such automatic audiometers are designed to determine threshold by following the logical pattern employed by a human tester. One such instrument that has had wide military use was described by Brogan, its designer.[83]

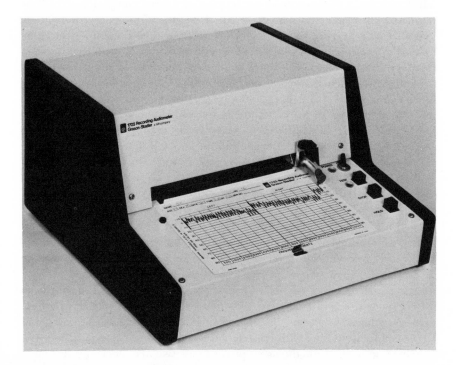

Figure 9-14.   The Grason-Stadler automatic audiometer. (Reproduced by permission of Grason-Stadler, a GR Company, Concord, Mass.)

[83] F. A. Brogan, "An Automatic Audiometer for Air Force Classification Centers," *Noise Control*, Vol. 2 (May, 1956), pp. 58-59; 67.

A Grason-Stadler automatic audiometer built on the Békésy principle is shown in Figure 9-14. This instrument tests at seven discrete frequencies: 500, 1000, 2000, 3000, 4000, 6000, and 8000 Hz. At the conclusion of the test on the second ear, it presents 1000 Hz again as a check on the test validity. At each frequency the rate of intensity change is rapid until the subject first responds. Then the intensity changes more slowly as threshold is approached. Thus the threshold region is reached quickly and more time is spent in defining the actual threshold hearing level.

Monitoring Audiometry

While threshold audiograms, whether obtained by standard procedures or by some form of automatic audiometry, are necessary for reference purposes, it is not essential that complete audiograms be obtained routinely in the monitoring program. A single-frequency type of screening test, such as that described by House and Glorig [84] and discussed in Chapter 8, is well suited to a rapid monitoring of the hearing of a large population. It will be recalled from Chapter 8 that the method consists of presenting a 4000-Hz tone first at a hearing level of 35 or 50 dB, and then presenting the same tone at a level of 20 dB. If the subject responds to the 20-dB tone in each ear, he is considered to be within the range of normal and no further testing is required. The test is based on the assumption that no other frequency will show a greater loss than that at 4000 Hz. If the subject fails to respond to the tone at a level of 20 dB, and his reference audiogram indicates that previously he had been able to hear 4000 Hz at this level, he would be referred for a complete audiometric examination. If, however, his reference audiogram indicated that his hearing level at 4000 Hz was somewhere between 20 and 35 dB, and in the single-frequency test he was able to hear the tone at the 35 dB level, again he would be dismissed as requiring no additional testing at that time. The same would be true if his reference audiogram showed a hearing level between 35 and 50 dB at 4000 Hz, and he demonstrated on the single-frequency test that he could respond to the tone at the 50-dB level in each ear. In other words, the single-frequency test is used to determine if there has been any shift in threshold at that important frequency (so far as reflecting noise-induced hearing loss is concerned). If a shift from the reference audiogram has occurred, than a complete audiometric examination is performed so that the monitoring audiogram can be compared frequency by frequency with the reference audiogram.

Some audiologists and otologists prefer to use two frequencies for screening or monitoring purposes instead of just the one. Ambco Electronics produces a battery-powered, transistorized instrument called the "Oto-Chek," which

[84] Howard P. House and Aram Glorig, "A New Concept of Auditory Screening," *Laryngoscope,* Vol. 67 (July, 1957), pp. 661-668.

generates only the frequencies of 2000 and 4000 Hz at hearing levels of 25 and 45 dB. This instrument was described in Chapter 8 and pictured in Figure 8-4.

NOISE SUSCEPTIBILITY

It has been generally recognized that there are individual differences in the susceptibility of ears to damage from exposure to noise. Many references have been made in the literature to "tough" ears and "tender" ears, referring to differences in degree of susceptibility. Because of the recognition of individual differences in susceptibility, considerable attention has been focused on the problem of identifying those individuals who, when placed in a noisy working environment, would be most susceptible to noise-induced hearing loss. The assumption has been that if such individuals could be identified, they could be assigned to less noisy working environments, or at the least could be provided with the best possible ear protection when they are working in noise. Attempts have been made, therefore, to devise tests for susceptibility that could be administered at the time the reference audiogram is obtained. Several such tests have been reviewed and evaluated by Summerfield, Glorig, and Wheeler [85] and by Rowland.[86]

Two general test methods have been proposed as having value in predicting which individuals in a population would sustain the most damage from exposure to noise. By far the most popular type of test is some measure of the temporary threshold shift (TTS). The method involves presenting a subject with a "fatiguing" stimulus that may be either a pure tone or a wide-band noise. After a prescribed period of exposure to the fatiguing stimulus, the degree of shift of the subject's threshold at some frequency— usually around 4000 Hz—is measured immediately following the cessation of the fatiguing stimulus. Predictions of susceptibility then are made on the basis of either the absolute amount of threshold shift observed, or the time required for the subject's threshold at the criterion frequency to return to normal, that is, its pre-stimulation level. The individual who incurs the greatest amount of threshold shift, or who requires the longest time for his threshold to return to its "normal" level, is then presumed to be the most susceptible to permanent, irreversible hearing impairment if placed in a noisy environment for his working life.

[85] Anne Summerfield, Aram Glorig, and D. E. Wheeler, "Is There a Suitable Industrial Test of Susceptibility to Noise-Induced Hearing Loss?" *Noise Control*, Vol. 4 (January, 1958), pp. 40-46; 54.
[86] Roy C. Rowland, Jr., "Tests for Identifying Noise-Susceptible Individuals," unpublished M. A. thesis, Stanford University, 1960.

The other type of test that has been suggested as having predictive value is the aural harmonics test of Lawrence and Blanchard.[87] This test attempts to determine the minimum intensity at which the response of the ear to a particular frequency becomes distorted or non-linear and produces harmonics. The assumption of the test is that at some point as intensity is increased the ear will "overload," that is, be unable to respond without distorting. Distortion is manifested by the production of aural harmonics (multiples) of the stimulating frequency. The presence of an aural harmonic is detected by introducing to the ear of the listener a second tone that is almost exactly twice the frequency of the original stimulus. If a harmonic is being generated within the ear, the second tone, called the *probe* tone, will interact with the aural harmonic to produce the sensation of beats. (See Chapter 2 for a discussion of the phenomenon of beats.)

For example, suppose that the stimulating tone was at a frequency of 1000 Hz. It is presented at some arbitrary level above the subject's threshold for that frequency, say 70 dB. A probe tone of 2004 Hz is introduced into the same earphone at a level of 60 dB above the subject's threshold for 2000 Hz. The subject is instructed to adjust the intensity of the stimulating tone and the probe tone up and down in relation to each other until he reports that he hears "best" beats, that is, until the beats he hears appear to be most pronounced. If he hears beats, they will occur at the rate of four per second, representing the difference in cycles between the probe tone (2004 Hz) and the aural harmonic (2000 Hz—the first overtone of the stimulus tone of 1000 Hz). The tester then gradually decreases the intensity of both tones until the subject reports that the beats have disappeared. The subject then adjusts the intensity of the probe tone alone to see if the beats recur. If they recur, then the tester again reduces the intensity of both tones until once more the subject reports the beats are no longer heard. Again the subject attempts to restore the beats by adjusting the intensity of the probe tone. This procedure is repeated until the beats have finally disappeared regardless of the adjustment of the probe tone in relation to the stimulus tone. The hearing level of the 1000 Hz tone at which the beats finally disappear is considered to be the threshold of non-linearity. The threshold of non-linearity is usually determined for two frequencies, 1000 and 2000 Hz, which would require the use of probe tones of 2004 and 4004 Hz, respectively.

Lawrence and Blanchard believe that when an ear is driven into non-linearity by high intensity stimuli and this condition producing distortion in the ear is allowed to persist for any considerable length of time, a breakdown in the auditory system will occur. The earlier non-linearity occurs, the lower the intensity of the stimulus required to produce breakdown in the auditory system. They make the assumption that subjects who have comparatively

[87] Merle Lawrence and Cyrus L. Blanchard, "Prediction of Susceptibility to Acoustic Trauma by Determination of Threshold of Distortion," *Industrial Medicine and Surgery,* Vol. 23 (May, 1954), pp. 193-200.

low thresholds of non-linearity or overload are therefore susceptible to noise-induced hearing loss. Their assumptions were based on laboratory experiments with guinea pigs. The animals that showed the lowest thresholds of non-linearity sustained the greatest losses after exposure to noise, while those that showed the highest thresholds of overload sustained the least losses following noise exposure.

After reviewing all of the tests that have been proposed as having usefulness in identifying those individuals who are noise-susceptible, Summerfield, Glorig, and Wheeler concluded that none of them was suitable in its present form for use in industry.[88] They suggest certain criteria that any test for susceptibility should satisfy if it is to be acceptable for use in industry. The equipment to be employed must be "simple and rugged." It must be sufficiently uncomplicated so that subjects and relatively naive testers can perform the test without difficulty. The test must not consume more than a brief portion of the time available for medical examinations of new employees. The test must be demonstrated to be both valid and reliable, that is, it must pick out those individuals who are truly noise-susceptible, and the results of the test must be repeatable within acceptable limits of variability. Also, the test results must be immediately classifiable into degrees of susceptibility that are meaningful to industrial personnel who have to assign employees to specific tasks.[89]

Summerfield, Glorig, and Wheeler urge that studies be undertaken to determine whether the number of individuals who are extremely susceptible to noise-induced hearing loss is sufficient to justify the expenditure of additional time and effort in attempting to refine existing measures, or design new ones, to identify them. They suggest that susceptibility to noise-induced hearing loss may be distributed normally throughout the population, so that the number of highly-susceptible ears may be only a very small proportion of the population. If this is in fact the case, then they suggest that research efforts might better be spent in learning how to achieve better protection of the hearing of the much larger numbers of workers who are moderately susceptible to noise-induced hearing loss.

NOISE POLLUTION

Recently a great deal of attention has been focused on the preservation of our environment. Ecologists have increased our awareness of the danger of destroying our environment by polluting the air and the water with the waste products of our technological civilization. As our civilization has become more "advanced," it has also become noisier. In 1961 it was esti-

[88] Summerfield, Glorig, and Wheeler, *op. cit.,* p. 45.
[89] *Ibid.,* p. 44.

mated that our urban noise levels were increasing by 1 dB a year,[90] which if true means that by 1970 the intensity (power) of urban noise had doubled three times. Obviously, without effective controls at various levels of government, our civilization will get noisier and noisier. As Vern O. Knudsen, a pioneer acoustic physicist, has said, "Noise, like smog, is a slow agent of death. If it continues to increase for the next 30 years as it has for the past 30, it could become lethal." [91]

In light of our present concern with pollution, it is natural to refer to the proliferation of unwanted sound as "noise pollution." While the consequences of uncontrolled noise pollution are not nearly as dire as the possible results of air and water pollution, they are quite properly of concern to an increasing segment of our population. Although life itself is not threatened by noise, certainly the quality of life can be affected by the noise environment in which we live. It is appropriate, therefore, to devote some attention to community noise problems and, hopefully, their control.

What are the principal sources of noise pollution within a community? Without any attempt to rank-order them either on the basis of frequency of occurrence or level of their noise, we can identify the following chief offenders: traffic noise—from automobiles, motorcycles and scooters, trucks, and buses; construction noises—from bulldozers, pile drivers, jackhammers, compressors, chain saws, etc.; subway or surface trains; sirens of emergency vehicles; power mowers; aircraft flyovers, including sonic booms; barking dogs; children's screaming; air-conditioning equipment or ventilating fans; garbage or trash collections. Such a list does not include industrial noises (assumed, not always correctly, to be confined within a factory or office) or noises within one's home or apartment from various kinds of equipment such as dishwashers, blenders, laundry equipment, vacuum cleaners, etc., and of course the ubiquitous TV and hi-fi sets. In all these examples of noise pollution we are concerned for the most part not about damage to the hearing (such as workers in a noisy industry might incur over a working lifetime), but about the invasion of our privacy and the threat to the tranquillity of our existence. And who is to say that the cumulative effects of all the daily environmental noises with which we are bombarded might not contribute substantially to the statistical curves of decreasing hearing sensitivity by decade of age that we term presbycusis, or more properly, sociocusis?

There is one possible exception to the statement just made that environmental noise is not a threat to one's hearing sensitivity, and that is the discotheque, or the rock concert. For some unexplainable reason, our youth today demand that their music be loud. And with electric guitars hooked to powerful amplifiers and all instruments and singers' voices boosted with public-address systems, the hundreds of hirsute rock groups give our youth

90 *Noise Control*, Vol. 7 (July-August, 1961), p. 39.
91 Quoted by W. H. Ferry, "The Citizen's View," in Ward and Fricke, eds., *op. cit.*, p. 303

what they demand. Newspapers and popular magazines have carried stories about the dangers of hearing damage in such environments, and sound-level meter readings in discotheques have confirmed that the audience is exposed to levels that greatly exceed industrial damage-risk criteria. Since the exposures are intermittent, however, with periods of days or weeks intervening between them, there is probably little or no danger that members of the audience will incur any NIPTS, although it is quite likely that many will demonstrate TTS's after attending a concert. The situation is different, however, for members of performing groups—at least those groups that are in such popular demand that they perform several times a week. Jerger and Jerger found that all members of such a group incurred TTS's ranging from 15 to 50 dB for frequencies of 2000 Hz and higher after playing for four and a half hours. Measurements made in the center of the group revealed octave-band levels in the 300–600 Hz and 600–1200 Hz bands ranging from 104 to 124 dB with occasional peaks as high as 130 dB. Three of the five musicians in this group had pre-exposure audiograms showing threshold hearing levels in at least one ear ranging from 30 to 70 dB for frequencies above 2000 Hz. Since the group had been playing about three nights a week for a two-year period, it is likely that at least some of their pre-exposure hearing levels represented NIPTS from their rehearsals and performances.[92]

Community noise control requires some means of measuring noise in terms of its nuisance or annoyance characteristics. Annoyance is a subjective judgment, and so a method must be used of equating judgments of annoyance with the physical characteristics of a noise, because regulations must be based on physical measurements. Since the jet aircraft is one of the noisiest objects to which a wide segment of our population is exposed, much time, effort, and money have been expended in trying to reduce the annoyance of airport operations to surrounding communities. Some of the measures of control attempted have been changing of flight patterns for landings and take-offs, and even relocation of major airports. In studying the reactions of listeners to aircraft noises, Kryter and his associates in a large consulting firm found it helpful to develop a new subjective measure, "perceived noisiness," expressed in units called "noys." [93] A scaling method for noisiness was developed in a similar manner to the way in which Stevens developed his scaling of loudness in sones.[94] The loudness scale indicates how loud a sound appears to a listener. A value of 1 sone is assigned to the loudness of a 1000-Hz tone that has a sound pressure level of 40 dB. Then a sound that is half as loud as assigned a value of 0.5 sone, and a sound that is twice as loud as the reference tone is assigned a value of 2 sones. Similarly, a value of 1 noy was

92 James Jerger and Susan Jerger, "Temporary Threshold Shift in Rock-and-Roll Musicians," *Journal of Speech and Hearing Research,* Vol. 13 (March, 1970), pp. 221-224.

93 Karl D. Kryter, "Scaling Human Reactions to the Sound from Aircraft," *Journal of the Acoustical Society of America,* Vol. 31 (November, 1959), pp. 1415-1429.

94 S. S. Stevens, "Calculating Loudness," *Noise Control,* Vol. 3 (September, 1957), pp. 11-22.

assigned to the perceived noisiness by listeners of a band of frequencies from 910-1090 Hz presented at a sound pressure level of 40 dB, and values of 0.5 noy and 2 noys were assigned to sounds of half the noisiness and twice the noisiness, respectively, of the reference sound.

Earlier in this chapter reference was made to the phon, which is the unit for measuring loudness level. The phon and the decibel are equated at the frequency of 1000 Hz by definition. When we say a sound has a loudness level of 50 phons, we mean that according to listeners' judgments it is equal in loudness to a 1000 Hz tone that has a sound pressure level of 50 dB. In audiometric work, phons and decibels are equated at 1000 Hz in terms of hearing level rather than sound pressure level. "Perceived noise level," measured in units called PNdB, was devised by Kryter as the analog of loudness level in phons. According to Kryter, the perceived noise level of a sound in PNdB is the sound pressure level of the 910-1090 Hz band of random noise that a listener judges to be as acceptable or unacceptable as the sound in question.[95] In 1960, Kryter published noys curves for bands of sound as a function of sound pressure level, tables for determining noisiness in noys for each of eight octave bands and each of twenty-two 1/3 octave bands once the band level in dB is known for each band, a formula for determining the total noisiness in noys for a given sound, and a table for converting noisiness in noys to perceived noise level in PNdB.[96] Kryter and his associates believe that these measures of noisiness and perceived noise level should contribute greatly to the development of quantitative methods of expressing the subjective effects of noise and thus will lead to methods of control to keep noise within acceptable limits. One example of the usefulness of this method of evaluating noisiness is in airport operation. One community specified that jet aircraft must not be noisier than propeller-driven aircraft, and it was possible to compare the noisiness of the two types of aircraft by means of PNdB values at various points along their flight paths. As a result of this study, airlines were forced to specify altitudes and power cutbacks for various kinds of jet aircraft to keep them within the prescribed noise limits at certain points along their flight paths in proximity to the airport.[97]

In the years since Kryter first proposed that PNdB be used as a measure of annoyance or the "unwantedness" of a noise dozens of articles have appeared refining the concept of perceived noise level and citing its usefulness not only in determining the acceptability of aircraft noise but, applying appropriate corrections or modifications, the acceptability of various environmental noises. These studies have been reviewed by Kryter.[98] No attempt

[95] Kryter, "Scaling Human Reactions to the Sound from Aircraft," *op. cit.*, p. 1425.

[96] K. D. Kryter, "The Meaning and Measurement of Perceived Noise Level," *Noise Control*, Vol. 6 (September-October, 1960), pp. 12-27.

[97] Laymon N. Miller, Leo L. Beranek, and Karl D. Kryter, "Airports and Jet Noise," *Noise Control*, Vol. 5 (January, 1959), pp. 24-31.

[98] Karl D. Kryter, "Psychological Reactions to Aircraft Noise," *Science*, Vol. 151 (18 March, 1966), pp. 1346-1355.

K. D. Kryter, "Concepts of Perceived Noisiness, Their Implementation and Application," *Journal of the Acoustical Society of America*, Vol. 43 (February, 1968), pp. 344-361.

to describe the various uses of perceived noise level will be made here. Suffice it to say that at the present time the scaling of noises in PNdB offers probably the best method available of setting community noise criteria. So far as measuring perceived noise level from aircraft flyovers, take-offs, and landings is concerned, a good approximation of PNdB can be made by adding 13 dB to A-weighted sound-level meter readings.[99]

Sonic booms represent a special kind of hazard to our environment resulting from flyovers of aircraft whose speed exceeds the velocity of sound. They have been known since the middle 1940's when high-performance fighter planes dived at supersonic speeds. Now with military aircraft commonly exceeding the velocity of sound (Mach 1), sonic booms are heard frequently during military maneuvers, or sometimes when a military plane accidentally exceeds the speed of sound. In the near future, supersonic transports (SST's) may be operational, in which case the potential for increasing the number of sonic booms to which the average person is exposed will be great. A boom is a shock wave generated by the "piling up" of air particles when a sound source moves at a greater speed than the velocity of propagation of the disturbance.[100] The shock wave can be likened to a bow wave from a speeding boat. When the shock wave hits the ground, a sudden increase in air pressure, called "overpressure," occurs, causing a booming sound like a single clap of thunder. In addition to the startling noise that disturbs and jolts unsuspecting listeners, the sudden overpressure from a sonic boom may cause damage to buildings. Many studies of sonic booms— both actual and produced in the laboratory— have been conducted for the purpose of determining the acceptability of the noise. The results are not encouraging. There is little evidence that most people can learn to adapt to sonic booms as they do to a certain extent to various other noxious sounds. A Citizens League Against the Sonic Boom has been formed to attempt to mobilize the public to influence legislators to squelch plans for the production of an SST in this country. According to a news release of the League, the Federal Aviation Agency's Director of SST Development admitted that "the boom from a single SST at cruising altitude will blanket an area 50 miles wide; thus a single SST flying across USA will 'bang' a region having an area ten times that of Massachusetts."[101] Although at present there is no known "cure" for the sonic boom, it is possible that supersonic aircraft in the future may be designed to minimize the intensity of the boom if not eliminate it altogether.

Other citizens' groups have been organized to protest the rising noise levels in our cities and suburbs and to attempt to persuade local governments to pass and enforce reasonable and realistic noise regulations. They argue that we have the technological knowledge now to reduce the noise levels of trucks, construction equipment, and such home noisemakers as power mow-

[99] Leo L. Beranek, "General Aircraft Noise," in Ward and Fricke, eds. *op, cit.,* p. 257.
[100] Harvey H. Hubbard, "Sonic Booms," *Physics Today,* Vol. 21 (February, 1968), pp. 31-37.
[101] *Sound and Vibration,* Vol. 2 (February, 1968), p. 4.

ers. All that is required, they say, is a large-scale protest on the part of the harassed citizen—and a willingness to pay the additional costs for quieter equipment—to convince governmental bodies of the need for noise regulations.

While, as we have seen, we are making progress in the development of measurement techniques that can form the basis of governmental regulations for community noise, we must not lose sight of the fact that measurements themselves will not solve the problem. As the leader of Citizens for a Quieter City, Robert Alex Baron of New York, said at a seminar held at the Miami Beach meeting of the Acoustical Society of America in 1967:

Why do we have to have such precise standards? Almost every community has an ordinance that prohibits disturbance by barking dogs. These ordinances do not specify the size of the dog, or the noise level of the bark. It is accepted that barking disturbs sleep, and sleep must be protected. Yet when it comes to jet planes or trucks or air conditioners, all of which can and do disturb sleep, we are asked to wait for the perfect measurement—or accept standards that do not abate the noise source. . . . The human receiver of noise must not remain low man on the totem pole. We must put our acoustical knowledge to work—for protective model codes, for silencing in design. It should be obvious the citizen noise receiver is no longer willing to put up with the lack of control of noise which assails his ears, offends his dignity, and could injure his health. . . . A quieter everyday environment is possible, reasonable, and long overdue.[102]

REFERENCES

Baron, Robert Alex, *The Tyranny of Noise* (New York, St. Mary's Press, 1970).

Burns, William, *Noise and Man* (Philadelphia, J. B. Lippincott, 1969).

Davis, Hallowell, and Silverman, S. Richard, eds., *Hearing and Deafness* (New York, Holt, Rinehart and Winston, 1970), Chaps. 5 and 9.

Kryter, Karl D., *The Effects of Noise on Man* (New York, Academic Press, 1970).

Ward, W. Dixon, and Fricke, James E., eds., *Noise as a Public Health Hazard* (Washington, D. C., The American Speech and Hearing Association, ASHA Reports 4, February, 1969).

Welch, Bruce L., and Welch, Annemarie S., eds., *Physiological Effects of Noise* (New York, Plenum Press, 1970).

Yerges, Lyle F., *Sound, Noise and Vibration Control* (New York, Van Nostrand Reinhold Company, 1969).

---

[102] Robert Alex Baron, "The Noise Receiver: The Citizen," *Sound and Vibration*, Vol. 2 (May, 1968), p. 9.

10

THE HANDICAP
OF HEARING IMPAIRMENT

In the previous parts of this book we have been concerned with the physiology and pathology of hearing, and with the measurement of hearing loss. Problems of hearing impairment have been considered thus far impersonally and hypothetically. Actually, of course, a hearing impairment cannot be separated from the patient who possesses it and has to live with it. Hearing is perhaps our most important sense, and naturally any marked interference with its functioning will produce difficulties in communication and in adjusting to our environment. Almost invariably, a hearing impairment produces psychological problems which add to the handicap imposed by the purely sensory dysfunction. The difficulties experienced will be proportional to the severity of the hearing impairment and related to the time of onset of the impairment, to cite two of the most important variables involved. It will be the purpose of this part of the book to analyze the handicap produced by a hearing impairment and to discuss the general principles of rehabilitation of persons with handicaps stemming from hearing losses.

It is difficult to discuss the rehabilitative needs of the hearing-handicapped generally because of the infinite number of possible variations of hearing loss, both in the severity of loss and in the configuration of the audiogram curve. It is difficult for hard-of-hearing persons themselves to recognize that their hearing problem is different from that of another hearing-impaired individual. Frequently the audiologist hears the complaint, "But Mr. Smith swears that Blank hearing aid makes it possible for him to attend lectures, and I can't understand why it won't do the same for me." What the complainer fails to realize, of course, is that his hearing loss may be entirely different from Smith's. Some patients will search for years for the "perfect" hearing aid, acquiring an imposing array of different makes and models in the process. They will be dissatisfied with each aid because it does not restore their hearing as they think it should, when the source of their difficulty is not the hearing aid but their own peculiar pattern of hearing loss, which cannot be helped by any hearing aid. Thus, in discussing the rehabilitative needs of the hard of hearing, it is necessary to differentiate somewhat on the basis of the degree and type of hearing loss involved.

SEVERITY OF HEARING IMPAIRMENT

The term *deafness* is used loosely to refer to any amount of hearing loss, but in planning a rehabilitative program for adults, or an educational program for children, it is necessary to make a distinction between the "deaf" and the "hard of hearing." In the mind of the layman, "deaf" means "completely without hearing." Actually, there are very few individuals whose auditory mechanism is completely dead. Most persons educationally classified as deaf have some shreds of hearing remaining, that is, some level of hearing that is demonstrable on an audiometric test. It is the *usefulness* of this residual hearing which determines whether a person is deaf or hard-of-hearing.

Some audiologists prefer to use more scientific terms to describe the degree of hearing impairment. *Hypacusis* (sometimes *hypoacusis*) means loss of hearing that is less than complete. *Anacusis* means deafness—literally "without hearing." Another scientific term is *dysacusis*, which designates an auditory disorder that is other than just a loss of sensitivity. Most frequently the term is applied to a central auditory dysfunction—a disturbance in the processing of auditory stimuli—although it can also refer to such phenomena as a loss of tonality and diplacusis. In this book we shall refer to hard-of-hearing and deaf individuals instead of to hypacusic and anacusic ones.

In 1937 the Committee on Nomenclature of the Conference of Executives of American Schools for the Deaf proposed the following definitions which are still valid:

1. *The Deaf:* Those in whom the sense of hearing is nonfunctional for the ordinary purposes of life. This general group is made up of two distinct classes based entirely on the time of the loss of hearing:

    a. *The congenitally deaf:* Those who were born deaf.

    b. *The adventitiously deaf:* Those who were born with normal hearing but in whom the sense of hearing became nonfunctional later through illness or accident.

2. *The Hard of Hearing:* Those in whom the sense of hearing, although defective, is functional with or without a hearing aid.[1]

[1] S. R. Silverman and H. S. Lane, "Deaf Children," in Hallowell Davis and S. Richard Silverman, eds., *Hearing and Deafness* (New York, Holt, Rinehart and Winston, 1970), p. 386.

Although it is not possible to draw firm boundaries between the deaf and the hard of hearing on the basis of the extent of loss shown on an audiogram, the following classification, based on pure-tone hearing levels through the speech frequencies, is a general guide to the degree of severity of hearing losses:

30–50 dB	Mild
50–70 dB	Moderate
70–85 dB	Severe
85–110 dB	Profound[2]

Conversational speech averages a sound pressure of about 70 dB, or a hearing level for speech of about 50 dB. The difference between "weak" and "loud" conversational speech is about 30 dB, covering a range of hearing levels for speech of 35 to 65 dB.[3] A person with a threshold hearing level for speech of 30 dB would just barely be able to hear conversational speech with the unaided ear. The weaker sounds in speech would be at about threshold level for him. He would miss a great deal of soft conversational speech. Such a person would benefit from the use of a hearing aid.

For many years it was a rule of thumb that unless a patient's loss for speech in his better ear was at least 30 dB a hearing aid would not be recommended. The advent of head-worn aids and "all-in-the-ear" aids has caused us to revise our thinking regarding the minimum loss for which an aid would be advised. There are many patients with losses of less than 30 dB for speech, and some with unilateral losses, who are at least part-time users of hearing aids—and satisfied users. As yet, the upper limit of hearing loss that can be benefited by a hearing aid has not been accurately determined. As aids have become more powerful, their benefit has been extended to a greater proportion of the hearing-handicapped population. Some patients with threshold hearing levels for speech of as much as 100 dB obtain "usable" hearing from a hearing aid. Others, with less extreme losses, are unable to utilize aids successfully. The factor of recruitment of loudness, which is characteristic of many cases of sensori-neural loss, may militate against a hearing aid. As was stated in Chapter 5, the configuration of the audiogram curve, as well as the extent of loss through the speech frequencies, is important in determining whether or not a given patient can benefit from amplification.

---

[2] Miriam D. Pauls and William G. Hardy, "Hearing Impairment in Preschool-Age Children," *Laryngoscope,* Vol. 63 (June, 1953), pp. 538-539. The hearing levels cited above have been changed from those presented in this article to conform to the ANSI–1969 audiometric calibration standards.

[3] Hallowell Davis, "The Articulation Area and the Social Adequacy Index for Hearing," *Laryngoscope,* Vol. 58 (August, 1948), p. 766.

TIME OF ONSET OF THE LOSS

The degree of handicap produced by a hearing loss depends to a considerable extent on its time of onset. This is true of the handicap of communication and of the problems of a psychological nature which accompany the hearing impairment. The effect of time of onset on the individual's ability to communicate is easy to understand. Language is learned through the auditory pathway. To learn to speak, the child must first understand or comprehend the speech that he hears. If a child is born with defective hearing, or incurs a hearing impairment in the first year to year and a half of life, his language development will be affected—to what extent depends, of course, on the severity of the loss and other factors such as his intelligence. If, however, a child's hearing is normal throughout the period when he is acquiring his basic language concepts, both receptive and expressive, the effect of an acquired hearing loss on his ability to communicate will be considerably less, again depending on the severity of the loss. The child with a severe congenital hearing impairment will have to be taught to recognize speech through minimal auditory clues and visual clues, and he will have to learn to speak laboriously on a word-by-word basis. Without the help of skilled teachers of the deaf, such a child would go through life deprived of oral communication.

On the other hand, the child who loses his hearing after he has learned to comprehend speech and to speak will in time lose his ability to communicate unless he is given special instruction. Nevertheless, the job of teaching such a child is relatively easy, since the teacher does not have to begin with basic language concepts. The problem here is to keep the child from losing what he has already acquired in the way of language ability, while helping him to develop a constantly increasing facility in language.

The problems of the adult who incurs a hearing impairment are usually quite different from those of children. In the first place, an adult seldom incurs a complete loss of hearing. Usually there is sufficient residual hearing present so that speech can be heard to some extent. In the second place, the adult has well-established language patterns. Although he may need help in learning to understand speech with his impaired hearing, he should have a minimum of difficulty with his own speech production.

PSYCHOLOGICAL PROBLEMS

A hearing impairment almost always produces some maladjustment in the individual. Sometimes, the psychological difficulties arising from the hearing loss are a greater problem for the hard-of-hearing person than the communicative disorder. Psychological difficulties are not always proportional to the severity of the loss, but they are usually related to the time of onset of the hearing impairment. According to some points of view, those who are born with impaired hearing or who lose their hearing early in life do not have as severe adjustment problems as those who suffer hearing loss after having had normal hearing well into adult life. The theory is that it is psychologically more difficult to lose one's hearing after having experienced a number of years of normal hearing than it is to be without hearing for all one's life. In other words, the congenitally deaf person does not realize what he is missing, and so it is easier for him to adjust to his situation. It should be emphasized, however, that there are many psychologists who disagree with the notion that the emotional adjustment of the congenitally deaf is superior to to that of the individual who loses his hearing later in life.

Ramsdell[4] refers to three levels of hearing, loss of any one of which would cause some phychological difficulty to the adult who has previously enjoyed normal hearing. The three levels are the *symbolic* level, the *warning* or *signal* level, and the *primitive* level. The symbolic level refers to the function of the hearing mechanism in the process of oral communication. Naturally, loss of the ability to communicate will cause the hearing-impaired individual to experience psychological difficulties. Not being able to talk easily with people leads to a tendency to withdraw from conversations, and eventually to withdraw from more and more social contacts. The hard-of-hearing person finds it difficult to enjoy meetings of the organizations to which he belongs, to attend plays or lectures, or to follow the minister's sermon in church. Thus, loss of hearing on the symbolic level may result in the individual's becoming increasingly withdrawn. Withdrawal in turn leads to feelings of depression, because the individual is cut off from his normal social life.

The *warning* or *signal* level of hearing refers to the function of the hearing mechanism in making us aware of dangers in the environment. For example, we hear the scream of a siren and are immediately alerted to look out for an emergency vehicle. The growl of a dog warns us to beware of patting him. The honk of an automobile horn tells us to be careful in crossing the street. Loss of the ability to utilize danger signals means that we must be more alert with other senses. Thus loss of hearing on the warning or signal level causes an individual to be more hesitant in his actions and increases his feelings of insecurity. In turn, increased feelings of insecurity tend to add to the feeling of depression.

In many respects, according to Ramsdell, loss of hearing on the *primitive* level creates more serious psychological problems than loss of hearing on the other two levels. The person with normal hearing is always situated in an environment of sound. Although we may not be conscious of the familiar daily sounds which surround us, they form an important part of our environ-

---

[4] Donald A. Ramsdell, "The Psychology of the Hard-of-Hearing and the Deafened Adult," Davis and Silverman, eds., *op. cit.*, Chap. 18.

ment. If we are suddenly deprived of the background of noises around us, we are aware of a feeling of discomfort and unease. It is awareness on the unconscious level of the environment of sounds surrounding us which is meant by the *primitive* level of hearing.

From a study of the psychological problems of servicemen who had been deafened during World War II, Ramsdell felt that loss of hearing on the primitive level was primarily responsible for the vague feelings of unrest and depression which were characteristic of this group of men. Many servicemen reported that they felt they were living in a "dead" world. Since the individual was no longer receiving the auditory sensations which had always been associated with his environment, he had the feeling that his environment was lost. Ramsdell thought that it was most important to explain to the deafened individual why he had these feelings of "aloneness" and restlessness, because with the understanding that they stemmed from loss of hearing on the primitive level the serviceman was better able to accept his feelings of depression and isolation.

Another frequently mentioned psychological characteristic of the adult who becomes hard-of-hearing is the exaggeration of any tendency the individual may have to be paranoiac. The hard-of-hearing person enters a room where people are talking. He sees them laughing together as he approaches them, but he cannot understand what they are saying. He may feel that the group has been talking about him, and for that reason will build up feelings of resentment toward them. It is difficult to communicate with a person who has a severe hearing impairment. One must speak carefully to him and frequently repeat what one says before the hard-of-hearing person can understand the conversation. It is perfectly natural for the members of the family of a hard-of-hearing person to talk among themselves in a normal manner without taking the trouble to explain to him what they are talking about. This person then feels "left out" of the conversation; he may even feel that the reason he was not included was because the other members of the family were making disparaging remarks about him.

Another psychological characteristic of the hard-of-hearing adult is his reluctance to admit that he has a sensory handicap. To some extent, of course, all handicapped persons have a natural aversion to advertising their handicap. The hard-of-hearing individual, however, manifests this tendency to a greater extent than is true of other handicapped people. The explanation is simple. The person with a handicap of hearing has no visible evidence of his handicap. In other words, his ear, the part that can be seen, looks just the same as that of a normal-hearing individual. Therefore, to the casual observer, the person with a hearing handicap appears to be the same as anyone else.

Further, the hard-of-hearing person exhibits merely exaggerated responses of the sort of which all of us are guilty. When we are listening to an anecdote but fail to appreciate the punch line because of missing an important word or two, our usual reaction is to laugh with the others instead of admitting that we did not get the point of the story. We apparently feel that such an admission would reveal to others that we were stupid. Thus we try to make the others believe that we, too, heard and understood everything. The hard-of-hearing person, who is in this position much more often and to a much greater extent, will attempt to bluff and give a response which he hopes is appropriate, rather than admit to a person with whom he is conversing that he did not understand a statement or a question. It is not unusual for a hard-of-hearing individual's friends to realize that he has a hearing impairment, although the victim believes firmly that no one is aware of his handicap. For example, it is not uncommon for older school teachers to develop sufficient hearing loss to cause them difficulty and embarrassment on many occasions. The students of such a teacher are sure to notice and to take advantage of his hearing handicap long before the teacher himself suspects that anyone knows that he is not hearing perfectly.

An individual who has a visual defect cannot successfully bluff his way through situations where good vision is required. Although he may dislike wearing spectacles, he will sooner or later accept them as a necessary part of his physical equipment, and so prevalent are they in our society that the person who must wear them is not penalized by others with whom he comes in contact. On the other hand, hearing aids are a relatively new development when compared with spectacles. Hearing aids are still sufficiently unusual to most people that they attract some attention. It is much more difficult to persuade a hard-of-hearing person to accept a hearing aid than it is to persuade a visually handicapped person to accept spectacles. Almost universally the hard-of-hearing adult will resist the acceptance of a hearing aid until he is driven to it through despair. Hearing-aid dealers maintain that it is necessary for them to "seek out" hard-of-hearing individuals by means of "come-on" advertising and door-to-door selling, because the hard-of-hearing person would never on his own initiative visit the hearing-aid dealer's office. There is some truth in the dealers' contention. Whereas the visually handicapped person goes to his opthalmologist, or to an optometrist, and then visits the optician to have the prescribed spectacles fitted, the hard-of-hearing person tends to procrastinate with regard to his hearing loss until he is forced to do something about it.

Very young children with hearing impairments do not have the psychological problems of older children and adults. Audiologists are aware that it is easier to persuade a child of five years of age to accept a hearing aid than it is to secure the acceptance of a child of eight or nine. Girls particularly are reluctant to wear hearing aids because they feel that they will be less attractive to the opposite sex. Boys tend to resist wearing aids because the hearing aid sets them off as being different from the rest of the "crowd." Of course, children who are in the "sensitive" period of their lives are prone to shy away from anything which marks them as different from their peers. Unfortunately, children are often cruel to one another, and any difference tends to become the focal point for ridicule. Thus it is especially difficult to persuade a child to accept a hearing aid when he is in the period of needing to conform. The child's psychological problems, therefore, stem largely from a dislike of admitting that he is different from his friends and schoolmates.

There are other reasons, of course, why the child may become maladjusted because of a hearing impairment. Difficulty in communication leads to trouble with school work and misunderstandings with family and friends. Thus the hearing problem heightens tensions within the child. As a result, the hard-of-hearing child is seldom perfectly adjusted. Usually he reacts to his frustrations either by withdrawing from situations that are difficult for him or by becoming overly aggressive in behavior. The parents of a hearing-handicapped child face the difficult task of assisting their child to find an adequate personal adjustment to his disability.

GENERAL CONSIDERATIONS IN REHABILITATION

Adults who have hearing problems generally can achieve a satisfactory adjustment to them through participation in a rehabilitation program. Children who are born with hearing impairments can be trained to get along with a minimum of handicap. Such training is not properly termed re-habilitation, since these children have never been "habilitated." Children who lose their hearing at some time after they have acquired language can be handled in the same sort of rehabilitation program that is appropriate for adults.

Rehabilitative work with the hard of hearing involves four primary steps. These are speechreading (lipreading), auditory training, speech training, and counseling. Whether the hard-of-hearing individual is child or adult, he will need all these basic rehabilitative approaches to some degree. For the child who is born deaf, or severely hard-of-hearing, a special education program which involves teaching *language* rather than correcting disabilities in oral communication is indicated throughout the child's school life. The remainder of this chapter will be concerned with the four primary facets of an aural rehabilitation program for the hard of hearing. Succeeding chapters will discuss in more detail programs of rehabilitation for children and for adults.

Speechreading

Historically, *speechreading*, or *lipreading* as it used to be called, is the oldest of the rehabilitative approaches to some of the problems of impaired hearing. By speechreading is meant the use of visual clues in determining what the speaker says. The newer term *speechreading* is preferred because visual clues come from watching the entire speaker rather than from concentrating solely on his lips. All of us engage in the practice of speechreading, although usually we are not conscious of the fact that our eyes are assisting our ears. It is a common observation, however, that we can more easily understand a lecturer whose face is clearly visible, and we can "hear" better in a well-lighted rather than a dark room. Many hard-of-hearing individuals stoutly maintain that they do not speechread. Nevertheless they will report that they seem to "hear" better when they can see the speaker. Teaching speechreading is really putting on a conscious level what the patient is already doing to some extent on an unconscious level.

Many people regard speechreading as a mysterious art which can be learned only after years of training and experience. The average normal-hearing person would probably answer a questionnaire by saying that he does not know anything about speechreading. The Hollywood idea of speechreading frequently is misleading. For example, the films will depict agents of the Federal Bureau of Investigation with a band of spies under observation in a hotel room across the street. They cannot tell what the conspirators are talking about; they therefore bring a well-trained speech-reader to the scene who watches the conversation through binoculars and reports accurately every word spoken by the conspirators. Speechreading is not that precise in real life. Actually, it is a poor substitute for hearing. At best, it is not possible to speechread 100 per cent of what is seen. The reasons are obvious. In English, only about one-third of our speech sounds are clearly visible, that is, are made with articulators involving only the front of the mouth. Sounds such as *k* and *r* are impossible to speechread, because the articulators that are involved in their formation cannot be seen. Even the best speechreader, therefore, is bound to miss a considerable proportion of what he sees. Moreover, many words which are different in phonetic content and in meaning appear alike from the standpoint of the visible movement made in uttering them. The word *mom,* for example, looks to the speech-reader exactly the same as the words *mop, mob, bob, bomb, palm,* and so forth, because the sounds *p* and *b* and *m* are all made with the lips and are in-distinguishable from each other by appearance alone. It is necessary, there-fore, for the speechreader to determine from the context of what he sees which particular word of the group looking alike the speaker is saying. This is a process which cannot be performed instantaneously; again, therefore, the speechreader is bound to miss a proportion of what he sees. Incidentally, words that look alike to the speechreader are called *homophenous* words. Practically every textbook on speechreading contains a section devoted to homophenous words.

Training in speechreading consists of the teaching of systematic observa-tion. The patient must be taught how to exercise his powers of observation most efficiently. Naturally, learning speechreading involves a considerable amount of practice. However great the facility that the speechreader attains, he can always learn to become even more effective through increased training and practice. At Stanford, a class in speechreading for adult hard-of-hearing persons was taught for a number of years. Many students who were originally enrolled in the class continued to attend year after year because they felt that it was possible to continue improving. This does not mean that instruction in speechreading requires a number of years of time. The average hard-of-hearing individual can achieve a working ability in speechreading in a period of about thirty lessons. Of course, many hard-of-hearing persons do an effective job of speechreading without having had any formal instruction. It is a skill that they develop through necessity, because of their inability to follow conversation through hearing alone. Curiously, it is difficult for a normal-hearing person to achieve a high degree of skill in speechreading. Apparently the motivation of having to depend on speechreading is a necessary prerequisite to becoming a proficient speechreader.

As stated above, speechreading is a poor substitute for hearing. Most hard-of-hearing individuals have residual hearing upon which they can rely to some extent. Speechreading supplements the residual hearing. It enables the individual to comprehend more conversation than would be possible through hearing alone. In fact, the total communication received through a combination of speechreading and hearing is considerably greater than could be obtained through either method alone.

Before hearing aids were invented, speechreading was the only rehabilitative technique available to persons with hearing handicaps. Speechreading classes have been conducted in this country for as many years as educators have been aware of the special needs of those with hearing handicaps. Some teachers of speechreading were resentful toward hearing aids when they first became common. It was as if the teacher considered the hearing aid a threat to his profession. Consequently, many teachers of speechreading refused to allow their pupils to use hearing aids while they were engaged in speechreading lessons. Their attitude was that the pupil was there to learn speechreading, and if he were able to use his ears at all he would not be motivated to learn speechreading. Apparently these teachers believed that learning speechreading for its own sake was a proper goal for a hard-of-hearing person. This attitude toward hearing aids manifested a shortsighted point of view on the part of the teachers toward their function, which must be defined as that of aiding the hard-or-hearing person to communicate more effectively. Since more effective communication can be achieved through combining sight and hearing, the teaching of speechreading should stress the use of both sensory avenues.

Actually, the development of the electronic hearing aid *has* constituted a threat to the old-time teacher of speechreading. Before the days of hearing aids, speechreading was the only rehabilitative avenue open to the hearing-handicapped individual. With the development of the individual, wearable hearing aid, the patient could combine his residual hearing with his powers of visual observation. Many people were able to get along satisfactorily by depending primarily on the hearing aid. For them, formal instruction in speechreading was not necessary. Thus as hearing aids became more popular, schools and individual teachers of speechreading served fewer and fewer hearing-handicapped individuals.

Various methods have been proposed for teaching speechreading. Historically, two of them represent somewhat opposing philosophies. On the one hand, there are the proponents of the *analytic* method, and, on the other hand, there are those who believe in the *synthetic* approach. Those who adhere to the analytic school believe that it is necessary to teach a patient, first of all, to recognize individual speech "movements" or sounds in isolation. From individual movements the patient proceeds to words, then phrases, sentences, and finally paragraphs. The synthetic approach operates on the principle that learning is accomplished by starting with wholes. In the synthetic method, the speechreader begins by learning to recognize the meaning of whole paragraphs. Theoretically, in the synthetic method, drilling on individual sounds or movements comes only when a breakdown in the comprehension of paragraphs has occurred. The analytic method is championed by Martha Bruhn, who brought to this country the techniques of Müller-Walle of Germany.[5] The synthetic approach was proposed by Edward B. Nitchie, who for many years operated a private school of speechreading in New York City.[6] Actually, when the lesson plans proposed by Bruhn and by Nitchie are closely examined, it is apparent that there is not as much difference between them as would be presumed from the opposing philosophies expressed by the authors.

The Kinzie sisters devised a method which attempted to incorporate the best of the Müller-Walle and the Nitchie systems.[7] Cora Elsie Kinzie herself was hard-of-hearing and had studied with both Martha Bruhn and Edward Nitchie. In addition to these two basic methods of teaching speechreading—the Müller-Walle and the Nitchie methods—a third method was proposed in Jena, Germany, by Karl Brauckmann. The Jena method, so-called from its place of origin, was brought to the United States by Anna Bunger.[8] Departing from the usual techniques of working with individual sounds, or with paragraphs of running speech, the Jena method proposes drill work on the rhythm patterns of English.

Auditory Training

As stated previously, there are very few individuals who are "deaf as a post." Even those who are educationally classified as "deaf" usually have

[5] Martha E. Bruhn, *The Müller-Walle Method of Lip-Reading for the Deaf* (Lynn, Mass., Thos. P. Nichols, 1920).

[6] Edward B. Nitchie, *Lip-Reading Principles and Practise* (New York, Stokes, 1919).

[7] Cora Elsie Kinzie and Rose Kinzie, *Lip-Reading for the Deafened Adult* (Chicago, John C. Winston Co., 1931).

[8] Anna M. Bunger, *Speech Reading—Jena Method* (Danville, Ill., Interstate, 1944).

some measurable residual hearing. The purpose of auditory training, with the deaf as with the hard of hearing, is to teach the hearing-handicapped patient to make the most effective use of his remaining hearing. Auditory training is usually given with the aid of amplification.

Before World War II, auditory training had been confined, for the most part, to teaching pupils in schools for the deaf to be aware of gross sound stimuli. Dr. Max Goldstein, founder of Central Institute for the Deaf in St. Louis, has described techniques for stimulating the hearing of such children.[9] Not until World War II, however, was much attention paid to the problems of teaching the hard of hearing how to make the most of their residual hearing. This is difficult to understand, because the person who is hard-of-hearing has a greater potential for drawing upon his residual hearing effectively than has the person who is deaf. To a considerable extent, however, the development of interest in auditory training of the hard of hearing followed the development of the wearable hearing aid. Hearing aids were not sold extensively, nor were they common before World War II.

Actually, then, the origin of auditory training as a rehabilitative technique was in the so-called "aural rehabilitation" centers operated by the armed services in World War II. Here, for the first time, specialists from many fields were drawn together with a common purpose: to plan and to administer a rehabilitative program which would enable the hearing-impaired serviceman to return to duty or to civilian life with a minimum of handicap. In these military centers, it was found that the "fitting" of a hearing aid was only one step in the rehabilitation of the hard-of-hearing patient. After the selection of a hearing aid, it was necessary to give the individual training in the proper adjustment of the aid for all situations, and how to interpret correctly what he heard with it. In addition to classes in speechreading and in "speech conservation," a class in auditory training was developed at each of the military centers. Some included in their program a "listening hour"; at that time patients would get informal practice in a variety of listening situations, thus supplementing on their own the formal instruction they received in class.

In Chapter 6, we discussed the measures in speech audiometry to evaluate a patient's loss of hearing for speech. One of them is an estimate of the patient's speech-discrimination ability, which is obtained by having him listen to phonetically balanced (PB) words at above-threshold levels. We have seen that some patients have excellent speech-discrimination ability, whereas other patients do poorly on the PB words, regardless of how loudly they hear them. The results of speech-discrimination tests determine the emphasis to be placed on auditory training in the rehabilitation program. The patient with good understanding of things that he can hear requires

---

9 Max Goldstein, *The Acoustic Method for the Training of the Deaf and Hard-of-Hearing Child* (St. Louis, Laryngoscope Press, 1937).

relatively little auditory training to learn to make effective use of a hearing aid. On the other hand, the patient who does poorly on the PB words may be able to improve his speech-discrimination ability by means of a concentrated program in auditory training. An analysis of the specific sounds that the patient confuses in the PB test will determine the training materials needed. Thus, if a patient consistently misses words with high-frequency voiceless consonant sounds in them, such as *s, th, f, k, t, p, sh, ch, wh, h,* the auditory training program should be designed to include practice in differentiating words containing these sounds. It should not be assumed that auditory training can teach the individual with a discrimination problem to make 100 per cent discriminations through hearing alone, but any improvement in the ability to recognize words by ear would be beneficial in terms of the total communication that the individual can receive.

For a child or an adult who has not used his hearing for some time, it may be necessary to institute a program of auditory training leading up to the application of a wearable hearing aid. In other words, if the patient has not been accustomed to hearing or having to interpret auditory stimuli, he must be taught how to *listen,* and taught that sounds convey meanings. This kind of training can be accomplished with an *auditory training unit,* a specially designed, high-fidelity, high-output amplifier which directs an auditory signal from a disc recording or microphone to high-quality earphones, the output of which is separately adjustable. Several models of auditory training units are commercially available. Some can be operated with several sets of earphones, so that a group of patients may receive auditory training simultaneously. Some models can be equipped with hearing-aid types of receivers, thus providing an easy transition to an individual hearing aid. Many auditory training units are of the stereophonic type, that is, have two microphones and two amplifiers, so that each earphone receives a separate signal. Such systems provide more "natural" hearing and a "depth perception" that is not possible with a unit that feeds the same signal to each earphone. Some educators of the hearing-handicapped use auditory training instrumentation of the "loop-induction" type. In this case, the signal from the amplifier is transferred to the telephone coil of an individual wearable hearing aid via a magnetic field. This arrangement has the advantage of permitting the child to move about the classroom freely without being hampered by wires connecting him with the auditory training unit. Another type of wireless auditory training unit consists of an FM transmitter worn by the teacher that broadcasts on a radio frequency to FM receivers worn by the children and tuned to the transmitting frequency.

An auditory training unit gives the patient the advantage of excellent sound reproduction, which stimulates his hearing to the maximum extent. Having learned to make use of high-fidelity sound, the patient can then transfer to the more limited amplification of the wearable hearing aid. If the patient cannot be taught to respond to the amplification of the auditory training unit, it is probably useless to expect him to be able to master an individual wearable aid.

Speech Training

Most individuals with severe or profound impairments of their hearing will require some speech training in addition to their other rehabilitative needs. It is obvious that a child born with defective hearing will have considerable difficulty developing intelligible speech, since it is a well-known fact that speech is learned largely by ear. It is not so obvious why an older individual who incurs a hearing impairment after the acquisition of language should need speech training. Generally, the onset of a hearing impairment is not sudden; rather, the progression from normal to profoundly impaired hearing is gradual over a period of years. Those of us who have normal hearing are able to monitor our own speech, thus to regulate the intensity of our voices to suit the noise conditions under which we are speaking, and to correct defects in articulation that arise from misuse of our articulators. This the person with a profound hearing impairment is unable to do. Thus it is common, as hearing loss progresses, for a person's voice and speech to show the effect of the hearing impairment.

As was stated in Chapter 3, a person with a conductive impairment may tend to speak too softly or with too little vocal intensity. The reason is that, by definition, a person with a conductive loss has good bone-conduction hearing. Since we hear our own voices to some extent through the mechanism of bone conduction, the conductively impaired individual may hear himself well whereas others may have difficulty in understanding him because of the softness of his voice. On the other hand, the patient with a sensori-neural loss of hearing may tend to speak too loudly since his bone conduction is affected along with air conduction, and he does not hear himself well unless he speaks loudly. Any severely or profoundly hearing-impaired person will likely have some difficulty regulating the level of his voice to suit unusual conditions of sound environment. Thus training is needed to teach these individuals how to regulate their voices by nonaural clues that they can perceive.

Many individual sounds of English require a rather delicate adjustment of the articulators in order to produce the correct acoustic effect. In the presence of a severe or profound hearing impairment, these sounds may deteriorate because we usually depend upon our auditory monitoring to tell us whether or not a change in articulator adjustment is necessary. In other words, we tend to make more or less automatic adjustment of our articulators in accordance with what our ears tell us. Two sounds which are most commonly affected by a hearing impairment are the *s* and the *r*. In both, the articulator adjustment is critical, and without a refined sense of auditory discrimination it is difficult to form these sounds in the correct manner. Generally, the sounds that require a precise adjustment of the tongue blade or the tongue tip will be affected most by a hearing impairment. Such sounds tend to become "thick" or "mushy."

Deterioration of speech can occur without the awareness of the patient. Others are much more conscious of a patient's speech deficiencies than he is. Since the deterioration of speech patterns, which have previously been well established, occurs gradually, the ideal time to commence speech training for the hard-of-hearing patient is before a marked deterioration has occurred. In the military aural rehabilitation centers in World War II, the term *speech conservation* was coined to refer to preventive speech therapy given to newly deafened individuals in order to keep their speech and voice disturbances to a minimum. In other words, the speech training was started before any marked changes in speech and voice patterns had occurred, in the hope that through such training the hard-of-hearing individual could maintain good speech.

Where the hearing loss makes it impossible for the patient to monitor his speech through the ear, he must be taught how to regulate his speech by other means. The usual method is that of teaching the patient to perform tactile monitoring, that is, to learn to control his speech and voice production through motor-kinesthetic sensations. Since a person with a profound impairment of hearing cannot hear the *s*, for example, he must be taught the correct articulator placement for it so that he can get the "feel" of the correct position while he is speaking. In speech-correction practice, there are two general methods of teaching the correct production of a sound. The preferred technique is the so-called stimulus or acoustic method, which is based on the fact that the individual can learn correct articulator placement by experimenting until he achieves what his ear tells him is the correct sound. The other technique is the "phonetic-placement" method, which involves teaching speech sounds by instructing the patient how he should place his articulators and teaching him to utilize kinesthetic sensations. It is this second method of speech correction that is required for the hard of hearing, since the first is ruled out by the nature of the handicap.

Psychological Counseling

Since the greatest handicap of a hearing loss is frequently the psychological problems that it produces in a patient, a rehabilitation program for the hard of hearing should provide for psychological counseling as needed. Frequently such counseling may well be the most important part of the rehabilitation program. The hard-of-hearing patient might be an excellent speechreader, he might be making maximum use of his residual hearing, and his speech patterns might be irreproachable, and yet he might be a rehabilitative failure unless he arrives at a satisfactory adjustment to his handicap.

The requirements of a counseling program for children differ from those of a program for adults. With a hard-of-hearing child, frequently the counseling must be directed toward the child's parents, since an improper attitude on their part will influence the child's point of view towards his own problems. As stated earlier in this chapter, children whose training begins after the age of eight or nine present more problems in learning to accept their disability. Then it may be helpful to approach the child's problems to some extent by counseling his associates and his teacher. An interested and skilled teacher can accomplish a great deal in determining the attitude of other children in the class toward the handicapped pupil.

The adult who incurs a handicapping hearing impairment faces a number of problems with which the counselor must cope. In the first place, he may have to be persuaded to accept the hearing loss as a problem. He must be willing to admit to himself, as well as to others, that he has a sensory impairment. Having admitted this, he relieves himself of the burden of trying to act in all situations as if his hearing were normal. He is not "keeping a secret," which he fears others may discover; instead, he has "confessed" his shortcomings and should find the relief from mental strain that confession brings. Once a patient has admitted his sensory deficiency, he can be guided to an intelligent approach to his problems. He can accept the wearing of a hearing aid without feeling a sense of shame, and he can advise others that they will have to take care in the way they speak to him.

It is likely that the hard-of-hearing adult will feel that he is not understood by the members of his family. As a matter of fact, the husband or wife and the children do often behave in an inconsiderate fashion in regard to the hearing-handicapped individual. Not infrequently, it is necessary for psychological counseling to extend to others in the family, so that they may be made to realize the patient's limitations and learn ways in which they can assist him.

Vocational counseling should be offered whenever the hearing impairment poses a problem in the work activities of the patient. Although hard-of-hearing individuals function effectively in countless professional and vocational activities, there are certain types of positions which cannot be filled properly by a person with faulty hearing. Sometimes, then, a hearing loss will make it impossible for a patient to continue in a position for which he was trained. Naturally, the longer a patient has been employed in a given job, the harder it will be for him to accept the need for changing to a different type of employment. The vocational counselor can help considerably in the psychological adjustment of the hard-of-hearing adult by guiding him correctly in the selection of a vocation or in a change from one type of position to another.

All of us need to feel liked and wanted by others. The adult who incurs a hearing loss which limits his ability to communicate is likely to become withdrawn and antisocial. Even with proper family acceptance and handling of the handicapped patient in his home situation, it is necessary that the patient have contacts outside the home and participate in activities in which he can forget himself. It frequently requires considerable "pushing" in a delicate way on the part of the patient's family and his counselor, but the maintenance of old social contacts and the development of new ones is necessary to a patient's mental health.

HEARING AIDS

No discussion of the rehabilitative needs of the hard of hearing would be complete without some information on hearing aids. The modern hearing aid is the descendant of such pre-electronic devices as the speaking tube or horn, which the hard-of-hearing individual held to his ear. The speaking tube provided "amplification" by concentrating or focusing the sound waves into the ear canal. The same effect can be achieved less efficiently by cupping the hand behind the auricle. The invention of the carbon microphone and amplifier revolutionized hearing aids. Actually, it was Alexander Graham Bell's search for a means of amplifying speech for the deaf which led to his invention of the telephone. For many years after their development, hearing aids were made with carbon microphones and sometimes carbon amplifiers. The development of the vacuum-tube amplifier, however, again revolutionized hearing aids, and when vacuum tubes were miniaturized, so that a small better-powered amplifier could be built, the vacuum-tube hearing aid quickly replaced the less efficient carbon type. More recently, transistors have superseded vacuum tubes in hearing-aid designs, resulting in increased efficiency and decreased size of hearing aids. Entire hearing aids are now built into the frames of spectacles. Some aids are designed to be worn behind the auricle, and some are so tiny that they fit into the ear canal.

All wearable, electric hearing aids, from the carbon type to the transistor model, have consisted of the following components: a microphone to change acoustic energy into electricity, a battery-powered amplifier to build up the strength of the signal coming from the microphone, and a receiver to change the amplified electric signal back to acoustic power. The receiver may be of the air-conduction or the bone-conduction type. An air-conduction receiver is connected to an ear piece, which is inserted in the patient's ear canal. Vacuum-tube aids required two batteries: an "A" battery to heat the filaments of the tubes, and a "B" battery to provide the amplification; transistor aids, not having any filaments to heat, require only a small "B" voltage.

The amount of amplification, or "acoustic gain," of the instrument depends in part upon the number of transistors, and the voltage of the battery that supplies the power. Most companies make several models of varying gain, suitable for different degrees of hearing loss. *Gain* is measured by determining the difference in decibels between the level of the input at the microphone and the level of the output at the receiver. Lybarger has described methods of measuring and expressing the performance of hearing aids which have been adopted by the Hearing Aid Industry Conference (HAIC) as the standard way for hearing-aid manufacturers to report performance data for their instruments.[10] The "basic frequency response" of an aid is determined by measuring the output of the hearing aid receiver in a 2 cc coupler when various frequencies are produced by a loudspeaker at a sound pressure level of 60 dB measured at the location of the hearing-aid microphone. The volume control of the aid is adjusted until the output of the receiver for a 1000-Hz input is 100 dB or 40 dB greater than the input (40-dB gain). The output for all other frequencies of the same input level is then measured, and the results are plotted on a graph, such as that shown in Figure 10-1. From such a graph, the frequency range of the aid is determined by averaging the output at 500, 1000, and 2000 Hz and drawing a horizontal line through a point 15 dB below the average output at these three frequencies. The frequency limits of the aid are the points where the response curve intersects the horizontal line. Thus in Figure 10-1, the frequency range would be from 350 to 4600 Hz.

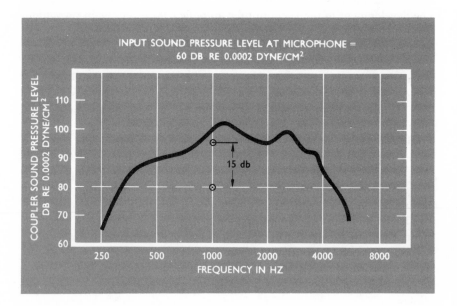

Figure 10-1.   Determination of frequency range from the frequency-response curve of a hearing aid.

[10] S. F. Lybarger, "Standardized Hearing Aid Measurements," *Audecibel*, Vol. 10 (March-April, 1961), pp. 8-10, 24-25.

HAIC defines the gain of a hearing aid as the difference between the average output of the receiver at the frequencies of 500, 1000, and 2000 Hz and the input sound pressure level at the microphone which, for this measurement, is specified as 50 dB for all frequencies. Output measurements of the receiver in the coupler are made with the instrument's volume control turned full on. Figure 10-2 illustrates the determination of gain by the HAIC method. In this hypothetical illustration, the average output at 500, 1000, and 2000 Hz is 116 dB. Since the input level was 50 dB, the gain is 66 dB.

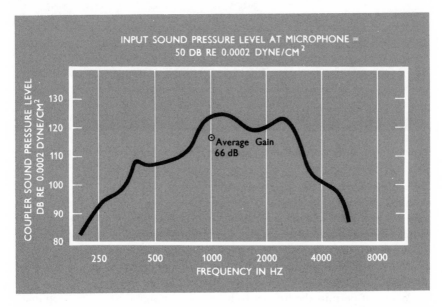

Figure 10-2. HAIC method of determining gain when hearing aid volume control is at the full-on setting.

The maximum acoustic output of a hearing aid, or simply "output" in HAIC terminology, is the average output of the receiver in the coupler for the frequencies 500, 1000, and 2000 Hz when the input at each frequency is adjusted to produce the maximum output at the receiver with the hearing aid's volume control in the full-on position. A graph of the maximum acoustic output at each frequency is called a "saturation curve." The output of the hearing aid whose saturation curve is shown in Figure 10-3 is 124 dB, the average output at 500, 1000, and 2000 Hz.

Hearing aids have built-in limiters of the maximum acoustic gain of the amplifier, so that, regardless of the level of the input, the output can never exceed a certain predetermined intensity, which is below the patient's

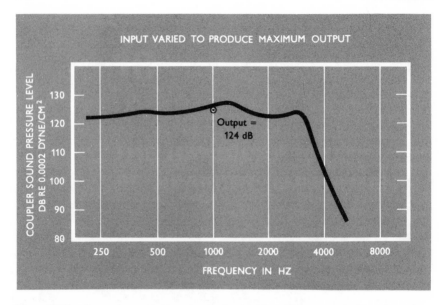

Figure 10-3.   Saturation output curve obtained with volume control of hearing aid at full-on position.

threshold of pain. The typical hearing aid has both a volume control and a tone control. These enable the wearer to adjust the output of the amplifier to his own particular needs. Some aids contain a telephone circuit. By flicking a switch, the user can disconnect the microphone and connect an induction coil which sends the signals from a telephone to the hearing-aid amplifier, thus bypassing the microphone of the hearing aid. Such an arrangement permits the listener to hear only the signal from the telephone; unwanted sounds in the listener's environment thus do not interfere with the signal from the telephone. When using the telephone, the patient switches on the telephone circuit and then places the telephone instrument next to the case of his hearing aid. With head-worn aids, the telephone would be held in the usual upright position but with the receiver of the telephone next to the hearing aid—not over the ear piece. With body-worn aids, the telephone instrument may need to be reversed, that is, held so the receiver of the telephone is close to the case of the hearing aid.

The air-conduction type of hearing-aid receiver connects to an ear piece, fabricated of acrylic or of a flexible plastic from an impression taken of the patient's ear. Amplified sound is delivered to the ear canal through a hole drilled through the ear piece. The purpose of the ear piece is to provide a tight seal at the ear, so that the amplified sound cannot "leak out" around the ear piece and reach the microphone of the aid, thus producing a "squeal" that is called *acoustic feedback*. With head-worn aids containing the receiver within the case of the instrument, the receiver is connected to the ear piece by a short length of plastic tubing. With body-worn aids, the receiver, which is connected to the amplifier with a fine wire, snaps on to a bushing imbedded in the ear piece.

Traditionally, a hearing aid would not be recommended for a patient unless his loss for speech in the better ear exceeded 30 dB. It was assumed that if a patient had one ear that was normal he would derive no benefit from amplification. Such an assumption was based on the observation in the audiology clinic that a patient's sound-field speech reception threshold and discrimination score tended to agree closely with the SRT and discrimination score of the better ear. Patients with unilateral impairments complain that they are handicapped in certain situations, however, particularly when people speak to them on the side of the impaired ear. In 1965, Harford and Barry reported their experience in providing patients with unilateral losses with specially designed head-worn aids that picked up signals through a microphone mounted on the side of the poor ear and transmitted them electrically to a receiver connected with the good ear. The receiver was coupled to the good ear by means of plastic tubing that was held in place in the outer part of the external canal by an "open" earpiece fitted to the concha. Since the earpiece did not occlude the canal, the good ear could still function normally while at the same time receiving amplified signals from the side of the poor ear. Harford and Barry called their arrangement CROS for "contralateral routing of signals." [11] While Harford and Barry utilized a headband for mounting the hearing aid and receiver on opposite sides of the head, the principle of their CROS arrangement was essentially the same as the eyeglass aid with microphone and receiver on opposite sides described by Wullstein and Wigand.[12] Harford and Barry reported that while it was not possible to demonstrate in the clinical testing of most of their experimental subjects that the use of a CROS fitting resulted in measurable improvement over the unaided sound-field listening situation, 85 per cent of their subjects "reported benefit from CROS hearing-aid use in their daily life activities after a minimum trial of CROS for one week." [13]

The CROS fitting resulted in an unexpected benefit to another group of hearing-impaired individuals for whom hearing aids had rarely been recommended. These are individuals whose hearing for the lower frequencies is excellent but whose sensitivity for the higher speech frequencies drops off abruptly. Patients with sloping audiograms above 1000 Hz generally have speech reception thresholds close to normal but poor discrimination. Since hearing aids amplify all frequencies through the speech range, they generally

11 Earl Harford and Joseph Barry, "A Rehabilitative Approach to the Problem of Unilateral Hearing Impairment: the Contralateral Routing of Signals (CROS)," *Journal of Speech and Hearing Disorders*, Vol. 30 (May, 1965), pp. 121-138.

12 H. L. Wullstein and M. E. Wigand, "A Hearing Aid for Single Ear Deafness and Its Requirements," *Acta Otolaryngologica*, Vol. 54 (1962), pp. 136-142.

13 Harford and Barry, *op. cit.*, p. 134.

could not use amplification successfully, because the amplified low frequencies tend to mask the weaker, high-frequency sounds. Dodds and Harford, noting that patients with unilateral impairments were able to benefit from CROS fittings even though their good ears had high-frequency losses, decided to experiment with CROS fittings and open earpieces with patients who had bilateral high-frequency losses. They hypothesized that the open earpiece would suppress low frequencies and thus result in less masking effect on the higher frequencies and improved speech discrimination. The CROS fitting—separating the microphone from the receiver—should prevent acoustic feedback from the open earpiece. Their results indicated that patients with high-frequency loss using open ear molds in CROS fittings were able to improve their speech discrimination scores significantly over the scores obtained in routine speech audiometry.[14] Green and Ross, utilizing sound-field Békésy audiometry, compared a subject's aided audiograms when he used a standard earpiece and when he used an open, or nonoccluding, earpiece with a CROS arrangement. The audiograms clearly indicate that the nonoccluding earpiece suppresses the lower speech frequencies while allowing the higher speech frequencies to be amplified to the same extent as with the standard earpiece. Further, Green and Ross demonstrated that the length of tubing connecting the receiver with the earpiece had a negligible effect on the frequency response of the aid, so that CROS fittings could be accomplished as efficiently by running the tubing across the head as by running an electrical wire, thus requiring less modification of a hearing aid to adapt it to a CROS fitting.[15]

The experimental successes of the CROS fitting for unilateral impairments and for patients with bilateral high-frequency losses resulted in the enthusiastic acceptance of this method of fitting by the hearing-aid industry and individual dealers. Modifications of the CROS principle have been introduced that provide the dealer with great flexibility in fitting a variety of patients that heretofore were difficult or impossible to fit. One modification is the BICROS aid that employs two microphones feeding a single amplifier and receiver mounted in a standard (occluding) ear piece in the better ear. The BICROS is useful for patients whose poorer ear is not suitable for amplification, so signals from both sides of the head are routed to the good ear. As Green and Ross suggest, the use of microphones of differing frequency-response characteristics should enable the wearer to obtain localization information from a BICROS fitting.[16] Dunlavy believes that the CROS fitting and its various modifications will almost double the number of individuals who can be helped with hearing aids. His preference is to use the

14 Elizabeth Dodds and Earl Harford, "Modified Earpieces and CROS for High Frequency Hearing Losses," *Journal of Speech and Hearing Research*, Vol. 11 (March, 1968), pp. 204-218.

15 David S. Green and Mark Ross, "The Effect of a Conventional Versus a Nonoccluding (CROS-type) Earmold upon the Frequency Response of a Hearing Aid," *Journal of Speech and Hearing Research*, Vol. 11 (September, 1968), pp. 638-647.

16 *Ibid.*, p. 646.

CROS principle in an eyeglass fitting with a short length of preformed polyvinyl tubing extending into the ear canal without the need for an open earpiece. The advantage of this procedure is the convenience of not having to insert or remove the earpiece when putting the aid on or taking it off, and the comparative invisibility of the tubing alone. Dunlavy reports that the amount of low-frequency suppression can be adjusted by varying the degree of penetration of the tubing into the canal.[17]

With the advent of head-worn aids, of either the behind-the-ear or the glasses type, the use of "true" binaural, that is, stereophonic, hearing became practicable. While binaural aids almost double the cost of monaural aids, there are many hard-of-hearing individuals who believe that the improved hearing abilities they obtain with stereophonic amplification are well worth the additional expense. In theory, binaural hearing aids should provide many advantages, such as improved localization of sound sources, better discrimination of speech in the presence of noise, and improved "quality" of sound. Many audiologists enthusiastically welcomed the appearance of binaural aids on the market and consistently recommended them to patients who presented problems in hearing-aid "fittings." Although standard methods of testing the performance of patients with hearing aids usually did not reflect an advantage of a binaural instrument over a monaural one, the assumption was made that new testing techniques needed to be developed for clinical use, and that such new techniques would demonstrate the advantage of binaural instruments.[18] Binaural aids were recommended frequently for young children with severe or profound impairments.

In the last several years there have been a number of research investigations comparing the performance of hearing-impaired patients with monaural and binaural hearing aids. Generally, these investigations have failed to demonstrate that patients perform appreciably better with binaural fittings.[19] Many patients who have purchased binaural aids after having owned monaural instruments report that they obtain superior benefit from the binaural aids, but it is difficult to determine whether they really are deriving acoustic advantages or are simply rationalizing their investment in more expensive instruments.[20] It seems important that audiologists continue

[17] Alfred R. Dunlavy, "CROS: the New Miracle Worker," *Audecibel*, Vol. 19 (Fall, 1970), pp. 141-148.

[18] Raymond Carhart, "The Usefulness of the Binaural Hearing Aid," *Journal of Speech and Hearing Disorders*, Vol. 23 (February, 1958), pp. 42-51.

[19] Louis M. DiCarlo and William J. Brown, "The Effectiveness of Binaural Hearing for Adults with Hearing Impairments," *Journal of Auditory Research*, Vol. 1 (September, 1960), pp. 35-76.

James Jerger and Donald Dirks, "Binaural Hearing Aids. An Enigma," *Journal of the Acoustical Society of America*, Vol. 33 (April, 1961), pp. 537-538.

James Jerger, Raymond Carhart, and Donald Dirks, "Binaural Hearing Aids and Speech Intelligibility," *Journal of Speech and Hearing Research*, Vol. 4 (June, 1961), pp. 137-148.

[20] Donald Dirks and Raymond Carhart, "A Survey of Reactions from Users of Binaural and Monaural Hearing Aids," *Journal of Speech and Hearing Disorders*, Vol. 27 (November, 1962), p. 321.

their investigations of binaural hearing-aid performance. It is quite possible that the tests which have been used to evaluate the performance of patients with binaural aids are not those which are most efficient in identifying differences that really exist. In the meantime, because of the lack of research evidence that binaural hearing aids are superior to monaural ones, audiologists are being more cautious in recommending binaural instruments.

Hearing-aid receivers may be of the bone-conduction type. These are small vibrators which fit on the mastoid process. When used with a body-worn aid, they are usually held in place by a narrow metal band which goes across the top of the head. A bone-conduction vibrator may also be built into the tip of the temple of a spectacles frame so that it makes contact with the mastoid process. In this way, bone-conduction hearing may be provided with the glasses type of hearing aid. In the early days of hearing aids, it was thought that any person with a conductive impairment should be provided with a bone-conduction receiver in preference to an air-conduction one. The reasoning was that, since the audiogram showed a loss by air but normal hearing by bone, the "better" of the two hearing methods should be improved. In theory this makes sense, but practically it does not work out. In the first place, the bone-conduction vibrator is a less efficient transducer than the air-conduction receiver. Second, because of the impedance of skin and bone, a considerable amount of power is required at the vibrator in order to produce an audible signal. If the same amount of power is applied to an air-conduction receiver, it is possible to "break through" the conductive block, and the signal which reaches the cochlea is a more faithful reproduction of the original stimulus. Hence, any patient who can successfully utilize a bone-conduction vibrator can usually make even more effective use of an air-conduction receiver, provided that his outer ear can accommodate an earpiece. The only patients who are provided with bone-conduction vibrators today are those who have permanently occluded canals, or who, for one reason or another, cannot tolerate an earpiece. Many older patients, most of them otosclerotics, have had bone-conduction vibrators since the early days of hearing aids, and through years of practice they have learned to make effective use of them. Thus, some of these people now refuse to try an air-conduction receiver with their aid, even though its frequency response is greatly superior and they could hear "more" with it than they can with their bone-conduction vibrators. Apparently, having become accustomed after many years to the distortion of the bone-conduction vibrator, these people are disturbed by the fuller range of amplification that the air-conduction receiver delivers to the inner ear. Since bone-conduction vibrators are seldom recommended now, the remainder of this chapter will be concerned only with the air-conduction type of hearing-aid receiver.

Among users of body-worn hearing aids, one of the most frequent complaints is that, when the aid is worn under clothing, the noise from the movement of the clothing over the microphone is almost unbearable. To avoid clothing noises, hearing aids have been designed with external micro-phones. The microphone can be worn as a tie pin by men, or as a lapel pin by women, with the case containing the amplifier concealed beneath the clothing. Fortunately, most hearing-aid users are able to utilize head-worn aids, and so clothing noise does not constitute a problem for them. It has been estimated by hearing-aid manufacturers that no more than 20 per cent of the hearing-aid users purchase body-worn aids. Dirks and Carhart reported that only 8 per cent of the 211 monaural aid users in their study had body-worn instruments.[21] The miniaturization of hearing aids and the con-sequent development of head-worn instruments have resulted in new markets for hearing aids. There are many part-time users today who have learned that a hearing aid can be useful in some listening situations. These people often have only slight losses but, with a hearing aid that can be put on and taken off easily and that is free from clothing noise, they become successful users. Individuals with very severe or profound impairments must still rely on body-worn instruments for best results, since with body-worn aids it is possible to provide a greater amount of amplification without producing acoustic feedback.

Selection of a Hearing Aid

Assuming that an individual needs a hearing aid and can benefit from it, what are the factors which determine his selection? In the order of their importance, so far as the audiologist is concerned, they are: acoustic efficiency of the instrument, its ruggedness of design, availability of service, initial cost, operating cost, and its attractiveness (size, appearance, and so forth). In the eyes of the purchaser, too often the first consideration is given to the factor of attractiveness. Sometimes, of course, it is only the initial cost which in-fluences the decision. Hearing-aid selection services are provided by many audiology clinics or hearing centers. Some centers are more specific in their recommendations than others, but in any event the prospective hearing-aid purchaser is well advised to visit the nearest audiology clinic. If an aid is recommended, he can then purchase one with confidence that it will be of benefit to him.

At the audiology clinic, the first question which demands an answer is: does the individual have a hearing impairment which will benefit from amplification? The question can be answered by a thorough audiometric evaluation by both pure-tone and speech testing. As stated previously in this chapter, the old rule of thumb that a hearing aid would not be advised until the loss for speech in the better ear exceeds 30 dB is no longer applicable. Each patient's suitability as a candidate for a hearing aid must be in-dividually evaluated, regardless of the degree of impairment he demonstrates on hearing tests. Of course it should be assumed from the outset that the

21 *Ibid.*, p. 315.

patient has been seen by an otologist, who determined that the patient's hearing loss is not of a temporary nature. As stated earlier, the upper limit of hearing loss which can benefit from amplification has yet to be determined. Even though it is not possible to understand speech through hearing alone, at any level of amplification, the profoundly impaired individual may still benefit from a hearing aid. The sounds that he hears with the aid provide some clues which assist him in speechreading, and with the aid he may be better able to control his own speech. Also, there is the advantage that his wearing the hearing aid does give evidence to other people that he has a hearing impairment, and so they are more careful in speaking to him.

The person who is likely to benefit most from a hearing aid is one who has a "flat" conductive loss of 30 to 60 dB in extent. This individual hears amplified speech with a minimum of distortion because his losses at each frequency are equal. Also he can tolerate high levels of amplification because of the protection to the inner ear which his conductive impairment provides and because of the absence of the problem of recruitment. The otosclerotic who is an ideal candidate for surgery is also an ideal candidate for a hearing aid. He needs only to have speech made louder for him to understand what he hears. The poorest risk for a hearing aid is an elderly individual who has a typical sensori-neural impairment with fairly good hearing in the low frequencies and hearing loss which increases by at least 20 dB an octave through the speech frequencies. Such a person would probably demonstrate lowered tolerance, which would limit the amount of amplification he could accept. Because of the uneven response of his hearing mechanism to the various frequencies which are most important to speech, even with amplification what he hears will be distorted. This is not to say that all people with sensori-neural losses cannot benefit from a hearing aid; the problem of selecting the aid simply becomes more difficult. Certainly with such patients the possibility of CROS fittings should be explored. With the elderly, the problem of hearing-aid selection is complicated by the various physical and psychological concomitants of old age.

At the audiology clinic, hearing-aid selection is based upon a number of tests which are conducted with the speech audiometer in a sound-field situation (testing through the loudspeaker). The benefit of the aid is measured by comparing the results when the patient is tested with the aid and without the aid. The tests with the hearing aid can be compared directly with the patient's unaided speech-audiometric scores. In many clinics the patient is tested with several aids under the same conditions, in order to determine if any one aid is markedly superior to all the others. The same measures obtained in speech audiometry are secured also in a hearing-aid evaluation: SRT, MCL, tolerance level, dynamic range, and speech-discrimination ability. In addition, speech discrimination in the presence of noise (recorded background noise) may be measured. The SRT is measured after the volume control of the hearing aid has been set at the point where the patient feels that it is "most comfortable" for him to listen to running speech at a particular level, usually at a hearing level of 40 dB. When this setting has been determined, the patient is instructed not to change the volume control throughout the testing. With each aid to be tested, the patient adjusts the volume control until the running speech of prescribed intensity is "comfortably loud." It is necessary to follow this procedure so that each aid will be tested at a comparable level of amplification with all the others. The objective of such a hearing-aid evaluation is to determine whether one particular hearing-aid and receiver combination will benefit the patient more than another combination.

Other things being equal—factors of cost, attractiveness, and so forth—the aid and receiver which help attain the lowest SRT, the highest tolerance level, and the highest speech-discrimination scores for the patient both in quiet and in noise will be the one selected. However, the "other things" are seldom equal, and frequently different combinations will bring a better score on some tests than on others, so that the selection of the "best" one for the patient may not be easy. Usually the selection represents a compromise which must take into account, too, the patient's own preferences. If the comparative tests of various hearing aids and receivers reveal no significant differences, the audiologist has the responsibility for telling the patient that he can apparently wear any of the combinations with equal effectiveness. It is the patient's responsibility, then, to make his own selection, also taking into consideration the secondary factors of availability of repair service, initial cost, size, and attractiveness of the instrument. In this situation, although the audiologist cannot tell the patient which aid he should buy, he can advise him on such matters as the gain requirements of the patient's loss, the type of ear piece he should get, and which ear should be fitted.

If the performance of the patient with the aid is not substantially better than his performance without the aid, a hearing aid is probably not indicated, although, as we have seen, the advantage of a hearing aid may not always be reflected in improved test scores. Perhaps the decision as to whether or not to recommend an aid cannot be made until after the patient has had a trial period of wearing one. Frequently the value to the patient of a hearing-aid evaluation at an audiology clinic is the discovery that an aid would be of little or no benefit to him. If he had gone directly to a hearing-aid dealer, it is possible that he would have been sold an aid; perhaps over a period of a few years he might have bought several aids, each time with the hope that "this was the one" which would accomplish what actually no aid could. By paying a modest fee to the audiology clinic, the patient is assured that if an aid is recommended his investment will be worthwhile.

Having determined that a patient will benefit from a hearing aid, the audiologist must decide which type of earpiece arrangement provides the most satisfactory results. Generally an analysis of the patient's monaural speech-audiometric scores will yield the information needed to make a selection of the ear to be "fitted,"[22] but sometimes experimentation is required. Other factors being equal, the ear which has the greater SRT, the wider dynamic range, or the better speech discrimination should be chosen. Three examples demonstrate the operation of these principles.

	Example 1		Example 2		Example 3	
	Left	*Right*	*Left*	*Right*	*Left*	*Right*
SRT	40	50	52	54	60	58
Tolerance	100+	100+	100+	88	96	98
Dynamic Range	60+	50+	48+	34	36	40
Discrimination	84%	84%	78%	80%	82%	54%
Ear to fit		Right		Left		Left

In Example 1, the only significant difference between the ears is in the SRT, and so the right ear should be selected for fitting. The logic here is that the patient's better ear can still be of some benefit to him without amplification, which does not hold true for the poorer ear. In Example 2, the only important difference between the ears is in the extent of the dynamic range. The left ear should be fitted, as with this ear the patient can have the advantage of a wider range of amplification. In Example 3, it is obvious that the left ear should be the choice because of its greatly superior speech discrimination. A BICROS fitting with the sound delivered to the left ear should be considered, although a head-worn aid might not provide sufficient gain for this patient.

As we have mentioned previously in this chapter, one can argue on a theoretical basis that binaural aids should provide definite advantages over monaural aids, such as improved localization of sound sources and improved discrimination of speech in the presence of background noise. Separate hearing aids on each ear should logically provide more "natural" hearing, because of the stereophonic effect the normal-hearing individual experiences by the separation of his ears. In 1958 Carhart anticipated the development of more refined tests of aided hearing that would reflect the superiority of binaural aids for some patients. Tests of localization involving sounds introduced through more than one loudspeaker, and tests of speech discrimination in the presence of recorded background noises and competing speech signals have been attempted in audiology clinics. There still are no tests the audiologist can apply that enable him with any degree of confidence to tell a patient that he should wear binaural aids. Some audiologists prefer to recommend a monaural instrument for a patient and, after a period of six months or so, when the patient has made a good adjustment to the aid, have the patient try a binaural fitting. Presumably, the difference between binaural and monaural listening might be more evident at this time than at the time of the initial evaluation. In the absence of any test evidence that a binaural

22 Unfortunately, the word *fit* implies that a hearing aid may be selected as precisely as a pair of shoes, or with the accuracy with which an eye doctor prescribes glasses. This is not true, but because there is no good substitute the word is sometimes unavoidable.

fitting is better for a patient, the audiologist must depend on the patient's subjective impressions and his preferences in regard to having a binaural instrument.

As a matter of fact, it is becoming increasingly necessary to depend on a patient's subjective impressions in arriving at a decision in hearing-aid consultations. Whether our tests are inadequate to point up differences in patients' performance with various hearing aids, or whether the differences that exist today from one aid to another are only of minor significance is a moot point. In any event, it is only rarely that the test results obtained in hearing-aid selection procedures point definitely to one particular instrument as being superior to all others. Shore, Bilger, and Hirsh studied the reliability of the measures obtained in hearing-aid evaluations with fifteen patients over a period of several days, using the same four aids with each patient. They concluded that the reliability of the measures of gain (comparison of aided versus unaided SRT's) and discrimination score in quiet and in noise ". . . is not good enough to warrant the investment of a large amount of clinical time with them in selecting hearing aids."[23]

Because of their dissatisfaction with hearing-aid selection procedures that attempt to specify the particular instrument a patient should purchase, the audiologists at Central Institute for the Deaf, where the Shore, Bilger, and Hirsh study was conducted, developed a different approach that aims not at giving a patient a specific "prescription" for a hearing aid but instead providing him with information on the basis of which the patient makes his own decision. The patient is not tested with a series of aids to obtain comparative scores of his performance. Instead, following pure-tone and speech audiometric tests, he is "tested" with two or three aids to permit him to experience amplification with actual hearing aids. The time that formerly was spent in comparative testing of aids is devoted to counseling the patient regarding his own hearing problems and advising him generally on his needs for amplification. An attempt is made to educate the patient on how to shop efficiently for a hearing aid. In other words, the burden for the selection of a specific aid is placed on the patient rather than on the examiner. After making a survey of patients' reactions to this more general type of "consultation," Shore and Kramer concluded that the new procedure was as effective as the old one that attempted to specify the make and model of the aid the patient was to purchase. They believe that ". . . time is being spent more valuably in counseling the patient than in trying many aids."[24] Resnick and Becker report satisfactory experience with a similar type of general counseling approach in hearing-aid evaluations.[25]

[23] Irvin Shore, Robert C. Bilger, and Ira J. Hirsh, "Hearing Aid Evaluation: Reliability of Repeated Measurements," *Journal of Speech and Hearing Disorders,* Vol. 25 (May, 1960), p. 167.

[24] Irwin Shore and Joan C. Kramer, "A Comparison of Two Procedures for Hearing-Aid Evaluation," *Journal of Speech and Hearing Disorders,* Vol. 28 (May, 1963), p. 165.

[25] David M. Resnick and Marshall Becker, "Hearing Aid Evaluation—A New Approach," *Asha,* Vol. 5 (August, 1963), pp. 695-699.

In certain instances, for example, referrals from agencies that purchase aids for their clients, the audiology clinic is obligated to provide specific recommendations. It can be anticipated, however, that in the future the trend will be toward a more general hearing-aid consultation service and away from specific "prescriptions" of hearing-aid fittings in audiology clinics. If for no other reason, the numbers of different makes and models of hearing aids have proliferated so that it is physically impossible to try more than a limited sample of available aids with any individual patient. The values of the hearing-aid consultation to the patient are in learning whether or not he can use any hearing aid, achieving an awareness of the limitations of his hearing with or without amplification, becoming educated to the proper way of shopping for a hearing aid, and learning to use it effectively after it is acquired. These are certainly sufficient benefits to make the hearing-aid consultation worth the patient's time and money.

REFERENCES

Berger, Kenneth W., *The Hearing Aid: Its Operation and Development* (Detroit, The National Hearing Aid Society, 1970).

Canfield, Norton, *Hearing: A Handbook for Laymen* (Garden City, N.Y., Doubleday and Company, 1959), Chaps. 9, 10, 11, and 13.

Davis, Hallowell, and Silverman, S. Richard, eds., *Hearing and Deafness* (New York, Holt, Rinehart and Winston, 1970), Chaps. 10, 11, and 18.

Levine, Edna Simon, *The Psychology of Deafness* (New York, Columbia University Press, 1960).

O'Neill, John J., and Oyer, Herbert J., *Visual Communication for the Hard of Hearing: History, Research & Methods* (Englewood Cliffs, N.J., Prentice-Hall, 1961).

Rose Darrell E., ed., *Audiological Assessment* (Englewood Cliffs, N. J. Prentice-Hall, 1971), Chap. 14.

Sanders, Derek A., *Aural Rehabilitation* (Englewood Cliffs, N. J. Prentice-Hall, 1971).

Victoreen, John A., *Hearing Enhancement* (Springfield, Ill., Charles C Thomas, 1960).

11

TRAINING THE
HEARING-IMPAIRED CHILD

The purpose of this chapter is to set forth a general approach to the training of children who have impaired hearing. For the most part, the emphasis will be on the hard-of-hearing child, not on the deaf child. There will be some mention, however, of the educational problems of the deaf, and special attention will be directed to the training of the preschool deaf child. There will be no attempt to give detailed information regarding the planning of lessons for hearing-impaired children. The reader who desires this kind of information is referred to the list of references at the end of this chapter.

The child with a hearing impairment almost always has some degree of language handicap, the extent of the handicap depending on such factors as the degree of loss, the time of onset of the loss, and so forth, as discussed in Chapter 10. The audiologist is concerned with the child's problems in communication, his ability to speak and to understand speech. Further, the audiologist has the responsibility of helping the parents to understand the problems of their hearing-handicapped child and teaching them how they can be of most assistance. Included in this chapter are discussions of the communicative skills which the child must develop. Although these skills are discussed separately, it must be understood that they operate in combination with each other and should be taught together.

SPEECHREADING

Speechreading is the one skill which has universal application to individuals with hearing problems, regardless of the patient's age or the extent of his hearing impairment. Whenever one sensory pathway is impaired, an individual compensates for it by developing an increased capacity to utilize his other senses. Thus, a blind person develops an increased ability to use the hearing sensitivity which he has always had. By the same token, the hard-of-hearing patient must learn to rely more on his visual sensations than is necessary for the person with normal hearing. The child who has a hearing loss naturally learns to concentrate on visual clues, even without special training. In fact, one of the diagnostic indications of an auditory impairment is the fact that a child watches speakers' faces with an intentness and concentration that signify his dependence on visual clues. The purpose of speechreading training for hard-of-hearing children is to develop their natural capacity for learning through the eyes to the maximum extent. Training in speechreading can succeed in quickening the child's powers of visual observation and systematizing his ability to comprehend speech through visual clues.

As stated previously, speechreading alone is not a perfect substitute for hearing. Because of the relatively large proportion of English sounds that are partially or completely invisible, it is impossible for any speechreader, no matter how skillful, to comprehend 100 per cent of what is said. Speechreading training, given in combination with auditory training, can usually yield better results in terms of the total communication the child receives than can either type of training alone.

Educators of the deaf stress the importance of teaching the young child how to "match." Initially, this training consists of teaching the child to match one object to another object which is exactly like it. Then, the child is taught to match one object to another object which is similar although not exactly the same. The next step is to teach matching of an object to a picture of the object, and then the matching of one picture to another picture. The aim of these matching procedures is to teach the child to be observant of similarities and differences, and to realize that symbols (pictures) relate to objects and may be substituted for the objects which they represent. This is the first rung on the ladder of abstraction. Finally, the child is taught to match words, as seen on the lips of the therapist or in printed form, with the objects for which the words stand, with the pictures of objects, and with other words. This is the next higher rung on the ladder of abstraction. Thus, through a series of matching experiences, beginning simply and becoming progressively more complex, the child is taught that things have names and that these names may be interpreted as movements of the articulators in a speaker or as combinations of written letters. Initially, the matching is on a concrete basis, that is, symbols which name objects are taught first. Eventually, of course, the child must realize that ideas in the abstract can be conveyed through spoken or written language, and he must learn to think with symbols—to "match" thoughts and concepts, and to express his thoughts to others in spoken and written form. This is the ultimate goal of procedures starting with the very simple matching of object to object.

With the hard-of-hearing child who can learn some language through the ear, it is not necessary to follow such a detailed step-by-step procedure in teaching speechreading. How closely the program for the hard-of-hearing child corresponds to procedures pursued with deaf children depends on the language abilities of the child, which in turn are affected by the severity of the loss, the time of its occurrence, and of course the intelligence of the child.

To be effective, a program of speechreading for children must be geared to children's interests. As in any kind of teaching of young children, speechreading lessons must be made entertaining and appealing by means of materials which are inherently interesting to the child. Various games may be devised to give the child the opportunity to practice speechreading without subjecting him to the stiffness and inflexibility of the formal lesson situation. For example, a lesson could be built around the theme of animals, which most children love. Attractive pictures of animals can be found in children's books, or in magazine advertisements, and these pictures can be mounted on colorful construction paper or cardboard. The child can be instructed to "find the cow," or to "place the horse in front of the sheep," and so forth.

In general, the object of speechreading lessons should be to give the child experience which will better equip him to get along in daily life situations. In the beginning, lessons should be restricted to the vocabulary with which the child is already familiar. As he learns to utilize this vocabulary in speechreading, new words can be introduced. Lessons should be planned to move from the familiar to the unfamiliar, so that the child is motivated to learn by proceeding from what he knows to fields of new information and experience. For the child of school age, lessons can be planned around the subject matter of his school studies.

Regardless of the subject matter on which the lesson is built, the therapist should observe certain principles in teaching speechreading. These are enumerated below:

1. Sit or stand so that the lighting is favorable for the child. The light should be on your face, and not in the eyes of the child.

2. Talk naturally. Don't exaggerate your articulation, and don't speak carelessly or too rapidly.

3. Don't "talk over the child's head." Phrase your thoughts in simple, easy-to-understand language, but always speak in complete sentences.

4. Because of the additional movements involved and the consequently greater opportunity for the child to observe, longer words or phrases are sometimes better than shorter ones. Thus it is better to say "It is lunch-time, and we must go eat our lunch," rather than "Time to eat."

5. Repeat what you say, still without exaggeration, until the child comprehends, or if necessary rephrase what you have said.

6. Spend little or no time in drill involving movements or nonsense syllables. Conduct the necessary drill work with phrases or sentences. In other

words, adopt a synthetic rather than an analytic approach to the teaching of speechreading.

7. Make your speechreading lessons happy and enjoyable experiences for the child with the aid of materials which are bright, gay, and interesting. Collect and organize your own materials; don't depend on lesson plans found in books.

8. Integrate speechreading work with auditory training and speech training. For the most part, your speechreading work should be done with natural voice, although on occasion, to sharpen the child's attention, a low-intensity voice or a whisper is desirable.

9. Always insist on the child's *watching* you while you speak, so that he may learn the importance of visual clues. Don't speak until you have the child's attention.

10. Be lavish with praise and reward for successful speechreading performances.

AUDITORY TRAINING

The kind and type of auditory training that a hard-of-hearing child needs depends upon the degree and type of hearing impairment. Naturally before a child is placed in a training program, a careful analysis should be made of his hearing loss. The way in which a child responds to speech audiometric tests will give an indication of what his auditory training needs are. As a result of the evaluation of a child's hearing, a decision can be made as to whether or not a hearing aid should be considered and what kind of earpiece arrangement would do best. If the loss is sufficient to warrant a hearing aid, the aid should be fitted at the earliest possible date. However, a period of some auditory training may be necessary before the child can make effective use of an aid. If he does not know how to interpret the speech sounds that he hears, he must be taught how to listen. Whether the auditory training precedes or follows the fitting of a hearing aid will have to be determined individually for each child. Some children will have hearing which is too good to necessitate an aid but still may have poor listening habits. What is more likely is that a child may have good hearing for the low frequencies but poor hearing for the higher speech frequencies and thus would need auditory training even though it may not be possible for him to use a hearing aid to good effect. The auditory training needs of these categories of children will now be discussed.

The Child Who Needs Training Before Getting an Aid

Generally, this type of child is one who has a profound loss and without amplification does not hear the ordinary sounds of life sufficiently well to pay attention to them. Such a child needs to be taught, first of all, that sound vibrations can be meaningful. At the start, it will be necessary to make him aware of the different sounds which exist in his environment and to acquaint him with the differences among these sounds that enable us to identify them. Carhart has described this process as the teaching of gross sound discrimination.[1] Thus the child should be taught that a bell and a horn make different sounds, and that these objects can be differentiated on the basis of their sounds. In the beginning, at least, this training will require amplification, that is, an auditory training unit. A good technique is to show the child two noisemakers, for example, a bell and a horn. While he wears the earphones, ring the bell and blow the horn alternately, so that he can see which noisemaker is making the sound each time. Then face the child away from you, and sound one of the toys in front of the microphone. Have the child turn around and indicate whether it was the bell or the horn that he heard. When he becomes adept at selecting which of two noisemakers he hears without watching, add a third, then a fourth, and finally a fifth noisemaker. When the child learns to identify consistently which of five noisemakers he is hearing, you are making progress in teaching him gross sound discrimination. Once the child learns to pay attention to sound, it may be possible to teach him some gross sound discrimination without amplification.

As soon as the child has learned that sounds may give him information about his environment, an individual hearing-aid fitting can be considered. Some audiologists feel that, as soon as it has been established that the child has a profound loss of hearing, he should be provided with an aid, in preference to waiting until he has received some training in recognizing and differentiating gross sounds. Their argument is that the child should be exposed to his sound environment throughout his waking hours and not just at the time of his auditory training lesson. They say that it is not fair to the child to deprive him of day-long amplification until he has received some training in differentiating gross sounds. Certainly it is important to supply the child with his own hearing aid at the earliest opportunity. Nevertheless, when you give it to him, you want it to be a pleasurable experience for him. Without any notion of what he is hearing, or previous experience with amplified sound, the child may reject the hearing aid. It would be better to prepare the child for it by furnishing him with carefully planned and controlled listening experiences with an auditory training unit. The child who has been introduced to amplification in this manner is much more likely to accept his own hearing aid from the start than if the aid were forced on him without any preparation at all.

After the child has learned to distinguish gross sounds, the next step in auditory training is that of teaching him to recognize the elements of speech. Preferably this training should be on the basis of whole words. If the child is

[1] Raymond Carhart, "Auditory Training," in Hallowell Davis and S. Richard Silverman, eds., *Hearing and Deafness* (New York, Holt, Rinehart and Winston, 1960), Chap. 13, pp. 374-376.

able to associate the word *ball* with the object for which the word stands, there is no need to spend time on the recognition of the separate sounds which make up the word. If, however, the child confuses the word *ball* with the word *bell*, it may be necessary to teach him the acoustic differences between the vowels *ah* and *eh*. If work on sounds is necessary, auditory training should start with the vowels, which are acoustically more easily distinguished than are the consonants. Before auditory training on meaningful words is possible, it may be necessary to spend time on the combination of sounds in nonsense syllables. Thus *baw* and *beh* must be differentiated before the words *ball* and *bell* have recognizable differences. Learning the difference between dissimilar speech sounds is referred to as gross speech discrimination, whereas learning the difference between similar speech sounds, such as *f* and *th*, for example, is known as fine speech discrimination.[2] A reasonably good mastery of fine speech discrimination is a prerequisite to the understanding of speech.

Auditory Training with the Hearing Aid

Seldom is it sufficient to give a child a hearing aid without providing him at the same time with some training in its operation. This is true even for the child who has received the kind of preparation for an aid referred to above. An auditory training unit provides high-fidelity amplification and usually has a built-in protection to the ears from too great intensity of sound —through compression or automatic volume control. The individual, wearable hearing aid, on the other hand, amplifies over a limited frequency range and even so introduces distortion. Moreover, very few aids have compression amplification, although all have some control over the maximum acoustic output. It therefore may require considerable adjustment for a child to transfer from an auditory training unit to an individual hearing aid. The problem of adjustment is even greater for the child who has never experienced amplification previously.

Teachers and parents are frequently frustrated in their attempts to get children to wear hearing aids. If a physician has told a family that they should obtain a hearing aid for the child, the parents quite naturally expect that the least he can do is to make use of the instrument on which they have spent a considerable sum of money. Frequently, the child will be sent to school with the hearing aid and a note to the teacher explaining that the child is to wear the aid throughout school. If the teacher has had no previous experience with children who wear hearing aids, he is inclined to regard the instrument with awe and to feel that it is his responsibility to see that the parents' instructions are followed. The poor child is thus badgered by both parents and teacher to wear an aid which he may be unable to accept at this time. If sufficient pressure is brought to bear, parents and teachers can

2 *Ibid.*, p. 376.

force children to wear hearing aids, but they cannot compel them to enjoy the process. What happens then is that the child takes off the hearing aid at the first opportunity. He learns to hate it because he associates it with the authority which insists that he wear it. The usual outcome is that the child does not benefit from it, and he may be so conditioned against the aid that, even with professional guidance, it will take considerable time to persuade him to accept it. It is far better to avoid this unpleasantness from the start by placing the child with a new hearing aid under the professional guidance of an audiologist. The audiologist will explain to the parents and teacher the difficulties that the child experiences in adjusting to the aid. The audiologist will instruct the parents and teacher not to force the aid upon the child but to help him to want to wear it by giving him praise and approval whenever he does.

Perhaps the first step in training the child to make effective use of his aid is to teach him how to operate the instrument's controls and to wear the aid most comfortably. The child should be shown how the volume control and tone control function, and how to change the battery. He should learn how to connect the receiver to the earpiece and how to insert and remove the earpiece. For the aid to be effective it is fundamental that he learn thoroughly the mechanics of operating it. If the child has a body-worn aid, generally it can be worn most comfortably in a pocket on a "sling," which is secured around the neck and chest. Adjustable slings may be purchased from hearing-aid dealers, but it is probably better for the child's mother to make one especially to fit him. The sling can be worn either under or outside the clothing. From an acoustic point of view, of course, it would be preferable to wear the aid outside. A child's auricles may be too small to support a behind-the-ear type of aid. Such aids can be mounted on headbands similar to those used with bone-conduction vibrators, however. If very much gain is required in the aid, a head-worn type may not be feasible, because of the problem of acoustic feedback. Incidentally, the child will require a new earpiece at regular intervals, because of the growth of his external ears. Even with a body-worn aid, it is necessary to have the earpiece fit snugly so that it effectively seals off the canal. Otherwise, sound leaking around the earpiece will reach the microphone and result in feedback which may frighten the child and condition him against wearing the aid.

A word of caution is in order regarding the setting of the volume control. If the child is allowed to make his own volume-control setting, there is a danger that he may turn the volume too high for the good of his ear. If the child has a sensori-neural hearing loss, his inner ear may be susceptible to additional loss from excessively high sound levels. The inner ear can incur damage from sound levels which are not high enough to produce pain or even physiological discomfort; the child may thus unwittingly cause further deterioration of his hearing by too high a volume-control setting. Some experimentation will be required to determine the best setting of the volume control, but it is better to err on the side of too little amplification than too much. The audiologist must assume the responsibility for showing the child where the volume control should be set.

The same procedures which are suitable for an auditory training unit may be applied in training the child with a hearing aid. Where to begin the auditory training program with the aid depends, of course, on the capabilities of the child. If the suggestions in the previous section of this chapter are followed, he will already have some awareness of sound and be able at least to differentiate various dissimilar sounds. Again the child would be asked to listen to various noisemakers and to select the one which the teacher sounds. It is even likely that by the time the child obtains his own hearing aid he will be able to recognize and understand certain words, and perhaps phrases or sentences. If so, training with the aid would consist of vocabulary building and work with more difficult words and sentences. Until the child has learned to make the transition from the high-fidelity amplification of the auditory training unit to the relatively poor-quality reproduction of the hearing aid, however, it would probably be best to limit the materials to those with which the child is familiar from his previous auditory training work.

The objectives of the auditory training program are, first of all, to persuade the child to accept the hearing aid, and then for him to learn to operate it so effectively that he will never want to be without it. As in any kind of educational training, the procedure is from the known to the unknown, from the simple to the complex. While for purposes of forcing the child to attend to auditory signals it may be desirable through some of his training to prevent his obtaining visual cues, the long-range objective is the development of the child's communicative abilities to their ultimate extent. Therefore, auditory training should usually be combined with speech-reading, and while the comprehension of speech is being taught emphasis must also be placed on helping the child to improve his own speech.

Auditory Training for the Child Who Does Not Need a Hearing Aid

Two groups of children do not need hearing aids and yet would benefit from a program of auditory training. One group includes the children who have losses less than the minimum loss for which a hearing aid is indicated. The other group consists of children who have sensori-neural impairments characterized by good hearing through 500 or possibly 1000 Hz, and severe drop in hearing sensitivity at higher frequencies. Of course some hearing-impaired children have such profound losses that even with a hearing aid it is not possible for them to respond to sound. In this chapter, however, we are concerned with the needs of the hard of hearing, as contrasted with those of the deaf. Another group which might be mentioned, but with which we shall not be concerned, consists of children whose hearing acuity as measured on the audiometer is normal but who have poor listening habits. In Chapter 8, mention was made of the fact that some children seem to be deficient in "auding," that is, in comprehending auditory verbal stimuli, even though their hearing sensitivity is normal. In the future, then, it may be necessary to establish "listening" classes for such children. This group is not dealt with in the present chapter since here we are interested only in children who have hearing losses.

In the first group of children mentioned above, the loss for speech as measured with the speech audiometer would be something less than 20 to 25 dB in the better ear. Such loss may be temporary in nature, or it may be permanent. In either event, the loss is not severe enough to warrant constant amplification, yet many situations arise in which the child with this mild loss is handicapped. For such children, auditory training should be directed toward the occasions that cause difficulty. For example, if the child consistently encounters problems in the classroom, the audiologist should help the child analyze why he has trouble hearing in the classroom and try to plan a program which will minimize his difficulties in these circumstances. As part of the attack on the problem, the child may be advised to experiment with different seating in the classroom. Of course the classroom teacher's cooperation would have to be secured in order to permit such experimentation. The child may find a desk-type hearing aid or portable auditory training unit helpful at least some of the time in the classroom. Many schools provide such instruments for the use of hearing-impaired pupils.

Instruction in speechreading may be all that the child with a mild loss requires. There are some auditory training procedures which may prove helpful, however, as an adjunct to speechreading. The emphasis in such auditory training is on teaching the child to pay close attention to speech which he can barely hear. When we are in difficult listening situations, the temptation is to let our attention wander and give up the attempt to listen. The child with a mild loss has the same tendency. He may learn to listen more effectively by participating in listening games. For example, the therapist can play a game of lotto with the child, who is not permitted to watch the therapist's face. Each time the child makes the correct response in the lotto game, the therapist speaks a little more softly. Thus, as the game nears the finish, the child has to "strain" to listen, but since the game is almost over, his motivation for listening carefully is excellent.

The child with a mild loss should be encouraged to ask for repetitions when he does not understand. This is easy to say but difficult for the child actually to practice. It is embarrassing for him to draw attention to himself by confessing that he did not hear, and the line of least resistance is to act as if he did hear. This requires considerable "bluffing," which usually leads to even more embarrassing situations in the long run than would the confession that he did not hear. Teachers and parents should be advised to speak a little more loudly and carefully to children with mild losses; yet the child still has a responsibility to himself to let them know when he does not understand. A child with any handicap has to develop a "thick skin" if he is to become well adjusted, and the one with a mild hearing loss is no exception.

The child with a sloping audiogram through the higher speech frequencies may be considerably handicapped. In some ways his plight is more difficult than that of the child with such a severe loss that he must depend on a hearing aid. The hearing aid does advertise to all who see him that the child has an impairment of hearing. There is nothing about the appearance of the child with a high-frequency loss which sets him apart from anyone else. Thus people tend to expect from him the same type of behavior as from a child who is normal in all respects.

The child with a loss for the higher speech frequencies has difficulty in understanding what he hears, yet because of his good hearing for the low frequencies he hears voices perfectly well. He may appear to be stupid because of his failure to comprehend what people are saying to him. His difficulty in comprehension comes from his inability to differentiate words with the same vowel but different consonants. Thus *think* and *sink* may sound the same to him. The voiceless consonants, which are *s, th, f, k, t, p, sh, ch, h,* and *wh,* are the sounds which are most frequently missed by the child with a hearing loss for the higher speech frequencies. In addition to their being high-frequency consonants, they are voiceless and have very little phonetic power. The combination of high-frequency characteristics of these sounds and their low phonetic power makes them particularly difficult. An example of how a child with this kind of loss might hear running speech demonstrates how difficult is his job of comprehending what he hears. For this example, we shall assume that the child hears vowels and voiced consonants in normal fashion, although in an actual case of a high-frequency hearing loss many other consonants would be heard by him with considerable distortion. The question "What time is it?" might be heard by the child as "—a— —ime i— i—?" Is it any wonder that the child says "Huh?" or "What?" Even if the speaker repeats the question in a louder voice, the distortion of speech is still present. The child will simply hear the lower-frequency sounds with greater power. Such a child must depend to a large extent on speechreading as a solution to his problems in comprehension, but teaching him to make the most of what he hears may be of assistance.

Paired words which differ only in the consonants present are a good technique for the child with a loss for the higher speech frequencies. A child who can read is able to point to the correct words in print. Pictures of objects can be substituted with the child who cannot read. A few examples of the type of paired words possible for this exercise follow.

stand	hand
tea	sea
mouse	house
tree	three
nose	toes

At the start, the therapist may have to say each word while he points to the printed word or to the picture which the word represents, and while the child watches for speechreading cues. After extensive practice, however, the child can learn to make many distinctions on the basis of his hearing alone. It is not known accurately by what mechanism the child with a severe loss for the higher speech frequencies learns to distinguish similar sounding words. Some research has indicated that vowel sounds are affected differently by different consonants, so that careful attention to the vowel will reveal subtle changes, which in turn point to the specific consonant preceding or following the vowel.[3] If that is so, certainly there is good reason for presenting auditory training work to children with loss in the higher speech frequencies in terms of complete words, rather than trying to drill on the consonant sounds for which the hearing is defective.

Hearing aids may be of little or no value to these children for the same reason it is useless to shout at them. They do not need amplification in order to hear voices or the low-frequency speech sounds. A hearing aid should not be ruled out, however, without extensive experimentation, particularly with the CROS type of fitting with an open or non-occluding ear piece that provides attenuation of the low frequencies. This type of fitting is described in Chapter 10.

SPEECH TRAINING

A hearing loss of greater than mild degree is almost always reflected in the child's own speech and voice patterns. For this reason, speech training is an important facet of the training program for the hard-of-hearing child. Speech disorders associated with a hearing loss may range from complete lack of oral language to the presence of only a single articulatory error. A frequent cause for the condition described by speech pathologists as "delayed speech" is a severe hearing disorder. The child with delayed speech will be slow in starting to use words. He may not begin to speak until he is three to four years of age. His vocabulary will be meager, and his grammar greatly simplified. He will omit many sounds and make substitutions for others, and

---

[3] Arthur S. House and Grant Fairbanks, "The Influence of Consonant Environment upon the Secondary Acoustical Characteristics of Vowels," *Journal of the Acoustical Society of America,* Vol. 25 (January, 1953), pp. 105-113.

he will rely greatly on gestures for purposes of communication.[4] All these symptoms may be explained on the basis of a hearing impairment, although there are other causes for delayed speech. If the child's hearing for speech is faulty, however, the speech he reproduces will be faulty since learning to speak is achieved through imitation of the speech that is heard.

Often, indeed, no one suspects that a child's hearing is not normal until he fails to develop an adequate oral language at the time when other children are learning to speak. Certainly in every case of delayed speech, the hearing of the child should be thoroughly studied. If he has a hearing loss which can be helped with amplification, a hearing aid should be tried at the earliest opportunity. Sometimes the introduction of amplification is all that is required to produce an immediate improvement in speech development. The author observed an almost miraculous development of oral language in a four-year-old boy with bilateral atresia of the external canal after he was fitted with a bone-conduction hearing aid. Usually, however, it is necessary to give extensive speech training to children even after they are fitted with aids.

With a severe hearing loss the child's voice will be affected. The most noticeable vocal characteristic is a marked deviation from normal voice quality to what can be described as a dull and lifeless quality. Pitch is usually monotonous, and it may be somewhat higher than desirable. There may be rapid and extensive changes in vocal intensity while the child is speaking, the effect being one of uncontrollable intensity. With lesser degrees of hearing loss, the vocal characteristics of the child are less noticeable. A mild or moderate hearing loss may have no noticeable effect on the voice.

Where vocal symptoms do occur, the therapist must cope with them and strive to achieve as normal vocal usage as possible. It is easier to effect changes in pitch and intensity than it is to produce improvement in vocal quality. Pitch and intensity can be controlled through kinesthetic sensations, but apparently vocal quality is almost entirely dependent on auditory monitoring. Variations in pitch, or inflections, may be taught by fairly mechanical means and through drill work. For example, the child can be taught to vary pitch upward or downward as the therapist raises or lowers a finger. Thus the therapist, in the manner of an orchestra leader, can direct the child's pitch so that his expression becomes more natural.

Control over intensity of voice requires an awareness of environment. In noisy surroundings, for example, a room crowded with talking people, individuals with normal hearing unconsciously increase the intensity of their voices to make themselves audible over the background noise. On the other hand, when they are in a quiet environment, people tend to speak with decreased intensity. The child with a severe loss of hearing is not able to judge the proper intensity of voice for a given situation except by a process of trial and error. He will have to depend largely on the reactions of the

4 Virgil A. Anderson *Improving the Child's Speech* (New York, Oxford, 1953), pp. 105-106.

people with whom he is talking. It is advisable, therefore, for the therapist to teach the child to be sensitive to the reactions of those around him, so that, if they seem to have difficulty hearing him, he can speak with somewhat greater effort in voice production. Since it is more difficult to judge when one is talking too loudly, it is better to teach the child to decrease the intensity of his voice until it is apparent that others are having difficulty in hearing him. Then he can speak at a slightly higher level of intensity, which should be just right.

Equipment has been designed and manufactured for the vocal training of the hard of hearing and the deaf. One such piece of equipment is a vertical bank of lights, which represent the intensity of the voice—the louder the voice, the more lights are illuminated. Another device consists of a vertical bank of lights behind different-colored panes of glass. With this, it is possible to obtain a rough "spectrogram" of a single speech sound, usually a vowel. The therapist demonstrates a speech sound while the patient observes the particular color pattern and the intensity of the colors produced on the instrument. The patient then attempts to produce a speech sound that will cause an identical pattern of lights to appear. Although such training devices have some clinical value, they do not by any means take the place of a qualified therapist. Some therapists even object to such training "aids," feeling that they serve to distract rather than to assist the patient.

Errors in articulation (sound formation) are commonly found in children who have even mild-to-moderate hearing losses. As was explained in the preceding chapter, certain English consonant sounds require very delicate adjustments of the articulators. Sounds that involve the precise placement of the blade or the tip of the tongue in relation to other articulators are particularly likely to be defective, for example, the s, r, l, sh, and ch sounds. Generally it can be said that the sounds which are less visible, more complex in their formation, and have important high-frequency characteristics are those most likely to be affected by a hearing loss. Sounds with these characteristics are also the last sounds to be mastered in the speech development of the normal-hearing child. As would be expected, sounds that the child hears least well because of his hearing loss would most likely be defective. Thus the voiceless consonants, which are both weak in phonetic power and contain important high-frequency components, are often defective, especially those which are also relatively invisible and complex in their formation.

The correction of defective articulation of hearing-impaired children requires an approach by the therapist which is largely visual and tactile. Depending on the extent of the hearing loss, an auditory approach is also possible, perhaps with amplification of an auditory training unit. With a severe or profound loss, however, primary dependence would have to be placed on nonauditory techniques. The therapist then resorts to a phonetic placement method, whereby he attempts to show the child where the articulators should be placed to produce a given sound. If the sound is at all visible, the therapist can demonstrate correct placement of articulators and encourage the child to imitate him. When the sounds are invisible, the therapist can show a cross-sectional drawing of the articulator placement and try to get the child to duplicate this placement with his own articulators.

It is frequently difficult to demonstrate to the severely impaired child the difference between voiced and unvoiced consonants that have the same articulator position, for example, *t* and *d*. The therapist can place the child's hand on his (the therapist's) larynx and show him that with the *d* there is vibration in the larynx, whereas for the *t* no vibration is felt. Plosives, that is, sounds that require the building up of breath pressure and then its sudden expulsion as in the *p, b, t, d, k,* and *g,* can be taught by the therapist's placing the child's hand in front of his (the therapist's) mouth, so that the child can feel the puff of air which results each time. Nasal consonants, the *m, n,* and *ng,* can be demonstrated by the child's feeling the vibration in the therapist's nose. Each time, after the child has felt the sound which the therapist has produced, he should try to imitate it and receive the same feeling when he places his hand on his larynx, in front of his mouth, and on his nose. When he experiences the same tactile sensations while imitating what he can see of the therapist's articulator placement, he will be producing the correct acoustic effect for whatever speech sound he is attempting. Even with children who do not have such severe impairments of hearing, tactile methods can be helpful in teaching correct sound production. At the end of this chapter, the reader will find references containing specific directions for speech-correction work with hard-of-hearing children. The child with impaired hearing has enough difficulty in communication and is sufficiently handicapped without being saddled with a speech handicap also. By teaching proper speech production, the therapist can do much to ease the way for the hard-of-hearing child.

THE HEARING-IMPAIRED PRESCHOOL CHILD

The audiologist is concerned with the hard-of-hearing child. The child who is deaf requires full-time, special education work, and generally the audiologist is not responsible for his training. An exception to this statement is that of the deaf child of preschool age. Public school education for deaf children usually is not available until the children are at least three years of age, and most of them are not actually enrolled until they are three-and-a-half to four years of age. If the child of preschool age is to receive any training before he enters school, he becomes the audiologist's responsibility. It is certainly desirable for the training of a deaf child to begin when his hearing handicap is first diagnosed. Normal-hearing children start to develop speech at twelve to eighteen months of age. At this age their nervous systems have developed to the point that they are "ready" for the unfolding of language concepts. Ideally the training of the deaf child should commence when his neurological and physiological system is "ready" for this development. If no training whatsoever is given until he becomes eligible for a public school special education program, much valuable time will have been lost during which the child might have made a good start on the road to the acquisition of language.

The needs of the preschool deaf child were brought to the attention of otologists, audiologists, and educators most forcefully by Mrs. Spencer Tracy, the wife of the late movie actor. Mr. and Mrs. Tracy's son John was deaf. They had a number of disappointing and discouraging experiences in their attempts to secure the advice and assistance they so desperately needed. Because of their unfortunate experiences, Mrs. Tracy determined to do all she could to help the parents of other deaf children understand what could be done to guide their children in the development of their full potentialities. Originally, she started a discussion group of parents of young children. Teachers of the deaf were enlisted to explain to the parents techniques that were feasible for stimulating the development of language in deaf children. The next step was the establishment of a nursery school for deaf children, where teachers of the deaf could demonstrate these techniques. As the work of the school became known, parents from all over the country wrote to Mrs. Tracy, asking how they could learn to become better parents of their deaf children. The outcome of these inquiries was a correspondence course, sent free of charge to parents of deaf children anywhere in the world. From the modest beginnings of a parents' discussion group, the John Tracy Clinic, as it is called today, has developed into an outstanding institution in Los Angeles, dedicated to helping parents of deaf children of preschool age, and thereby, of course, helping the children themselves.

Although work with deaf children of preschool age was not entirely unknown before the opening of the John Tracy Clinic, its influence is largely responsible for the development of most of the training programs for the preschool deaf which today are to be found in scores of cities in the United States. Most such programs follow the Tracy Clinic policy of concentrating on parent education, because it is realized that parents have the responsibility of training the preschool child. Although the children can work in groups for a limited time, they are the mothers' responsibility for the greatest part of each day. The mother, therefore, must learn how to become a teacher in order to help the child develop language.

In addition to training parents to become teachers of their children, the training programs for preschool deaf serve another, equally important function: that of helping the parents to accept and understand their hearing-handicapped children. It is frightening to parents to find that they have a handicapped child, and their reactions are likely to be extreme in one direction or another. They may reject the child completely, or at the other extreme they may be inclined to overindulge him. Either way, of course, the effect on the child is unfortunate. By observing a group of hearing-handicapped preschool children under the direction of a competent teacher, parents can learn that the children are first of all *children*, and only secondarily are they *deaf* children. It reassures parents to see that other children are behaving in the same way as their own child. When the parents of preschool deaf children meet in discussion groups, they can share their fears and frustrations, and their awakening awareness of their child's assets, with the result that all of them benefit from sharing their experiences.

Some preschool programs operate a nursery school, which to outward appearances is the same as any other nursery school. A trained nursery school teacher supervises the children's play and socializing experiences. Language-stimulating activities are provided at every opportunity. There is an audiologist or sometimes a teacher of the deaf on the staff who is responsible for supervising the language stimulation of the children. The audiologist takes them singly and in groups for auditory training work, and he determines when each child is ready for his own individual hearing aid. The audiologist also explains to the parents what he is doing and his reasons for doing it. In addition to the audiologist and/or teacher of the deaf, the nursery school staff may consist of a clinical psychologist, a child psychologist, or a medical or psychiatric social worker. The function of this staff member is to teach the parents about child development, and to help them better understand their own children's periods of development. Also, within the limitations of his training and capabilities, this staff member can serve as a general counselor to the mothers in their personal and family problems. The parents of handicapped children frequently have many such problems. The counselor can serve as a liaison between the mothers and whatever professional people are involved, for example, psychiatrists. The counselor must be careful not to assume more responsibility for guidance than his capabilities fit him for. He should be familiar with various sources of referral for the kinds of additional help that the parents need.

The mothers of the children participate cooperatively with the nursery school teacher and the audiologist in all phases of nursery school activities. In this way, the mothers become familiar with methods of handling children, their own included, and they learn at first hand how to administer auditory training and other language-stimulating activities so that they can apply these techniques at home.

The children in this kind of program benefit tremendously. They learn to play with other children, to share, and to discipline themselves, and they are in an atmosphere in which oral language is used and encouraged. They learn to accept their hearing aids gracefully, because others in the group wear them. By the time these children reach school age, they already have a substantial background in some aspects of the school work that they will perform during their first year. Teachers of the deaf in public school systems are quick to praise the work of the preschool programs for the results that are evident in the "graduates" of the programs. Children who have had the advantage of preschool training develop their capabilities in school much more quickly than do other children who have not had the training. Teachers of the deaf will supervise the training of the child for all his school years. The audiologist can take pride, however, in what he has accomplished through the preschool training program—in sending these children to school with an excellent preparation.

COUNSELING FOR PARENT AND CHILD

As stated in the preceding chapter, the bulk of the counseling required with the hearing-impaired child should be directed to the parents, as the attitudes of the parent toward the handicap are most important in influencing the child's own attitudes. The audiologist has the duty of counseling the parents, and to some extent the child, as to the best ways of coping with the problems produced by the hearing loss. The audiologist must take care, however, not to undertake more counseling than the situation calls for, and not to attempt to handle problems of deep-seated psychological maladjustment. It is the audiologist's responsibility to establish the limits of his counseling, and to refer to proper professional people the cases that require help with personal or family problems. In other words, the audiologist must guard against the temptation to assume the role of a psychiatrist or clinical psychologist. The final section of this chapter on training the hearing-impaired child will deal with the most important areas in which the audiologist's counseling is required.

Acceptance of the Child

Parents of a handicapped child frequently find it difficult to accept the child for what he is. It is the hope of all parents that their children will be perfect in all respects. The presence of a handicap means that the parents' hopes have not been realized. Because of this failure to achieve the ideal of perfection, the parents may feel bitter and antagonistic towards the child. Usually the feelings are submerged, and the parents do not admit even to themselves that they have difficulty in accepting the child. As a matter of fact, their unconscious rejection of the child may result in their protesting vigorously that they want to do everything possible to help the child realize his full potentialities. Because it is not socially acceptable to reject one's children, the parents may be motivated in their actions by deep-seated feelings of guilt. Those who protest too loudly that they love and accept their children may be expressing only surface feelings. It is a blow to the ego to produce an imperfect child, and many parents blame the child, albeit unconsciously, for being imperfect. On the other hand, some parents feel that their having produced a handicapped child is punishment for their "sins," and their relations with the child are colored by their own feelings of guilt.

Although the audiologist has no business "psychoanalyzing" the parents or trying to interpret their feelings or motivations, he can assist them to a proper acceptance of the hearing-handicapped child through positive actions and statements. Perhaps his most important contribution is that of adopting an optimistic and encouraging attitude toward the child's problems. He should emphasize the child's assets and minimize his liabilities. He can explain to the parents that it is possible to educate him, even if he is deaf. If it is likely that the child will be able to utilize a hearing aid, the audiologist can emphasize the positive connotations of this fact. What must be avoided in dealing with parents is the attitude that their child has a problem for which nothing can be done. Diagnosticians are too prone to pass on their findings to parents without any mention of what can be done in the way of overcoming or minimizing the handicapping condition discovered. We know today that the hearing-handicapped child can usually be taught to speak and understand speech, he can be educated, and he can be vocationally trained. By pointing out the positive aspects of the situation, the audiologist may be answering some questions which the parents have been afraid to ask even themselves.

The audiologist can help allay fears and guilt feelings by explaining everything he can to the parents about the nature of the hearing loss and its cause. For information concerning the diagnosis and etiology, he will have to rely, of course, on the otological findings. Usually the otologist will have explained his findings to the parents, but even so the audiologist's repetition and explanation will be helpful to them. Frequently they are in such a state of shock upon first discovering they have a handicapped child that they cannot comprehend what the otologist is saying to them. Also, some otologists, unfortunately, do not take the time needed to explain fully to the parents just what the child's situation is. By interpreting the otological findings, the audiologist can do the otologist, as well as the parents, a service.

Frequently, hearing loss or deafness is a complete mystery to parents. In that event, the audiologist can help the parents better understand their child's problems by explaining how we hear and what can happen to cause interference with the normal hearing process. The difference between the hard of hearing and the deaf should be explained, and the child placed in his proper classification, so far as it is possible to determine it at that time. Parents can be referred to books on the subject of hearing loss and deafness which will also contribute to their better understanding of their child's problems and what can be done about them.[5]

The audiologist can perform a considerable service to parents by informing them of the existence of the John Tracy Clinic correspondence course

[5] Helmer R. Myklebust, *Your Deaf Child: A Guide for Parents* (Springfield, Ill., Charles C Thomas, 1970).

and by putting them in touch with the nearest preschool training program. He can also refer them to other parents of hearing-handicapped children, who have "been through the mill" and who can help and guide these parents from their own experiences with the problem.

The dangers of overprotection are almost as great as those of rejection. The healthiest home environment for the hearing-impaired child is one in which he is treated the same as other children in the family, with appropriate allowances, of course, for his communicative difficulties. Above all, the environment should be an *oral* one. The parents and other children in the family should talk with the child at all times and also encourage him to talk. It is only through constant exposure to speech that the child is motivated to want to understand what is said to him and to express himself through speech. He may be receiving the best possible school training in oral language, but if he is given no opportunity at home to exercise his communicative skills the school training will be to little avail.

The child who acquires his hearing loss some time after birth requires acceptance just as much as does the child with a congenital hearing problem. Frequently the problem of fitting a hearing aid to a child with an acquired loss is based on the parents' refusal to accept the situation. Some feel that the wearing of a hearing aid advertises to others that their child is defective, and they will go to any lengths to avoid this stigma. With such parents the audiologist must demonstrate, by whatever means he can, the help that the hearing aid gives the child. Parents of other children who wear hearing aids can be of considerable assistance at this point. If the parents can be brought to acceptance of the aid, with a sensible attitude toward it, it is much easier to convince the child. At the same time, as mentioned in the preceding chapter, parents must be cautioned against exerting too much pressure on the child to wear a hearing aid when the child is not yet convinced that he should do so. They must realize that it usually takes time for a child to adjust to a hearing aid. They must be patient and understanding in order to be helpful to him.

Some parents feel that a hearing aid will restore their child's hearing to normal. Naturally, they are bitter and disappointed when they learn that he still is handicapped, even with the hearing aid. Thus, the audiologist has the responsibility of explaining to them how hearing aids work and what they can and cannot do. He must give the parents a realistic notion of hearing aids.

Not only must the parents be realistic about what a hearing aid can accomplish; they must also be realistic about the extent of their child's handicap. Some parents do know the difference between the deaf and the hard of hearing but refuse to admit to themselves that their child is deaf. They nurse the hope that, with proper instruction and the use of a hearing aid, the child will be able to make his way in a regular classroom. When he experiences difficulty in trying to keep up with the other children, the parents blame the teacher for not giving their child the "special attention" that he deserves. The author remembers one such example very vividly. At the age of four, a little girl whom we shall call Ruth was found to have a profound impairment of hearing. She gave no indication of responding to sounds of high intensity when they were presented close to her ear. Ruth was enrolled in the Stanford Speech and Hearing Clinic for experimental therapy, to see whether with training she would give any indication of responding to sound. Instruction in speechreading and other techniques of language stimulation were started. Ruth's parents were urged to enroll her in a special class for the deaf conducted in a county school. This the parents refused to do; instead the mother enrolled Ruth in a regular kindergarten. Because of the character of kindergarten activities, Ruth was able to get along reasonably well during her first year. No demands were made on her to respond to speech or to speak, and she was able to color, to handle scissors, and to engage in most kindergarten activities. Meanwhile, the mother kept Ruth enrolled at the Speech and Hearing Clinic. She was sure that with the special help Ruth was receiving at the clinic, she would be able to make her way successfully at regular school.

The next fall, Ruth was enrolled in the first grade at the school she had previously attended, although both the kindergarten teacher and the principal of the school recommended her enrollment in the county class for the deaf. Within a few weeks after the beginning of the fall term, in the first grade, it was clear to the teacher that Ruth was wholly unable to profit from the instruction given. In this grade, Ruth was competing with about thirty youngsters whose hearing was normal, and day by day she became more withdrawn and sullen. Finally, everyone concerned with the case cooperated in insisting that Ruth attend the special class for the deaf. The principal of the school that she had been attending refused to let her continue, and the directors of the Speech and Hearing Clinic refused to continue work with her, since as long as Ruth attended the clinic two or three times a week the mother could continue to maintain that Ruth was receiving all the language-training instruction that she needed. It was obviously unfair to Ruth, to the teacher, and to the other children in the class to have her continue any longer in the first grade. Thus Ruth's parents were finally forced to face the true extent of their child's handicap. It can be added that in the county classes for the deaf Ruth made excellent progress and a good psychological adjustment. How much better for her it would have been had her parents faced squarely the true extent of her handicap and permitted her enrollment in a class for the deaf in the first place.

Educational Counseling

Parents need the audiologist's guidance in planning the proper educational program for their hearing-handicapped child. The audiologist is limited in his advice, of course, to the types of educational programs that are available to the parents in the communities in which they live. It goes without saying that the audiologist must be thoroughly familiar with all the educational facilities for hearing-impaired children which are available to the people whom he is advising.

Educators are now agreed that deaf children cannot be educated properly in the same classes with normal-hearing children, as was demonstrated with Ruth. Possible school placements for deaf children, dependent on the area, now include: a city school for the deaf, a county school with classes for the deaf, a state-supported residential school, and private residential schools. The city and county schools are *day* schools, in contrast with the state-supported and private residential schools. The advantage of the day school is that the children live at home, which is desirable from the standpoint of maintaining the child's security in his family relationships. The advantage of the residential schools is that the children enrolled there obtain a more concentrated program of special education which continues throughout their waking hours.

Although it is not the purpose of this book to discuss and evaluate methods of training the deaf, some mention should be made of the educational conflict which has persisted for centuries between the *oralists* and the *manualists*. The oralists maintain that with proper teaching methods the deaf can be taught to talk and understand speech, so that it is possible for them to communicate with normal-hearing people in the usual fashion. On the other hand, the manualists maintain that the results of oral teaching do not justify the tremendous effort required on the part of the child and his teachers. They say that it is unrealistic to expect that the deaf will ever be able to compete on equal terms with people with normal hearing, and that little advantage is therefore gained from the time and effort required to teach them speech. The manual method of communication, by means of finger spelling and conventional signs, is relatively easy to teach. By this means, the deaf can communicate easily with each other and with their teachers. Thus more school time is available for subject matter. The manualists admit that without speech the deaf adult is limited in the vocations that he can follow and his contacts with normal-hearing people. They stress vocational training, therefore, in such fields as baking, shoe repair, carpentry, machine work, and so forth, where the need for communication is minimal. Their attitude is that the deaf are going to have to look primarily to other deaf people for companionship anyway; thus it does not matter if they cannot communicate readily with those who have normal hearing.

Some schools teach what they call the "combined method" of communication. This is supposed to consist of both oral and manual methods of communication. Unfortunately, however, the manual system is easier to learn and use, and in schools where any students are permitted this system most prefer it to speech. Graduates of the combined-method schools are usually able to do some speechreading, but rarely are they able to speak with real intelligibility. Generally speaking, the city and county schools, the "day" schools, have adopted the oral approach in education, whereas the state-supported residential schools cling to the manual or combined methods. It was in protest against the manual method that the private residential schools for the deaf were founded. The accomplishments of the graduates of such private schools as Central Institute for the Deaf in St. Louis, Clarke School in Northampton, Mass., and Lexington School in New York in establishing themselves in professions and business are a tribute to the oralists' belief that with proper training the handicap imposed by deafness can be minimized and the deaf can make their way in a hearing world.

Quite apart from educational differences of opinion, there is a good reason why deaf children should attend day schools rather than residential ones—the genetic implications of segregating the deaf. Some cases of deafness are due to heredity, and if the social contacts of the deaf are limited to others who are deaf the problem of hereditary deafness will not only be perpetuated, it will increase as the deaf intermarry. Thus from the geneticist's point of view, it is a mistake for deaf children to attend residential schools. It would be much more sensible from the standpoint of the future of the race if deaf children could be educated in public schools where they would mingle with hearing children both on the school playgrounds and at home.

The parents of deaf children must plan for their children's education, and in this they will need the help of the audiologist and otologist. For the reasons stated above, the audiologist and otologist are prejudiced in favor of day schools and the oral method of educating the deaf. All factors in a given case must be carefully weighed and evaluated, however. A day school is to be preferred if there are enough deaf children to constitute several classes, each with a narrow age range. In some sparsely settled communities, day school classes have been established in which there is an age range of six or seven years. It is not possible for a teacher to do effective work with deaf children under these circumstances, even though there may be only six children in the class. Deaf children require such concentrated work in language, in addition to the subject matter, that all members of a class should be of about the same age and in the same stage of development. Faced with a choice between this day school situation and sending their child to the state residential school, parents may well decide that it is better to send the child to the state school. The alternatives would be to move to a community which does have a strong day school program or to send their child to a private residential school.

The educational opportunities for the hard of hearing are in some ways more extensive, and in others more limiting, than the opportunities for the deaf. Since by definition the hard of hearing have hearing which is functional with or without a hearing aid, presumably they should be able to profit from the same kind of instruction that normal-hearing students receive. Within the category of hard of hearing, however, there is a wide range of mental abilities as well. Even though a child is classified educationally as hard-of-hearing, he may not necessarily be able to make his way in regular classes. In the larger cities, and in some counties, there are special education programs for the hard of hearing as well as for the deaf. There may be special "contact" classes for the hard of hearing, in which the children are given instruction in speechreading, auditory training, and speech for part of the day, while they attend classes with normal-hearing children the rest of the time. In most public school situations, however, the child would have to attend regular classes all the time. If he is fortunate, the school system may employ speech and hearing therapists who travel from school to school and who could give him special oral language instruction two or three times a week outside the classroom. By and large, therefore, the hard-of-hearing child must get along as best he can in the regular classroom. If this is the situation, the help that the parents can give to the child assumes tremendous importance.

Parents cannot expect that every teacher their child has will be familiar with the problems of the hard of hearing, and so they must assume the responsibility for "educating" the teachers as to their child's needs. At the beginning of each school year, the child's mother—and father, too, if possible—should meet with the teacher and discuss the child's abilities and disabilities. The experience of his previous teachers should also be helpful in guiding the new teacher to an understanding of the child's problems. If he wears a hearing aid, the parents should explain to the teacher how the aid operates and what its limitations are. If he is embarrassed at wearing an aid, the parents can give helpful suggestions as to how the teacher can help the child to overcome his self-consciousness and make a better adjustment to his situation. The teacher, of course can do a great deal to determine the attitudes of the other students toward the hearing-handicapped child and particularly toward the hearing aid question. Throughout the school year, the parents should keep in close touch with the child's teacher; any problems arising can then be handled promptly through the cooperative action of the parents and the teacher. It goes without saying, of course, that in these parent-teacher conferences the child's mother and father must exercise tact and understanding, so that it does not appear that they are dictating to the teacher what she can and cannot do. Teachers most naturally resist overbearing and oversolicitous parents, and the parents must tread a narrow path between showing too much concern on the one hand and failing to give the teacher enough help and support, on the other.

For the child's sake, too, the parents must beware of becoming too solicitous, lest the child be "overprotected." Some parents find an emotional "release" in crusading for the betterment of hard-of-hearing children. This is fine so long as the child does not become a pampered, spoiled, incompetent "victim" of his parents' zeal. The hearing-handicapped child will have to make his own way eventually, and it is doing him a disservice to overprotect him. The audiologist can help the parents keep their "crusading" activities in proper focus. Of course, the better informed the parents are on hearing problems in general, and the situation of their own child in particular, the better able they are to assist the child's teachers in a proper handling of the child in school, and to help the child in and out of school in better adjusting to his problems.

Children with hearing impairments and their parents must give careful consideration to the choice of a vocation. The effect of the hearing impairment must be placed in proper perspective. The child's intelligence, aptitudes, and abilities must be considered, as well as the limitations imposed by the hearing problem. One important factor in the choice of a vocation is whether or not a college education is feasible or possible. The hard-of-hearing child who has been able to make his way successfully in public school programs can certainly continue to make his way educationally in college, provided that he has the intelligence and the motivation to do acceptable academic work. There are very few deaf individuals, however, who can do college work successfully, because of the tremendous emphasis on communication skills at the college level. Even the deaf person with excellent intellectual equipment finds it almost impossible to compete in college with normal-hearing students without an assistant to take notes in lectures. A good background in oral education methods is a prerequisite to attending regular college, of course. There is only one college in the United States exclusively for deaf students, Gallaudet College in Washington, D.C. Gallaudet College is supported by the federal government, and it is the only college which graduates of manual systems of education can attend without being faced with a virtually insurmountable communicative handicap.

Deaf or hard-of-hearing college graduates naturally have a wider vocational choice than do hearing-handicapped individuals who cannot attend college. So, in planning for the future, parents of hearing-impaired children must consider whether or not a college education is a possibility. For children who cannot attend college, some kind of vocational training must be planned. There are countless occupations in which a hearing impairment is of secondary importance. The choice of vocation, therefore, should depend primarily on the child's aptitudes and abilities, always keeping in mind, of course, the limitations imposed by the hearing handicap. The parents should be advised to consult with a competent vocational counselor at least by the time the child reaches high school age. In the matter of choice of vocation, the parents must be willing to accept the child and his handicap, just as they must accept the child wholeheartedly when his hearing impairment is first discovered.

REFERENCES

Bender, Ruth E., *The Conquest of Deafness* (Cleveland, The Press of Case Western Reserve University, 1970).

Berg, Frederick S., and Fletcher, Samuel G., eds., *The Hard of Hearing Child* (New York, Grune & Stratton, 1970).

Davis, Hallowell, and Silverman, S. Richard, eds., *Hearing and Deafness* (New York, Holt, Rinehart and Winston, 1970), Chaps. 12, 13, 14, 16, and 17).

DiCarlo, Louis M., *The Deaf* (Englewood Cliffs, N.J., Prentice-Hall, 1964).

Harris, Grace M., *Language for the Preschool Deaf Child* (New York, Grune & Stratton, 1963).

Johnson, Wendell, Brown, Spencer F., Curtis, James F., Edney, Clarence W., and Keaster, Jacqueline, *Speech Handicapped School Children* (New York, Harper & Row, 1967), Chap. 8.

McConnell, Freeman, and Ward, Paul H., eds., *Deafness in Childhood* (Nashville, Tenn., Vanderbilt University Press, 1967), Chaps. 16, 17, 18, and 19.

Myklebust, Helmer R., *The Psychology of Deafness* (New York, Grune & Stratton, 1964).

Proceedings of International Conference on Oral Education of the Deaf, Vols. I and II (Washington, D.C., The Alexander Graham Bell Association for the Deaf, 1967).

Ronnei, Eleanor C., *Learning to Look and Listen* (New York, Columbia University Bureau of Publications, 1951).

Streng, Alice, Fitch, Waring J., Hedgecock, Leroy D., Phillips, James W., and Carrell, James A., *Hearing Therapy for Children* (New York, Grune & Stratton, 1958).

Travis, Lee Edward, ed., *Handbook of Speech Pathology and Audiology* (New York, Appleton-Century-Crofts, 1971), Chaps. 15 and 16.

West, Robert, and Ansberry, Merle, *The Rehabilitation of Speech* (New York, Harper & Row, 1968), Chap. 17.

Whitehurst, Mary W., *Auditory Training for Children* (Armonk, N.Y., Hearing Rehabilitation, 1966).

Whitehurst, Mary W., *Integrated Lessons in Lipreading and Auditory Training* (Armonk, N.Y., Hearing Rehabilitation, 1964).

12

REHABILITATING THE
HARD-OF-HEARING ADULT

The therapeutic problems presented by the adult who develops a hearing impairment are in most respects simpler than those of children. The principal difference is that the adult has well-developed language concepts and presumably throughout his life has been "auditorily minded." Thus the therapist can assume that the adult has a memory for sounds, and vocabulary building is not a necessary part of the rehabilitation process. In the area of psychological adjustment, however, the adult presents a more challenging problem to the therapist. As stated in Chapter 10, it may be more difficult to adjust to a hearing disorder after having experienced normal hearing for a number of years than it is when there is no memory or knowledge of normal hearing. Counseling, therefore, is a necessary and important part of the rehabilitation of the hard-of-hearing adult. Not infrequently, counseling must precede all other aspects of rehabilitation. Before the individual can benefit from instruction in speechreading, auditory training, or speech training, he must be motivated to want to help himself. Persuading him to accept a hearing aid, for example, may be a trying ordeal for the patient, the patient's family, and the therapist. Rehabilitative work with an adult is rewarding, however, for once the patient has accepted the situation and decided that he should make an effort to help himself he can make rapid progress under instruction, which of course is gratifying to the therapist.

As in the previous chapter, no attempt will be made here to develop specific lesson plans for the adult. Rather, a general view will be taken of ways to meet the patient's rehabilitative needs. Again, the reader seeking more specific information is referred to the bibliographic listing at the end of the chapter.

SPEECHREADING

Regardless of the extent of hearing loss or whether or not the patient can profit from a hearing aid, instruction in speechreading will be beneficial. As a matter of fact, those of us with normal hearing can improve our communicative abilities through understanding and practicing the skill of speechreading. One of the first tasks of the therapist is to convince the patient that speechreading is not an esoteric art which requires years of training. It is advisable in the beginning to build up the patient's confidence by demonstrating that even without instruction he is capable of doing some speechreading. This can be done by asking the patient a number of questions about himself—questions of the type that he would be asked in many common situations, such as applying for a driver's license, a marriage certificate, or a passport. To make the demonstration more convincing, the therapist should use no voice, that is, the normal rate, rhythm, and articulation of speech should be maintained without audible speech, so that the patient cannot claim that he had auditory clues.

The questions should be on the order of the following:

What is your name?
How do you spell your name?
Where do you live?
What is your telephone number?
Are you married?
What is your wife's (or husbands') name?
Do you have any children?
What are their names?
How old are they?

It is easier for the patient to understand when each question follows logically from the preceding one. It may be necessary to ask a particular question two or three times before the patient comprehends it, and on occasion the therapist may have to rephrase the question. For example, it may be easier for the patient to understand the question "What is your address?" although he does not comprehend at all your question "Where do you live?" With skill, the therapist can make this question-and-answer game a rewarding and motivating experience for the patient. Moreover, the way in which the patient responds to this kind of questioning can yield valuable information for the therapist in planning the program of speechreading instruction. If the patient answers quickly and easily, the therapist knows that he will probably be an excellent student, and the speechreading lessons can progress rapidly. On the other hand, if the patient has difficulty with these simple questions, the prognosis for his making rapid progress in the training program is not too good. In any event, personal questions of the type referred to can be helpful in establishing a friendly working relationship between the therapist and the patient. Besides the insight into his facility in speechreading, the therapist can quickly learn a good deal about the patient from the factual answers which he gives to the questions.

It is well in the beginning to explain to the patient what the object of speechreading instruction is and to give him some specific suggestions for becoming an effective speechreader. The purpose of the training in speechreading is, of course, to quicken the patient's powers of visual observation; it does not teach him a new skill so much as it systematizes what he already does on a more or less unconscious level. The patient should be informed at the outset that speechreading is not a perfect substitute for hearing. He himself will realize after the initial practice work that he cannot possibly speechread all that he sees. The therapist must stress the fact that the patient should not attempt to get every word but should keep up with the pace of the person's speech. If the speechreader dwells on a particular word which he did not comprehend, he loses out on what the speaker is presently saying; thus, at all costs the speechreader must keep pace with the speaker. Another important suggestion concerns the development of a flexible mind. To be an effective speechreader, one must not have too firmly set, preconceived notions of how things should be said. The speechreader should realize that there is more than one way of expressing a thought, and he should keep alert to what the speaker is saying instead of trying to put words into his mouth.

It is the author's feeling that a synthetic method of teaching speechreading is preferable for adults. At least it should be given first choice. As long as the patient is able to do a reasonably good job of speechreading sentences and paragraphs, there seems little point in spending time on an analysis of individual sounds. It has been the author's experience that the adult who cannot do well with a synthetic approach will likewise have difficulty with analytic procedures. The only time that work on individual sounds is justified is when it becomes clear that a particular sound is causing the patient difficulty. Even then the sound usually can be demonstrated in words or phrases more effectively than in isolation.

As in working with children, speechreading for the adult should be approached as one of several related communicative skills, which are combined to compensate for a hearing loss. The therapist must keep the over-all objectives of the rehabilitative program in mind and not succumb to the temptation to regard ability in speechreading as a goal in itself. At the same time that he is receiving instruction in speechreading, the patient should be encouraged to utilize his hearing as well. The therapist then should strive to teach the adult to combine speechreading with whatever auditory ability he has. Some voice should be employed during the speechreading lessons, so that the patient can make use of hearing, as well as vision. If, however, the therapist speaks in such a manner that the patient can understand every word by hearing alone, he will develop little or no ability in speechreading *per se*. It is preferable, therefore, for the therapist to speak in a voice which is barely audible to the patient and which presents a difficult listening situation for him. This is the kind of practical, everyday communicative condition in which the patient will experience difficulty. The therapist can vary the difficulty of the speechreading lessons on occasion with whispered voice or some of the time with no voice at all. These techniques should be applied sparingly. By and large, the patient should be given experience in meeting situations which he will confront in the normal course of events.

Numbers are a good way to start speechreading instruction. They are important to all of us in our daily living. We live by the numbers on the clock and the calendar, and we pay for our living with the numbers on money. It is easy to plan lessons around them. For example, a patient may be asked to set the hands of a clock to the time which the therapist designates. To start, the therapist should talk about the various ways of stating times: "Twenty minutes before ten" is the same as "nine-forty"; "twelve o'clock" may be "noon" or "midnight"; and so forth. Then the therapist should give practice to the patient in speechreading numbers from one to sixty. When the patient is able to do this successfully, his ability can be put to the test by having him set the hands of the clock.

Working on dates provides an opportunity for the patient to learn the days of the week and the months of the year as well as both ordinal and cardinal numbers. In the first place, the patient should be given an opportunity to learn the days of the week as the therapist goes over them in sequence. The months of the year can be practiced and learned in the same way. Then dates in the form of the day of the week and the day of the month can be practiced, for example, "Tuesday, September 9." Finally, the days of the week and the month should be combined with the four digits of a year, for example, "Friday, January 27, 1956." Holidays which occur every year provide interesting ways of practicing on dates. Thus, the therapist can give a date, such as "December 25," and ask the patient to reply what holiday it is. If the patient is at all proficient in history, the dates of famous historical events can be employed in the same way, as a test of the patient's ability to speechread months, days, and years.

Further practice on numbers is possible by planning lessons around money. As with time, there are various ways of talking about money. A dime may be spoken of as "ten cents"; a quarter as "twenty-five cents," or "two bits"; and a dollar may be referred to as a "buck," or any of several additional slang terms. The prices of articles in the grocery store can be practiced in numbers from one cent to ten dollars. Items of clothing permit practice on prices from one to a hundred dollars, and other commodities from washing machines to yachts provide the opportunity to practice on the higher-numbered prices. In dealing with prices, the therapist must point out to the patient that "two ninety-eight" is the same as "two dollars and ninety-eight cents," or, depending on the commodity being discussed, "two hundred and ninety-eight dollars."

In work dealing with numbers, certain ones will consistently give difficulty. The numbers "eight" and "nine" are almost indistinguishable from each other in speechreading. Numbers such as "thirteen" and "thirty," "fifteen" and "fifty," and so forth, are frequently confused. The patient must learn that he cannot always rely on speechreading with these numbers. In a "real" situation, he should always repeat the number that he thinks he has seen in order to check himself. Thus, if, in reply to a question about train schedules the ticket agent says something which the patient reads as "9:17," he should ask the agent, "Did you say "9:17?" It might just as well have been "8:17," and, without asking, the patient can never be sure.

Speechreading instruction can be made interesting to adult patients by planning lessons around so-called life situations. In the preceding paragraph, mention was made of a conversation between a patient and a ticket agent. The therapist can prepare a dialogue between a hypothetical ticket agent and the patient, involving questions and answers about particular trains, their schedules, and the price of tickets. Again, instead of drill work on prices alone, a dialogue could be prepared on a shopping visit to the grocery or a visit to the shoe store or any of dozens of situations which involve the pricing of objects. Situations in which the patient is most likely to find himself should be selected for these dialogues. After explaining to him what the situation is, the therapist should proceed with the complete dialogue between the two characters involved, while the patient speechreads both parts of the conversation. With this kind of material, the therapist should first go through the complete dialogue without stopping and then ask the patient questions about what was said. After the questions, which will disclose how much of the dialogue the patient is able to speechread on his first attempt, the therapist should go back over the dialogue on a sentence-by-sentence basis, asking the patient to repeat each sentence as he speechreads it. It may be necessary at this point for the therapist to repeat a given sentence two or three times or perhaps to rephrase the sentence before the patient can comprehend it. The therapist should accept the patient's version of a sentence, even if it should not be word-perfect, if the patient has succeeded in understanding the thought. As a final step, the therapist should then repeat the whole dialogue without stopping, in order to give the patient an opportunity to synthesize what he has just gone over on a sentence-by-sentence basis.

Situations such as those mentioned above should be fairly easy speechreading experiences for the beginner. As the patient develops facility in this kind of situation, the therapist should provide more difficult speechreading experiences. Short anecdotes, such as those which appear in the *Reader's Digest,* provide good material for speechreading lessons. Since they are written for the silent reader, it is usually desirable for the therapist to rewrite the story in an oral style. Anecdotes usually contain a "punch line" at the end. The test of the patient's speechreading ability is whether he "gets the point" of the story on his first attempt. The same procedure should be followed as with the life-situation dialogues. The therapist should give the story as a whole to begin with, then ask questions about it, repeat it on a sentence-by-sentence basis, and finally give the story in its complete form again.

It is helpful and stimulating for patients to obtain some experience in a group situation. Ideally, groups should be organized so that all members have similar interests and similar speechreading abilities. Group speech-reading experiences help the patient to realize that other hard-of-hearing individuals have difficulties of the same type as his. Group work may stimulate the individual to greater effort because of the spirit of competition. Finally, the members of the group may help each other to achieve a better speechreading ability and also a healthier attitude toward their hearing handicaps. In group work, each member should take his turn being a speaker, so that the members of the group may have the practice of speechreading a number of different speakers. As the members of the group become more proficient, more difficult experiences may be provided, like setting up actual dialogues so that the speechreaders must shift their attention from one speaker to another, and giving the speechreaders the opportunity to view speakers from various distances and angles. Group work does not take the place of individual instruction in speechreading, but it can supply an interesting and profitable means of putting speechreading ability to practical use.

AUDITORY TRAINING

The hard-of-hearing adult does not require as extensive auditory training as does the child because of his previous experience as a normal-hearing individual. Thus, with the adult it is not necessary to start with gross auditory discriminations or even with gross speech sound discriminations unless, of course, he has suffered almost a complete loss of hearing. Generally, it is with the consonant sounds that the adult has difficulty, and usually it is the high-frequency, low-powered voiceless consonants that give him the most trouble. Whether or not the adult will require any auditory training depends, of course, on the severity of his loss, the length of time that he has been hard-of-hearing, and also the audiometric configuration of his loss. The adult with a hearing impairment which is easily compensated for by a hearing aid may require no auditory training, whereas an individual with a typical sensori-neural impairment, who has considerably better hearing in the low frequencies than in the high ones, will probably benefit from auditory training whether or not he wears a hearing aid. The test of whether or not auditory training is indicated is the individual's ability to *understand* speech with or without amplification. If he has difficulty in understanding speech even when he hears it well, he would probably benefit from auditory training. The candidate for a hearing aid may profit from auditory training administered with amplification such as that provided by an auditory training unit. The person who cannot successfully utilize a hearing aid should receive auditory training without amplification, for the most part, although on occasion an auditory training unit may be employed for the purpose of focusing his attention.

As with speechreading instruction, a worthwhile starting technique in auditory training is the use of numbers. The therapist starts with two-digit numbers, such as "four-six," and asks the patient to repeat them or to write them down. As the patient gains facility in recognizing two-digit numbers, three-digit numbers can be introduced, and eventually four- and five-digit numbers.[1] Numbers are good because the choices which the patient has to make are limited, and since many numbers can be differentiated on the basis of vowels alone the patient can do well with a minimum of auditory clues.

As was suggested in auditory training for children, practice with paired words which differ only in their initial or final consonant is a good technique for adults. The therapist gives the patient a written list of paired words and then says one word in each pair while the patient checks the word that he thinks the therapist said. This can be extended to as many as five words, all of which are similar, such as *fear, dear, near, cheer, beer*. The therapist says one word, and the patient must check which of the five possible words it was. This type of auditory training material is available in recorded form.[2]

The word lists customary in speech audiometry for obtaining thresholds (spondees) and speech-discrimination scores (phonetically balanced words) are useful also for auditory training work. The spondee words, being easier, should be practiced first. Whenever the patient misses a spondee word, it should be noted and put on a list which will then serve for extensive drill. The phonetically balanced words are more difficult, because they are monosyllables and thus contain a minimum of auditory clues. As was suggested with spondee words, lists should be kept of the PB words that are consistently missed by the patient, and they can serve also for drill work. Because of the difficulty of the words in the phonetically balanced lists, it cannot be expected that the patient will be able to understand 100 per cent of them, no matter how extensive his training. In other words, an individual who has a loss for the higher speech frequencies is bound to make some mistakes on the PB word lists, and it is advisable not to set too high standards of performance for the patient on these words. Other tests for speech discrimination described

[1] J. C. Kelly, *Clinician's Handbook for Auditory Training* (Dubuque, Iowa, Wm. C. Brown, 1953).

[2] Laila L. Larsen, *Consonant Sound Discrimination Recordings and Manual* (Bloomington, Ind., Indiana University, 1950).

in Chapter 6, such as the Rhyme Test, the Modified Rhyme Test, and the CNC word lists, are useful for auditory training purposes.

From single words, the therapist should progress to sentences and paragraphs. Davis and Silverman reproduce several sentence tests that have been used at various times for testing intelligibility.[3] In one test, prepared at the Harvard Psycho-Acoustic Laboratory, each sentence contains five key words. The patient is asked to repeat the sentence or to write it down. He must hear each of the five key words correctly for the sentence to be scored correct. An example of the sentences is the following one, in which the key words are italicized: "The *birch canoe slid* on the *smooth planks.*" The sentences may be repeated a number of times for the sake of practice, but once the patient becomes familiar with them they lose their value for auditory training.

The therapist may prepare paragraphs which deal with simple subjects such as "how to sew on a button." For each paragraph a number of questions should be prepared that test the patient's ability to follow the running-speech material. The therapist can also adapt for auditory training the materials which are suitable for speechreading practice. Although it is frequently necessary to spend time drilling on words in auditory training, the object should be to increase the patient's ability to understand running speech.

One of the objectives of an auditory training program for adults may be to increase the patient's tolerance for speech of high intensity. In conditions of sensori-neural loss characterized by recruitment, there may be such a narrow range between the threshold of speech reception and the threshold of discomfort that a hearing aid is contraindicated. With training it is possible to increase the patient's tolerance level and thus make a hearing aid feasible for him. Such training requires equipment with amplification which can be carefully controlled, such as an auditory training unit. Recorded-speech materials are possible, with the auditory training unit set at a volume level that corresponds with the patient's present ability to tolerate intense speech. He is permitted to increase the volume himself and to discontinue the listening whenever the process becomes unbearably annoying to him. With many patients, very little practice in listening to intense speech enables them to accept more amplification than formerly. With some patients, a low-tolerance level is the result of living for years without hearing very intense speech. In the beginning they are unable to tolerate amplification because, having gradually become accustomed to their defective hearing, they are disturbed at the experience of hearing speech loudly again. As they become more familiar with amplified speech, they are gradually able to accept higher and higher levels of amplification. The only purpose of training to increase the usable range of hearing for speech is to enable the patient to benefit from a hearing aid.

[3] Hallowell Davis and S. Richard Silverman, eds., *Hearing and Deafness* (New York, Holt, Rinehart and Winston, 1970), pp. 489-495.

HEARING-AID ORIENTATION

Even the patient who does not require auditory training will frequently benefit from a program of instruction after he is fitted with a hearing aid. Hearing-aid orientation consists both of instruction in the mechanics of operating the instrument and a psychological strengthening of the individual's resolve to help himself. Hearing aids are expensive instruments, and it might be expected that once a patient had invested in one he would force himself to learn to operate and adjust to it. A large proportion of hearing aids sold directly to patients without preparation or orientation end up in the proverbial dresser drawer. The military aural rehabilitation programs demonstrated that, with proper hearing-aid selection procedures and a period of orientation, patients fitted with hearing aids would continue to wear them. Therefore, it is certainly worth a few dollars of the patient's money and a few hours of his time to learn effective mastery of it.

Before he purchases an aid, the patient should be made to realize that any hearing aid has its limitations. Too many patients expect that the hearing aid will be the answer to all their hearing problems, and that once they start wearing the aid they will be able to hear just as well as they did when their hearing was normal. Unfortunately, this is not true. As we have seen in Chapter 10, a hearing aid is an amplifier system, and not a very high-fidelity one. The patient who has speech-discrimination problems, as demonstrated by poor scores on the discrimination tests in speech audiometry, may still have discrimination problems with the hearing aid. However, if the patient needs amplification in order to hear speech, the hearing aid will be of assistance to him even though he does not understand 100 per cent of what he hears. Therefore, the first step in a hearing-aid orientation program is to discuss with the patient the limitations of his own hearing and the limitations of the benefit he can expect from the hearing aid.

Most patients will be disappointed with the comparatively poor quality of the speech reproduction that they receive with the hearing aid, particularly if they have had previous experience with an auditory training unit. At present, patients will have to be satisfied with the limited quality of reproduction that hearing aids provide. It is to be hoped that in the near future it will be possible to design and manufacture hearing aids that reproduce speech more faithfully. If the patient is told what he can expect in the way of quality of reproduction, he is prepared for the ensuing disappointment when he wears the hearing aid. It should be pointed out to the patient, however, that the quality of reproduction of the hearing aid is sufficient to cover the principal speech frequencies, so that with the aid it will be possible for him to understand speech even though it may not sound as natural to him as he thinks it should. We are all accustomed to the limited frequency response of the telephone and the way in which it distorts voice quality. Yet, with the telephone we are able to achieve extensive comprehension, and excellent communication is possible. The hearing-impaired individual can learn to communicate successfully with the limited frequency response and distortion of the hearing aid also.

The patient must be told that it will take time for him to become accustomed to hearing with the aid, and that for the first several days, or even several weeks, he will have discouraging experiences. In the beginning, the patient should not attempt to wear the aid throughout the day but should start by wearing it only a few minutes at a time. Each day, the time can be increased, as he becomes used to the amplification received. The goal eventually, of course, is for the patient to reach the point of wearing the aid throughout the day, just as he would wear spectacles if his vision were impaired. Some adults find it difficult to adjust to bifocals or to false teeth. A hearing aid is a prosthetic device also, and it requires time to become used to wearing it. When an individual has gone for a number of years without hearing normally, the sudden introduction of amplification can be a startling experience.

A common complaint of hearing-aid users is the amount of noise that the aid delivers to the ear. The noise may be from two sources: the environment of the individual, and then it is heard by everyone else as well; or the instrument itself, for example, in the case of a body-worn aid, from the movement of clothing across the microphone grill. Patients must learn to accept the noise, whether it is external or internal in nature, and to ignore it while concentrating on what they want to hear. Those of us who have normal hearing must go through this process of selecting what we want to hear from the surrounding noise, which is undesirable but which we have to tolerate. The person with a long-standing hearing loss may have forgotten that our environment is so noisy, and it will take time for him to adjust to the background noises surrounding him.

The new hearing-aid user must not expect to obtain good results with his aid in difficult listening situations. Examples of difficult situations are: a play, a lecture, or a church service, a meeting in which many people are speaking at a distance from the listener; and conversation outdoors in the presence of loud traffic noises. Generally, a situation which is difficult for people with normal hearing will be one in which a hard-of-hearing patient will experience special difficulty in using his aid to good effect. A play on the legitimate stage is an extremely difficult listening situation, because of the fact that a number of people with unfamiliar voices are speaking rapidly and perhaps not too carefully, and the listener is seated in an auditorium filled with people coughing, moving their feet, rustling their programs, and otherwise making noise which tends to mask out the words of the actors. At the movies, the listener's problem is further complicated by the presence of people who enjoy eating popcorn and other "noisy" food. The individual with a hearing aid in any of these circumstances may be getting excellent reception of the sounds close to him, that is, the noises made by members of the audience, and will have considerable difficulty "tuning in" the dialogue on the stage or the screen. What the hearing-aid user frequently does not realize is that in these difficult listening situations the person with normal hearing also may be missing a considerable amount of what is said. It is not advisable for the hearing-aid wearer to attempt to use his aid in difficult listening situations until he has become thoroughly accustomed to it in easier situations. In any event, he should be warned that the results in these difficult situations are likely to be very disappointing. The reason that the aid should not be worn out of doors at the outset is that loud traffic noises will cause the patient extreme annoyance and may discourage further attempts with the aid. Again, once he has learned to make effective use of the aid indoors and in easy listening situations, he can then wear the aid outdoors if he wants to. The easiest situations are those in which there is a minimum of background noise and a limited number of speakers. Thus, even the beginning hearing-aid user should be successful with the aid at home with members of his family.

An important part of the hearing-aid orientation program is to teach the patient how to wear his aid most effectively and how to take proper care of it. As was mentioned in Chapter 10, best results can be obtained with a body-worn hearing-aid when it is worn outside the clothing, so that there is no brushing of clothing across the microphone grill, and when the receiver is attached to a standard ear piece. Some patients will accept the hearing aid only if they can effectively conceal it. Women are able to conceal hearing aids effectively by employing appropriate hair styling, but men cannot hide the fact that they have something in the ear. The therapist must understand the problems of adjustment faced by the patient when first wearing a hearing aid and be patient and sympathetic. It is to be hoped, however, that as the patient becomes adjusted to the idea of wearing the aid he will accept the wearing of it in the most efficient manner. The therapist has the responsibility at least to inform the patient how he can obtain the best possible service from the aid.

Adult patients frequently are timid about turning the amplification to the degree desirable. Some patients constantly adjust the volume control, turning it up when they cannot hear well and down if someone speaks a bit too loudly. It is difficult for a patient to benefit from his hearing aid when he is constantly fiddling with the controls. The therapist should encourage the patient, therefore, to select a volume-control setting which is adequate for his needs and to leave the control at that setting regardless of changes in the levels of voices around him. People with normal hearing must adjust to varying levels of loudness, and the person with a hearing aid can learn to do the same. If there is a tone control it should normally be set to give the full range of the amplifier. The quality of hearing-aid reproduction is not too good to begin with, and it is undesirable to reduce the frequency-response characteristics of the aid still more by adjusting the tone control to any point other than full-amplification range. The patient should learn to insert and remove his ear piece with facility, and he must also learn how to change the battery in the instrument. He should be instructed to carry extra batteries with him at all times, so that in the event of a battery failure his aid is not put out of commission.

A part of the hearing-aid orientation program should be instructing the patient how to locate the source of difficulty when the aid is not functioning properly. The commonest cause of difficulty, with the exception of a dead battery, is a broken cord which connects the receiver with the amplifier, or a broken connection between the case of a head-worn aid and the ear piece. The cords are made of extremely thin wire and are easily broken. Unless the aid and the receiver have been dropped, it is not likely that they will develop faults. Sometimes the canal piece of the ear insert becomes clogged with wax, which of course interferes with the transmission of sound from the receiver to the ear. The patient should be instructed to keep the ear piece clean by washing it in soap and water and by running a pipe cleaner through the hole at frequent intervals.

The patient needs instruction in manipulation of the aid with the telephone. If his aid has a telephone circuit, he can be shown how to operate the switch and how to hold the telephone next to the hearing aid in order to utilize the telephone circuit. Incidentally, patients sometimes complain that their hearing aids are not functioning correctly, when the difficulty proves to be that the microphone has been switched off and the telephone circuit switched on. Patients should be reminded, therefore, that after a telephone conversation they must return the switch on the aid to the microphone position. Where no telephone circuit is contained in the aid, the patient may still use the hearing aid with the telephone by placing the receiver of the telephone next to the microphone of the hearing aid. In the case of body-worn aids, the telephone must be held upside-down, with the receiver against the microphone of the hearing aid and the transmitter in front of the patient's mouth. It is sometimes difficult for hearing-aid users to realize that their "ear" is the microphone of the hearing aid. Incidentally, some patients who wear hearing aids are able to hear over the telephone successfully with the unaided ear. For people who prefer to use the telephone without their hearing aid the telephone company has available a special phone with a built-in amplifier which can be adjusted for intensity. Also, amplifiers are available on the market which clamp onto the receiver of the telephone. The hard-of-hearing person can carry this kind of amplifier in his pocket and have it ready for a conversation over any telephone.

The patient who has had the limitations of his hearing explained and demonstrated to him, who has been guided through a series of graded experiences with his hearing aid, and who has thoroughly learned the mechanics of operating it is in a position to become a good hearing-aid user. The first few weeks with it are the difficult ones. Assistance in the form of hearing-aid orientation at this point can be of untold benefit to the patient in his lifelong "career" as a hearing-aid user.

SPEECH TRAINING

The adult who has a mild-to-moderate hearing loss, who has no problems of speech discrimination, and who can derive benefit from a hearing aid will probably have no observable speech symptoms of hearing impairment. On the other hand, the individual who has a severe-to-profound degree of hearing loss and who does have speech-discrimination problems will usually demonstrate through his voice quality and articulation the effects of the hearing impairment. Since the quality of our speech depends largely upon auditory monitoring, our speech production may deteriorate if our auditory monitoring becomes faulty. A hearing aid assists in the monitoring process, particularly in helping the individual to achieve proper voice control, but when there is a severe or profound loss, even a hearing aid cannot wholly prevent some deterioration of speech. The therapist must keep in mind therefore that, in addition to whatever speechreading instruction and auditory training the individual needs, some work on speech will frequently be indicated.

In the military aural rehabilitation centers of World War II, one of the rehabilitative services provided was termed "speech conservation," as has been previously mentioned. Here, hearing-impaired service personnel were made aware of the danger that their speech might deteriorate because of the hearing loss and were taught techniques which, it was hoped, would prevent serious speech deterioration. In other words, the work in speech conservation was a kind of "insurance" for the future. Speech conservation, as it was taught in the military centers, is probably not a practical procedure for a civilian population. Although the hard-of-hearing adult may be convinced of his need for speechreading and training with a hearing aid, it is difficult to persuade him that he should spend time and money working on his speech when currently he has no speech problems.

The effects of a severe or profound loss are reflected in the patient's lack of proper voice control and in a general "mushiness" of articulation. The voice-control problem consists of an inability to judge the proper intensity of voice needed in a given speaking situation. The commonest example of the effect of a hearing loss on the voice is the hard-of-hearing individual who shouts. It was explained in Chapter 3 that the hard-of-hearing person who shouts or speaks too loudly is probably evidencing one symptom of a sensorineural hearing loss. He speaks loudly because he cannot hear his own voice well. If the hearing loss is of long duration and is severe in extent, vocal quality will be affected. The voice will lose its vitality and tend to develop a "deadness" of quality, such as we find in the congenitally deaf individual. In an adult with this severe impairment of long duration, monotony of pitch will probably also be present. The first sounds to deteriorate in the speech of the adult with a hearing problem are those which require the most delicate adjustment of the articulators and the greatest amount of auditory monitoring. As with the child, referred to in the preceding chapter, these sounds include most prominently the *s, r, l, sh,* and *ch* consonants.

The correction of the voice and of articulation disorders, which the adult demonstrates as a result of his hearing impairment, is based on principles discussed in the preceding chapter dealing with hearing-impaired children. The therapist can teach the adult patient to control the intensity of his voice by being conscious of the muscle tensions in his larynx. Carhart suggests that the individual learn to talk at each of four or five levels of intensity, judging by the kinesthetic sensations in the larynx at which level he is speaking. He will then have to judge by the reactions of the people with whom he is talking whether or not he is at the proper level of laryngeal tension to meet the needs of the situation.[4] Difficulties of inflections can be handled in the same manner as was suggested for children in the preceding chapter. The correction of articulatory difficulties is based on an analysis for the patient of the way in which his faulty sounds can be corrected, relying on his knowledge of phonetic placement and his learning to utilize kinesthetic sensations. Sometimes the patient's attention can be focused on correct articulation by means of an auditory training unit. As mentioned previously, the hard-of-hearing adult's hearing aid also will be of benefit in regulating his speech and voice usage.

For the most part, instruction in speech should be integrated with instruction in speechreading and the auditory training program. The therapist must be alert to seize every opportunity to correct speech difficulties in the patient as they occur.

COUNSELING

In Chapter 10, the psychological problems of the hard-of-hearing individual were discussed, and the need for counseling the patient was stressed. There is little that can be added here to what has already been covered in Chapter 10, except to emphasize again the fundamental principle that the hearing-impaired individual must be willing to accept and admit his handicap before he can profit from the rehabilitative procedures discussed.

The hard-of-hearing adult who presents the greatest challenge to the therapist is the person with a typical sensori-neural impairment, who has

---

[4] Raymond Carhart, "Development and Conservation of Speech," in Davis and Silverman, *ibid.,* Chap. 14, p. 370.

such good hearing in the low frequencies that he may not be able to utilize even a CROS-type hearing aid successfully, but whose hearing for the higher speech frequencies is so impaired that he has severe speech-discrimination problems. This is the person who says, "I can hear you, but I don't understand what you are saying." He can usually benefit little from auditory training but will have to rely primarily on speechreading. This individual, for whom so little can be done in the way of compensating for his hearing impairment, may be bitter toward the therapist and the otologist who are relatively powerless to help him. He observes other hard-of-hearing people deriving satisfactory results from hearing aids, and he resents his inability to secure similar assistance. Since he does not wear a hearing aid, he bears no outward sign of being handicapped, and so people with whom he comes in casual contact do not realize that they must take special pains in speaking to him.

The therapist can only hope that such a patient will eventually arrive at an acceptance of his disability and a thankfulness that he still has some hearing abilities. The only salvation for this type of individual is to admit freely to all with whom he comes in contact that his hearing is faulty. It is necessary for him to develop a "thick skin" and to take the initiative in helping himself by telling other people how they can most effectively communicate with him.

As was mentioned in Chapter 10, there is a tendency for the hard-of-hearing adult to become withdrawn and psychologically depressed. The therapist must make every effort through counseling the patient and if necessary, through counseling the patient's family, to keep him from withdrawing from social contacts. Somehow he must be brought to the realization that although his hearing loss is an inconvenience it is not a tragedy. He is the same individual he was before his hearing problem developed, and there is no need for him to abandon his former activities and interests because of the change in his hearing ability. Some adjustments may be necessary in his vocational and avocational pursuits, but they are usually of a minor character and need cause him no great concern. Patients who have major problems of psychological adjustment should be referred for psychiatric or psychological guidance, and those who are faced with difficult vocational problems should be directed to a vocational counselor.

It is helpful to individuals who become handicapped to be reminded of others who were able to surmount their handicaps and live happy and useful lives. There are several inspiring autobiographies to which the hearing-handicapped person can be referred.[5] The best cure for the person who feels sorry for himself is to realize that others even more severely handicapped have succeeded in spite of their handicaps. The supreme example, of course,

[5] Examples of such autobiographies are: Marie Hays Heiner *Hearing Is Believing* (Cleveland, World, 1949); Frances Warfield, *Cotton in My Ears* (New York, Viking, 1948); and George W. Frankel, *Let's Hear It!* (New York, Stratford House, 1952).

is the late Helen Keller, who was able to rise above the double handicap of deafness and blindness.

REFERENCES

Davis, Hallowell, and Silverman, S. Richard, eds., *Hearing and Deafness* (New York, Holt, Rinehart and Winston, 1970), Chaps. 12, 13, and 14.

Heller, Morris F., Anderman, Bernard, and Singer, Ellis, *Functional Otology* (New York, Springer, 1955), Chaps. 13, 14, 15, and 16.

Montague, Harriet, *Lip Reading Lessons for Adult Beginners* (Washington, D.C., Volta Bureau, 1945).

Nitchie, Elizabeth H., *New Lessons in Lip Reading* (Philadelphia, Lippincott, 1950).

O'Neill, John J., *The Hard of Hearing* (Englewood Cliffs, N.J., Prentice-Hall, 1964).

Ordman, Kathryn A., and Ralli, Mary P., *What People Say* (New York, The Nitchie School of Lip Reading, 1949).

Oyer, Herbert J., *Auditory Communication for the Hard of Hearing* (Englewood Cliffs, N.J., Prentice-Hall, 1961).

Whitehurst, Mary W., *Train Your Hearing* (Washington, D.C., Volta Bureau, 1947).

Whitehurst, Mary W., and Monsees, Edna K., *Auditory Training for the Deaf* (Washington, D.C., Volta Bureau, 1952).

13

THE PROFESSION OF AUDIOLOGY

The previous chapters have been designed to give the reader some acquaintance with the subject matter of the field of audiology. In the author's mind, one purpose of this book is to interest students in audiology as a profession. This final chapter, therefore, will be concerned with professional opportunities in audiology and the preparation necessary to become a professional worker in the field. Since the development of the profession of audiology has been closely related to the evolution of the hearing center, and since many of the employment opportunities in audiology are in hearing centers of various sorts, the first section of this chapter will deal with the hearing center.

THE HEARING CENTER

The modern hearing center is an outgrowth of two developments: the military aural rehabilitation center of World War II and the prewar university speech clinic. There are at present approximately 750 hearing centers in the United States.[1] These are variously sponsored and offer a variety of services, but basically their purpose is the same: to provide diagnostic and rehabilitative services for individuals with hearing impairments. The term *hearing center*, as it appears in this chapter, refers to any nonprofit professional agency, regardless of its name, which offers diagnostic and rehabilitative services to the hard of hearing.

[1] *A Guide to Clinical Services in Speech Pathology and Audiology 1971* (Washington, D.C., The American Speech and Hearing Association, 1970).

History of the Hearing Center

As indicated in Chapter 1, historically audiology is the progeny of two parents: otology and speech pathology. The two were united in the aural rehabilitation centers of World War II, which were established by the medical departments of the armed forces to provide the medical and rehabilitative services required by servicemen and women who incurred hearing impairment. The Army established three such centers: Borden General Hospital at Chickasha, Okla.; Hoff General Hospital at Santa Barbara, Calif.; and Deshon General Hospital at Butler, Penn. The Navy established an aural rehabilitation center at the Naval Hospital in Philadelphia. By the end of World War II, all these centers had proved their tremendous value in rehabilitating hard-of-hearing service personnel.

To establish the services necessary to operate an effective program of rehabilitation for the hard of hearing, the military sought help from college and university speech clinics, from teachers of lip-reading, teachers of the deaf, and from psychologists. Since the aural rehabilitation programs were the responsibility of medical departments, they were put under the command of physicians—ear, nose, and throat specialists. The medical and nonmedical specialists together planned a program which would meet the needs of aural casualties. Naturally, the first responsibility of the aural rehabilitation center was to determine whether a given casualty would benefit from medical or surgical care. In evaluating the type and degree of hearing loss that a patient presented, a thorough audiometric examination was required. Some specialists in speech became classified as "acoustic physicists," charged with the responsibility of developing and administering adequate tests of the hearing function. Today such specialists would be referred to as "audiologists." Patients who could not be helped by medicine, or whose hearing loss was of a permanent, nonreversible nature, were placed in the rehabilitation program, which included determination of the need for and selection of an individual hearing aid; speechreading, auditory training, and speech training as needed; and psychological and vocational counseling.

The military aural rehabilitation centers were so successful in returning hearing-handicapped service personnel to duty, or to civilian life with a minimum of handicap, that all who were concerned with these wartime programs were impressed with their effectiveness. Thus, when the war was over and the various specialists returned to civilian life, many were of the opinion that similar aural rehabilitation programs should be organized for the civilian population. It was primarily the otologists who were responsible for initiating action in their own communities to establish programs for the hearing-handicapped. However, although the otologists were the "sparkplugs" of the new activities, they did not have the time nor the desire to perform all the services required. Thus, otologists turned for help to the group of specialists who had developed the audiometric techniques and rehabilitative services in wartime—primarily specialists in speech—to administer and perform the clinical work in the newly established civilian centers. Since the war, otologists have assumed more of an advisory than a directive role in the development of hearing centers. To the otologist, however, belongs the credit for the initial interest which prompted the establishment of the first postwar civilian centers.

One of the outstanding contributions of the military aural rehabilitation center was the development of procedures to determine whether or not a patient needed a hearing aid and, if so, to select the hearing aid for him. An integral part of the hearing-aid selection was training with the aid which the patient received. The military programs established an enviable record in the percentage of hearing aids used by patients who were provided with them. Previous to World War II, studies had revealed that as many as 50 to 60 per cent of the hard-of-hearing individuals with hearing aids did not use them after the first week or two. The studies of graduates of the military aural rehabilitation programs revealed that as high as 94 per cent of the individuals receiving hearing aids continued to use them several months after their discharge from the center.[2] The civilian hearing centers which began to spring up after the war were usually created primarily for the purpose of bringing systematic hearing-aid selection services to the civilian population. In addition, other services were offered as required, but the major emphasis was on hearing-aid selection. Many civilian centers attempted to establish training programs similar to those which had been in effect during the war. These civilian centers soon discovered, however, that most civilians were not willing to devote several weeks to a training course, and, being civilians, they could not be ordered to do so. Thus, the transfer of aural rehabilitation procedures from a military to a civilian setting required many adjustments.

A word of credit should be given here to the Veterans Administration for helping to develop the concept of the civilian hearing center. Immediately after the war, there were thousands of veterans with service-connected hearing impairments who required services of the sort that had been available to them as servicemen and women in wartime. Also, of course, veterans of previous wars needed help with hearing problems. The Veterans Administration met the various needs by establishing audiology clinics in some regional offices and veterans hospitals, and by contracting for these services elsewhere with college and university speech clinics and with other types of hearing centers. At present, there are relatively few "contract clinics," since the Veterans Administration has greatly expanded its own audiology and speech pathology program. The earlier necessity for handling hearing-handicapped veterans on a contractual basis, however, served as a tremendous impetus to colleges and universities to develop training programs and clinical services in the field of audiology. Also, the Veterans Administration contracts lightened the burden of financial support for many community hearing centers. Anderman has described the details of the Veterans Administration audiology program.[3]

Types of Hearing Centers

Hearing centers are of many types so far as sponsorship and organizational structures are concerned.[4] In point of number, hearing-center activity sponsored by colleges and universities accounts for the greatest percentage. For the most part, colleges and universities merely added aural rehabilitation services to an already existing speech clinic. Before World War II, college speech clinics had been concerned primarily with the speech problems of children and adults, including such disorders as stuttering, aphasia, cleft-palate speech, vocal problems, and articulatory difficulties. Some speech problems handled by the clinic were related to hearing disorders, but the speech clinic, as it existed in prewar days, as a general rule did not offer any services for the hard-of-hearing individual except speech training.

It is interesting to note the influence of hearing-center activities on college and university programs. Until 1947, most clinic programs in connection with the training of students in speech pathology were called "speech" clinics. In 1947, the American Speech Correction Association changed its name to the American Speech and Hearing Association and the name of its official publication from the *Journal of Speech Disorders* to the *Journal of Speech and Hearing Disorders*. Concurrently, in colleges and universities around the country, there was a movement to change the name *speech clinic* to *speech and hearing clinic*. By 1950, training programs in audiology were in existence in practically all the colleges and universities where any previous training in the field of speech correction had been offered. Thus, five years after the termination of the war, the importance of audiology as a related but separate discipline from speech correction had been recognized.

The primary purpose of the college- or university-sponsored hearing center is to provide a laboratory in which students of audiology may observe and obtain experience in handling patients. Just as the medical student must learn to diagnose and treat illnesses in patients by obtaining supervised experience in medical clinics, so the embryo audiologist must also "learn by doing." Service to the public is therefore only incidental to the training purpose of the college- or university-sponsored hearing center.

A second type of hearing center is one which operates as part of a hospital or rehabilitation center and serves only the patients referred by physicians connected with that institution. Generally, the audiology program in a

---

[3] Bernard M. Anderman, "The Veterans Administration Audiology Program," in Hallowell Davis and S. Richard Silverman, eds., *Hearing and Deafness* (New York, Holt, Rinehart and Winston, 1970), Chap. 19, pp. 449-456.

[4] Jack L. Bangs, "Speech and Hearing Centers," in Nathaniel M. Levin, ed., *Voice and Speech Disorders* (Springfield, Ill., Charles C Thomas, 1962), Chap. 26, pp. 899-929.

hospital is associated with a department of otolaryngology, whereas in a rehabilitation center it may be part of a department of physical medicine. In either event, this kind of hearing center provides a specialized service to only a limited number of physicians and their patients.

In contrast to the two types of hearing centers just discussed, there are activities which we shall designate as "community" hearing centers, because they serve the entire community and not just a segment of the hard-of-hearing population. In the community hearing center, the emphasis is on providing professional services to all who need them, provided that they are properly referred through medical channels. Some community hearing centers are affiliated with local chapters of the National Association of Hearing and Speech Agencies (NAHSA), formerly the American Hearing Society, and some were created as separate, nonprofit, privately sponsored agencies. Most community hearing centers, whether or not they are affiliated with NAHSA or a local hearing society, receive some aid from the community chest or united fund, although they also require a considerable amount of private underwriting. Most such centers also depend somewhat on fees collected from patients. For community hearing centers to be successful in securing the support needed to continue in existence, they must prove themselves through the high quality of professional services which they offer the community.

A fourth type of hearing center is the government-sponsored one, which provides audiological services for personnel of the armed forces and for veterans. The Army maintains audiological services in a number of hospitals in this country and abroad. The Air Force and the Navy have their own audiological facilities, although they are more limited than the Army as to number of locations. The Veterans Administration audiology and speech pathology services or clinics are geographically distributed throughout the country. These clinics, together with other hearing centers with which the Veterans Administration contracts, serve the needs of approximately 100,000 veterans who are service-connected for hearing loss and/or otological disease. The Veterans Administration clinics provide hearing aids to eligible veterans and are responsible for conducting the examinations on which compensation for service-connected hearing disabilities is based.

The four types of centers mentioned above account for the vast majority of clinical audiology programs that are in existence today. There are some miscellaneous programs, however, which do not fit into these categories. For example, a hearing center may be sponsored by a religious organization, by the Junior League or other service organization, or by a school for the deaf. Also, in some cities there are so-called hearing centers which are actually the activities of a single audiologist in private practice. Although of course no one has a monopoly on the term *hearing center*, such individual projects do not meet the definition of the term given earlier in this chapter, that a hearing center is an activity which is nonprofit in character. In a hearing center, fees may be charged for services rendered, but patients who cannot pay fees are also served. Obviously the individual who is in private practice must operate at a profit in order to make a living.

It is interesting to see how quickly hearing-aid dealers have set out to capitalize on the success of the hearing-center idea. One has only to leaf through the yellow pages of a city's telephone directory to find listed several "hearing centers," which are actually hearing-aid dealer's offices. The dealer who uses the name *hearing center* as part of the title of his business operation is obviously trying to capitalize on the professional success of the nonprofit hearing center.

Services of the Hearing Center

As stated above, initially the most important service offered by a hearing center was hearing-aid selection. This service is still one which is fairly universally offered by hearing centers, regardless of their type or sponsorship. With so many makes and models of hearing aids commercially available at a wide range of prices, the hard-of-hearing person in need of a hearing aid is bewildered as to how to make a choice. He requires objective consideration of his problem, which the average hearing-aid dealer is not equipped to give him. The hearing center is the place where the patient can obtain the objective approach that he is seeking.

The services of a hearing center may generally be divided into two main classifications: diagnostic services and rehabilitative or training services. Under the first classification would come such services as diagnostic audiometry, pre- and postoperative audiometry, and hearing-aid selection. Diagnostic audiometry refers to the measurement of a patient's hearing and an analysis of his hearing problems for the purpose of assisting the otologist toward proper diagnosis. Diagnostic audiometry with young children has assumed increasing importance as techniques have been developed to make hearing measurements with very young patients more valid and reliable. With very young children it is important to discover the hearing impairment at the earliest possible time, so that medical attention can be given to the disability and adequate training procedures can be initiated. The sooner the training of the hard-of-hearing child starts, the better is the prognosis. Thus diagnostic audiometry with children is a particularly valuable service of the hearing center. Included under the heading of diagnostic audiometry also is the differentiation of hearing problems from other types of auditory disorders. Children who do not develop an understanding of oral language or an ability to speak are frequently classified as deaf, when in fact their ability to respond to pure-tone test stimuli may be perfectly normal. The differentiation of hearing impairment from other types of disorders such as brain injury, mental retardation, and emotional difficulty is important in order to discover with what problem or problems the physician and therapist are dealing, and in order to permit the planning of an adequate medical and rehabilitation program.

With adults, diagnostic audiometry is concerned with establishing a hearing loss as being organic or functional, and in determining the relation between air conduction and bone conduction as an indication of whether the loss is conductive or sensori-neural in nature. Also, in sensori-neural loss, the determination of the site of the lesion is an important part of diagnostic audiometry. In the case of contemplated surgery on the middle ear, it is important to the otologist to have an accurate assessment of the patient's cochlear reserve.

The remaining diagnostic activity—the selection of hearing aids—was discussed in Chapter 10. When the civilian hearing centers were first established, this activity was almost their sole *raison d'être*. In the early postwar days, however, hearing aids were crude and somewhat unreliable. Differences from aid to aid could easily be demonstrated in test situations. As hearing aids became more refined and their parts standardized, it became harder to establish differences on the basis of test-room situations. Although some hearing centers still test a patient with six to eight different aids and then tell him which aid he should purchase from a dealer, today many centers offer a more general type of hearing-aid selection. Some centers have changed the name of their service from "hearing-aid selection" to hearing-aid consultation, in line with their de-emphasis of comparative tests of hearing-aid functions.

The selection of hearing aids continues to be an important service in government-sponsored audiology clinics. At these clinics, the patient who needs a hearing aid is provided with the particular aid with which he has performed best in the test situation. Furnishing the patient with a hearing aid is part of the responsibility that the government assumes for those who are eligible for the services of a military or Veterans Administration audiology clinic. Since so many thousands of patients are involved in these government programs, it is economically more advantageous to the government, and of course eventually to the taxpayer, to contract for hearing aids on a large-lot basis, and to assume the responsibility for dispensing these aids, than to send each patient to a hearing-aid dealer for an aid of the recommended type. Moreover, with this method of distributing hearing aids, the patient is assured that the instrument selected for him is the very one with which he performed best. In spite of quality-control measures applied by hearing-aid manufacturers, no hearing aid is exactly like every other aid of the same make and model. Unfortunately (for the patient) it is not possible for most non-government-sponsored hearing centers to make hearing-aid selections in this manner, and so their hearing-aid "consultations" are of necessity "watered-down" varieties of the type of hearing-aid selection program to be found in the government clinics.

The rehabilitation services offered by hearing centers usually include the following: group and individual instruction in speech-reading, auditory training, speech training, and hearing-aid orientation. In addition, some centers provide special training programs for preschool-age deaf and hard-of-hearing youngsters and their parents. These rehabilitative services have been discussed elsewhere in this book and need no further elaboration here.

Accreditation of Hearing Centers

In 1959 the American Speech and Hearing Association established the American Boards of Examiners in Speech Pathology and Audiology. One of the constituent boards of this organization is the Professional Services Board, which is charged with the responsibility for processing applications for accreditation of clinical services and making recommendations to the Directors of the American Boards of Examiners regarding the accreditation of those clinical services that have applied. When the Directors approve a clinical service activity, a certificate of approval is issued and the name of the activity is added to a registry of approved clinical services which is published regularly. A clinical activity may be approved for services in audiology, in speech pathology, or in both areas. A clinical activity must meet high standards in regard to personnel, equipment, organizational structure, range of services, and relations with other agencies and professional personnel in order to be recommended for approval by the Professional Services Board. Thus the public and referring physicians and agencies can be assured that they are receiving the best of clinical services when they make use of a hearing center that has been approved by the American Boards of Examiners in Speech Pathology and Audiology.

EMPLOYMENT OPPORTUNITIES FOR AUDIOLOGISTS

As long as there is a demand for trained audiologists there will be a need for college and university teachers of audiology, and so the field of higher education provides one very important employment opportunity for audiologists. For practical purposes the doctoral degree is an essential requirement for the audiologist who has academic aspirations. University teaching in the field of audiology is far from being an "ivory-tower" type of existence, however. Audiology can be learned only through a combination of work with patients and "book learning," and therefore a necessary part of the university training program in audiology consists of clinical practicum. The audiologist in charge of a training program thus becomes a clinic supervisor and administrator while performing a considerable amount of clinical work himself. The university teacher of audiology must of necessity keep up with new developments in all aspects of his field, and ideally he should participate to some extent in research activities. Certainly one of his duties, if he is involved in a graduate training program, is that of directing the research of his students, and reading and criticizing theses and dissertations. Thus, a teacher of audiology at the university level will undoubtedly have as busy a day and as fully occupied a work year as any other professional person. The audiologist-teacher receives all the satisfactions of any teacher in vicariously experiencing the professional successes of his students. In addition, of course, the teacher of audiology himself has ample opportunity for reaping the pleasure of working with patients who benefit from his help.

The increasing popularity of the community hearing center presents a stimulating professional challenge to the audiologist who is more interested in clinical work than in teaching. Since most such hearing centers are directed by professional audiologists, they offer the added opportunity of administrative experience. The director of a community hearing center must combine the talents of a successful clinician with the abilities of a public relations expert, a personnel counselor, and a fund raiser. Although a doctoral degree is not a necessity to the director of a community hearing center, it certainly is an advantage to him in representing a professional status, particularly in dealings with the medical profession. Other clinical workers in the community hearing center should have a least a master's degree in audiology.

Government positions in audiology represent another opportunity for professional employment. The Veterans Administration employs many audiologists as clinicians and administrators in its audiology and speech pathology clinics throughout the country. A master's degree is required for employment as a staff audiologist, while directors (chiefs) of V.A. clinics must have doctorates. Civil service appointments in the military audiology clinics are on a basis comparable to the Veterans Administration positions. Individuals with a master's degree and at least the academic requirements for clinical certification in audiology from the American Speech and Hearing Association (as described in the following section) are eligible for commissions in the Medical Service Corps of the Army and the Biomedical Science Corps of the Air Force.[5] As of the present writing there are no provisions for commissions in the Navy for audiologists. Opportunities for enlisted personnel with some training in audiology exist in all three branches of the armed forces.

Another employment possibility for the audiologist is in a hospital or medical-school setting. Such positions usually constitute appointments in a department of otolaryngology, and the audiologist works closely with ear, nose, and throat physicians. Generally, the qualifications for such a position would be at least a master's degree in audiology.

[5] Jerry L. Northern and James E. Endicott, "Military Opportunities in Speech Pathology and Audiology," *Asha*, Vol. 10 (August, 1968), pp. 325-330.

At the present time, there is a growth of rehabilitation centers, which consist of various medical and allied medical specialists working as a team. Since a communication disorder represents a handicapping impairment, most rehabilitation centers must provide for dealing with problems of speech and hearing. In the setting of a rehabilitation center, the person in charge of the audiology program should have at least a master's degree.

Public school work in speech and hearing represents perhaps the area of greatest personnel need. Although few public school systems can afford an audiologist to supervise the entire hearing program, most school systems do require audiometrists. In addition to employment opportunities as audiometrists, public schools provide opportunities for work as speech and hearing therapists or as teachers of special classes for hearing-handicapped children. Since the schools have accepted the responsibility for the "whole" education of their pupils, they must attempt to meet the needs of those who are handicapped in hearing. In most public school situations, a credential issued by the state department of education, or for audiometrists, a certificate from the state department of health, is a requirement for employment. Thus a master's degree in itself may not be required, although a speech and hearing therapist with a master's degree will command a larger salary.

As yet, very few opportunities exist for the audiologist in industry, although some companies concerned with the manufacture of hearing aids and audiometers have begun to attract audiologists as desirable places of employment. It is conceivable that at some time in the future hearing aids may be dispensed by individuals who have been professionally trained in audiology, especially if most states should pass legislation requiring the licensing of those who deal in hearing aids. The field of hearing-aid selling is one which could provide an opportunity for the person who has only a bachelor's degree in audiology. At present, hearing-aid dealers are usually not required to have any formal academic training in audiology, and as a result many dealers are merely salesmen, without knowledge of the special problems of the hard-of-hearing people with whom they are dealing.

Another industrial opportunity for audiologists lies in organizing and directing hearing-conservation programs in noisy industries. As our civilization becomes a noisier one, both employers and employees are becoming aware of the hazards to hearing from noise exposure. Claims for noise-induced hearing impairment are becoming more and more common, and insurance carriers and employers alike are alarmed at their increasing frequency. Several years ago, the American Academy of Ophthalmology and Otolaryngology established a Subcommittee on Noise in Industry within its Committee on Conservation of Hearing. The subcommittee has a staff with laboratory and research facilities. The purpose of the subcommittee is to investigate the incidence of noise-induced hearing problems in industry and to recommend programs of noise control in the hope that the programs will prevent damage to hearing. As we saw in Chapter 9, one of the recommendations of this committee is that employees be given regular audiometric tests for the purpose of (1) detecting the presence of any hearing loss as soon as it occurs, and (2) preventing further loss of hearing by proper placement of employees within an industry. At present, most routine testing in industries is conducted by nurses under the supervision of the medical director of the company. Hearing-conservation programs in large factories, however, generally require more specialized supervision than the average company physician can provide. In all likelihood, therefore, we shall see "industrial audiologists" performing these services in the near future. It is preferable for them to have doctoral degrees. In any event, the field of industrial audiology presents opportunities for consultation by professionally qualified audiologists, if not full-time employment.

Audiologists are now employed as full-time consultants in departments of health and education in state governments. In these positions, it is the responsibility of the audiologist to consult with local health or school officials on problems of hearing impairment, and to take the responsibility for organizing hearing-conservation programs on the local level. These consultants also confer with other branches of their state departments of health and education in such matters as planning special education programs in the public schools and health education. This type of position calls for a person with at least a master's degree in audiology and with a considerable amount of organizational ability.

Finally, there is a limited opportunity for audiologists to engage in private practice. This vocational possibility presents a number of problems, not the least of which is the necessity for maintaining close liaison with a physician or physicians. The audiologist who attempts to do hearing evaluations independently of a medical diagnosis is headed for trouble. Of course, if the audiologist restricts his activities to training and rehabilitation of hearing-impaired children and adults, he does not have to work under medical direction. Private practice presents economic hazards, and few audiologists are sufficiently intrepid to engage in private practice, because of its financial pitfalls. Some otologists with extensive practices engage audiologists to provide diagnostic and rehabilitative services in their offices.

In summary, the requirements of existing positions in the field of audiology demand training at least through the master's degree, except for the area of hearing-aid sales, and the doctorate is a necessity in many work environments, particularly in college and university teaching. The doctorate is a definite advantage to the audiologist who is working in any medical setting.

Thus far in this discussion, we have been concerned with employment for audiologists in clinical environments. Research career opportunities exist for individuals who have received special preparation in laboratory research methods. In past years most research in audition and on the ear and its function has been performed by specialists whose training was in fields other than audiology. Now, however, departments that produce clinical audiologists are also graduating research audiologists who are joining physiologists, physicists, experimental psychologists, and representatives of other scientific disciplines in making important contributions to our knowledge of normal and disordered hearing. As more individuals complete their professional preparation in audiology, which is primarily a clinical discipline, it may be expected that more of them will become interested in pursuing a career in research. Also, if more government and private funds become available for research into audiological problems, and more hearing centers of various sorts expand their facilities to include laboratories, many more opportunities should arise for research-minded audiologists to follow their inclinications. Thus, in each of the employment possibilities mentioned above, there should be opportunities for research audiologists. Since a Ph.D. is a research degree, it is reasonable to assume that a research position should be filled by an audiologist with a doctorate.

ACCREDITATION REQUIREMENTS FOR AUDIOLOGISTS

The professional organization to which audiologists belong, and which provides certification of clinical competence for its members who qualify, is the American Speech and Hearing Association. This organization is for the professions of audiology and speech pathology what the American Medical Association is for physicians and what the American Psychological Association is for psychologists. The American Speech and Hearing Association was founded as the American Academy of Speech Correction in 1925. It has experienced steady growth since then. In its history the organization has been known by various names, the current name having been adopted in 1947 as a recognition of the importance of work in hearing. Previously the organization was composed primarily of speech pathologists and speech correctionists. The purposes of the American Speech and Hearing Association, as stated in its by-laws, are as follows:

The purposes of this organization shall be to encourage basic scientific study of the processes of individual human communication, with special reference to speech, hearing, and language, promote investigation of disorders of human communication, and foster improvement of clinical procedures with such disorders; to stimulate exchange of information among persons and organizations thus engaged; and to disseminate such information.[6]

To be eligible for full membership in the American Speech and Hearing Association (ASHA), an individual must hold at least the master's degree or

6 By-Laws of the American Speech and Hearing Association, Article II, *Directory* of the American Speech and Hearing Association (1970), p. ix.

its equivalent with major emphasis in speech pathology, audiology, or speech and hearing science, or have at least the master's degree or its equivalent and present evidence of active research, interest, and performance in the field of human communication. Each year a selected group of members are chosen as Fellows of the Association in recognition of their professional or scientific achievements. The Association publishes the *Journal of Speech and Hearing Disorders* and the *Journal of Speech and Hearing Research,* both of which appear quarterly, and two monthly publications: *Asha,* which gives news and announcements and carries articles dealing with professional matters, and *Trends,* which is an employment bulletin. The Association's national office is in Washington, D.C.

The American Speech and Hearing Association assumes responsibility for awarding clinical certification to those of its members who meet the published requirements. Clinical certification is granted either in speech pathology or in audiology. There is provision for dual certification for those who qualify in both fields. Certification is granted on recommendation of the Certification Committee of the Association upon application and submission of credentials and upon passing an examination. The current requirements for clinical certification may be obtained by writing to the executive secretary of the American Speech and Hearing Association, 9030 Old Georgetown Road, Washington, D.C. 20014.

Generally, the requirements for clinical certification in audiology are a minimum of sixty semester hours of course work at accredited colleges or universities, including at least eighteen semester hours in courses that provide fundamental information applicable to the normal development and use of speech, hearing, and language, and at least forty-two semester hours in courses that provide information about and training in the management of speech, hearing, and language disorders and supplementary information. The major portion of this course work must be in the area of audiology. Also required for certification are the completion of at least 275 clock hours of supervised, direct clinical experience as part of the training program, and an academic year's full-time, "satisfactory" professional employment under supervision following completion of the training program.

The Association publishes a Code of Ethics, to which all members must subscribe. The Code of Ethics outlines the professional responsibilities of the person performing clinical work in speech and hearing. It is similar to the code of ethics subscribed to by other professional groups. Incidentally, the Code of Ethics prohibits members of the Association from engaging in sales or promotional activities of products related to their professional field.

As the gap between the number of positions to be filled and the number of fully qualified audiologists available for employment has narrowed as a result of increased enrollments in training programs, it is becoming increasingly necessary for an individual seeking employment as an audiologist to hold the ASHA certificate of clinical competence. The best guarantee that the public will receive competent professional services is a strong national organization with the power to determine which individuals are qualified to practice the specialties of audiology and speech pathology. There is a trend now toward state licensing of individuals who wish to practice either as audiologists or speech pathologists. It seems likely that at some future date most or all of the states will require licensing of professional personnel in audiology and speech pathology just as with physicians, dentists, clinical psychologists, and many other professions. Until that day, however, the certification authority must remain with the national organization, and every audiologist and speech pathologist should give this organization his full support.

Since certification by the American Speech and Hearing Association should be the primary goal of every student training in the field of speech and hearing, training institutions must take into account the course requirements that the Association has established. The specific course requirements published by the American Speech and Hearing Association may change from time to time, and training programs must be sufficiently flexible to adapt to the changing requirements of a growing professional field.

THE PREPARATION OF AUDIOLOGISTS

In 1970, almost two-hundred master's degree training programs in speech pathology and audiology were listed by the American Speech and Hearing Association.[7] It is estimated that about half of these programs provide sufficient course work and supervised clinical practice in audiology to qualify graduates for the ASHA certificate of clinical competence in audiology.

Training programs in audiology are usually found in departments of speech in colleges of arts and sciences, although some programs are situated in colleges of education, and a few are in schools of medicine. In many of the larger universities separate departments have been established under such titles as speech pathology and audiology, audiology and speech sciences, communicative disorders, speech and hearing science, and so forth.

The American Boards of Examiners in Speech Pathology and Audiology of the American Speech and Hearing Association established the Education and Training Board for the purpose of accrediting master's degree programs in speech pathology and/or audiology. The National Commission of Accrediting has recognized the American Speech and Hearing Association as the official accrediting body in this field. As of December 15, 1970, some forty-four university and college programs had received accreditation in speech pathology and/or audiology.[8] Many more programs are in the process

[7] *A Guide to Graduate Education in Speech Pathology and Audiology* 1970-1971 (Washington, D.C., American Speech and Hearing Association 1970).

[8] "Accredited Training Programs, Education and Training Board," *Asha*, Vol. 13 (January, 1971), pp. 22-23.

of applying for accreditation. To receive accreditation, a training program must submit an application describing its academic and clinical program in detail. Following a site visit, the Education and Training Board submits its recommendation to the directors of the American Boards of Examiners in Speech Pathology and Audiology. Approved programs are awarded certificates by the American Boards of Examiners and are appropriately identified in various directories and brochures issued by the American Speech and Hearing Association.

The content of a training program must depend upon the professional job requirements of positions in audiology, as well as upon the certification requirements of the American Speech and Hearing Association. No attempt will be made here to specify every course which the audiologist-in-training should take. Rather, suggestions will be made concerning the breadth of knowledge which it is desirable for the audiologist to have in various areas. Naturally, the numbers and types of courses that an individual takes would depend upon the degree for which he was working and upon his professional goals. A complete training program which extends through the doctoral-degree level should, in the opinion of the author, cover all the course work indicated in the areas enumerated below. No significance should be attached to the order in which these areas are discussed. It is assumed that courses in various areas would be taken concurrently.

Audiology

Naturally, it is necessary for the student to have a solid grounding in the theoretical and practical aspects of audiology. In addition to a survey course in audiology, he should take courses in basic and advanced audiometry, hearing aids, experimental audiology, speechreading, auditory and speech training for the hearing-handicapped, and methods of teaching the deaf child. Also, he should take seminars which enable him to become more thoroughly acquainted with topics that can only be touched on in the formal courses. There should be ample provision for supervised clinical practice, which is equally distributed among all aspects of audiology, that is, not limited to testing, for example. As a minimum, the student should obtain the number of clock hours of clinical practice required for certification by the American Speech and Hearing Association.

Speech Pathology

The specialty of audiology is closely related to the field of speech pathology, just as speech and hearing are related communication skills. Both require similar clinical techniques. The audiologist who knows nothing of speech disorders other than those directly associated with a hearing impairment is too narrowly specialized to be able to perform his functions as an audiologist satisfactorily. The American Speech and Hearing Association recognizes the necessity of the audiologist's receiving some training in speech pathology and correction by requiring at least six semester hours of course work in this field for certification in audiology. In the author's opinion, even more course work and clinical practice in speech pathology should be required. The audiologist-in-training should take courses in speech pathology, organic disorders, voice and articulation disorders, language disorders, and a seminar in speech pathology. He should also have extensive, supervised clinical experience with various types of speech problems.

Speech and Hearing Sciences

In point of chronological order, courses in this field should precede at least the advanced courses in audiology and speech pathology. Just as the medical student must take courses in sciences that are basic to clinical medicine, so the student audiologist should be thoroughly grounded in the sciences that are basic to clinical work in the field of speech and hearing. He should take such courses as descriptive phonetics, experimental phonetics, basic and advanced speech science, language development, linguistics, acoustics, bioacoustics, psychoacoustics, speech and hearing instrumentation, and research methods in speech pathology and audiology. Some of these courses, acoustics, for example, may be taught in other departments within the university.

Psychology

Psychology is the discipline perhaps most closely related to the fields of speech and hearing. The student audiologist should take courses in statistics, child psychology, sensation and perception, physiological psychology, abnormal psychology, experimental psychology, learning, and mental hygiene. Course work and experience in intelligence and personality testing are also highly desirable.

Other Fields

Because audiology is also closely related to medicine, it is to be hoped that the student will have the opportunity to obtain some course work which is taught in a school of medicine. Ideally, there should be close liaison and cooperation between the department in which audiology is taught and the school of medicine, so that courses specifically for students in speech pathology and audiology can be arranged. One of these courses should cover the anatomy, physiology, and neurology of the communicative mechanism. Of course this could be taught also by the nonmedical specialists in the student's major department, but it would be preferable to have the course taught by specialists in anatomy, physiology, and neurology. Another desirable course is one dealing with the medical backgrounds of speech and hearing disorders, that is, the pathology underlying disorders of the type with which the audiologist and the speech pathologist will be concerned. Such a course should be taught by the medical specialists concerned with particular disorders, for example, a neurologist or neurosurgeon, a pediatrician, a physiatrist, and an otolaryngologist.

The student who is preparing for a career as a speech and hearing therapist in the public schools should take a number of courses in general and special education, so that he will be prepared to work cooperatively with teachers and other personnel in the school system. For the student preparing to be a clinician in a hearing center of some type, courses in education would not be required.

Clinical Internship

The training of audiologists is not complete without some provision for supervised professional experience. As stated previously, certification by the American Speech and Hearing Association requires an academic year's professional experience. If employers are to be educated to hire only audiologists who have been certified by the Association, a dilemma is created. Where can the beginning audiologist secure the experience which is prerequisite to his being certified? The solution to this problem lies in the affiliation of training institutions with nonacademic hearing centers. The affiliation serves two purposes: first, it provides the university with an outlet for its products—a chance to put new audiologists into an internship situation; and, second, it enables the hearing center to obtain additional help at a minimum of expense. There is an additional benefit to the hearing center: the prestige attached to an academic connection, tenuous though the latter may be. It is difficult to attract highly trained personnel to a working situation which is purely clinical. If the chance to develop an academic affiliation on a "clinical staff" basis is offered to a promising audiologist, a position at a hearing center becomes more attractive. For many years, a large number of medical schools have obtained the part-time services of a clinical teaching staff merely by granting an academic status to practicing physicians who gain only in increased prestige. Clinical audiologists, too, are hungry for the prestige that a university appointment bestows.

Just as no medical school in the country can consider the training of physicians as complete without a year's internship, so the departments in which audiologists are trained should consider it necessary to arrange for a year's internship for audiologists before considering their training complete. Such internship, under proper professional supervision, would satisfy the professional experience certification requirement of the American Speech and Hearing Association. With certification, the audiologist can then accept a position with confidence that he is equipped by training *and* experience to handle the job.

Appendix

MATERIALS FOR
SPEECH AUDIOMETRY

WORDS LISTS FOR C.I.D. AUDITORY TEST W-1[1]

List A

1. greyhound	10. duckpond	19. baseball	28 oatmeal
2. schoolboy	11. sidewalk	20. stairway	29. toothbrush
3. inkwell	12. hotdog	21. cowboy	30. farewell
4. whitewash	13. padlock	22. iceberg	31. grandson
5. pancake	14. mushroom	23. northwest	32. drawbridge
6. mousetrap	15. hardware	24. railroad	33. doormat
7. eardrum	16. workshop	25. playground	34. hothouse
8. headlight	17. horseshoe	26. airplane	35. daybreak
9. birthday	18. armchair	27. woodwork	36. sunset

List B

1. playground	10. railroad	19. toothbrush	28. eardrum
2. grandson	11. baseball	20. mushroom	29. greyhound
3. daybreak	12. padlock	21. farewell	30. birthday
4. doormat	13. hardware	22. horseshoe	31. hothouse
5. woodwork	14. whitewash	23. pancake	32. iceberg
6. armchair	15. hotdog	24. inkwell	33. schoolboy
7. stairway	16. sunset	25. mousetrap	34. duckpond
8. cowboy	17. headlight	26. airplane	35. workshop
9. oatmeal	18. drawbridge	27. sidewalk	36. northwest

[1] These word lists are reproduced with the permission of the Veterans Administration, Dr. Ira J. Hirsh of Central Institute for the Deaf, and the Chairman of the Publications Board of the American Speech and Hearing Association.

List C

1. birthday	10. woodwork	19. farewell	28. sunset
2. hothouse	11. stairway	20. mousetrap	29. cowboy
3. toothbrush	12. daybreak	21. armchair	30. duckpond
4. horseshoe	13. sidewalk	22. drawbridge	31. playground
5. airplane	14. railroad	23. mushroom	32. inkwell
6. northwest	15. oatmeal	24. baseball	33. eardrum
7. whitewash	16. headlight	25. grandson	34. workshop
8. hotdog	17. pancake	26. padlock	35. schoolboy
9. hardware	18. doormat	27. greyhound	36. iceberg

List D

1. hothouse	10. duckpond	19. playground	28. greyhound
2. padlock	11. baseball	20. oatmeal	29. mousetrap
3. eardrum	12. railroad	21. northwest	30. schoolboy
4. sidewalk	13. hardware	22. woodwork	31. whitewash
5. cowboy	14. toothbrush	23. stairway	32. inkwell
6. mushroom	15. airplane	24. hotdog	33. doormat
7. farewell	16. iceberg	25. headlight	34. daybreak
8. horseshoe	17. armchair	26. pancake	35. drawbridge
9. workshop	18. grandson	27. birthday	36. sunset

List E

1. northwest	10. greyhound	19. headlight	28. eardrum
2. doormat	11. cowboy	20. airplane	29. mushroom
3. railroad	12. daybreak	21. inkwell	30. whitewash
4. woodwork	13. drawbridge	22. grandson	31. hothouse
5: hardware	14. duckpond	23. workshop	32. toothbrush
6. stairway	15. horseshoe	24. hotdog	33. playground
7. sidewalk	16. armchair	25. oatmeal	34. baseball
8. birthday	17. padlock	26. sunset	35. iceberg
9. farewell	18. mousetrap	27. pancake	36. schoolboy

List F

1. padlock	10. baseball	19. mousetrap	28. mushroom
2. daybreak	11. woodwork	20. workshop	29. armchair
3. sunset	12. inkwell	21. eardrum	30. whitewash
4. farewell	13. pancake	22. greyhound	31. hotdog
5. northwest	14. toothbrush	23. doormat	32. schoolboy
6. airplane	15. hardware	24. horseshoe	33. headlight
7. playground	16. railroad	25. stairway	34. duckpond
8. iceberg	17. oatmeal	26. cowboy	35. birthday
9. drawbridge	18. grandson	27. sidewalk	36. hothouse

C.I.D. AUDITORY TEST W-22 (PB WORD LISTS)[2]

List 1A

1. an	14. low	27. as	40. jam
2. yard	15. owl	28. wet	41. poor
3. carve	16. it	29. chew	42. him
4. us	17. she	30. see (sea)	43. skin
5. day	18. high	31. deaf	44. east
6. toe	19. there (their)	32. them	45. thing
7. felt	20. earn (urn)	33. give	46. dad
8. stove	21. twins	34. true	47. up
9. hunt	22. could	35. isle (aisle)	48. bells
10. ran	23. what	36. or (oar)	49. wire
11. knees	24. bathe	37. law	50. ache
12. not (knot)	25. ace	38. me	
13. mew	26. you (ewe)	39. none (nun)	

List 2A

1. yore (your)	14. now	27. young	40. off
2. bin (been)	15. jaw	28. cars	41. ill
3. way (weigh)	16. one (won)	29. tree	42. rooms
4. chest	17. hit	30. dumb	43. ham
5. then	18. send	31. that	44. star
6. ease	19. else	32. die (dye)	45. eat
7. smart	20. tare (tear)	33. show	46. thin
8. gave	21. does	34. hurt	47. flat
9. pew	22. too (two, to)	35. own	48. well
10. ice	23. cap	36. key	49. by (buy)
11. odd	24. with	37. oak	50. ail (ale)
12. knee	25. air (heir)	38. new (knew)	
13. move	26. and	39. live (verb)	

[2] These word lists are reproduced with the permission of the Veterans Administration, Dr. Ira J. Hirsh of Central Institute for the Deaf, and the Chairman of the Publications Board of the American Speech and Hearing Association.

List 3A

1. bill	14. oil	27. when	40. on
2. add (ad)	15. king	28. book	41. if
3. west	16. pie	29. tie	42. raw
4. cute	17. he	30. do	43. glove
5. start	18. smooth	31. hand	44. ten
6. ears	19. farm	32. end	45. dull
7. tan	20. this	33. shove	46. though
8. nest	21. done (dun)	34. have	47. chair
9. say	22. use (yews)	35. owes	48. we
10. is	23. camp	36. jar	49. ate (eight)
11. out	24. wool	37. no (know)	50. year
12. lie (lye)	25. are	38. may	
13. three	26. aim	39. knit	

List 4A

1. all (awl)	13. my	26. darn	39. few
2. wood (would)	14. leave	27. art	40. jump
3. at	15. of	28. will	41. pale (pail)
4. where	16. hang	29. dust	42. go
5. chin	17. save	30. toy	43. stiff
6. they	18. ear	31. aid	44. can
7. dolls	19. tea (tee)	32. than	45. through
8. so (sew)	20. cook	33. eyes (ayes)	(thru)
9. nuts	21. tin	34. shoe	46. clothes
10. ought	22. bread (bred)	35. his	47. who
(aught)	23. why	36. our (hour)	48. bee (be)
11. in (inn)	24. arm	37. men	49. yes
12. net	25. yet	38. near	50. am

List 1B

1. carve	14. twins	27. stove	40. could
2. wire	15. isle (aisle)	28. ache	41. them
3. felt	16. ace	29. us	42. high
4. thing	17. deaf	30. him	43. or (oar)
5. knees	18. she	31. not (knot)	44. low
6. poor	19. none (nun)	32. me	45. jam
7. owl	20. mew	33. it	46. ran
8. law	21. skin	34. see (sea)	47. east
9. there (their)	22. hunt	35. earn (urn)	48. toe
10. give	23. up	36. true	49. bells
11. what	24. day	37. bathe	50. yard
12. chew	25. an	38. you (ewe)	
13. as	26. dad	39. wet	

List 2B

1. way (weigh)	14. air (heir)	27. chest	40. too (two, to)
2. by (buy)	15. that	28. thin	41. flat
3. smart	16. does	29. gave	42. new (knew)
4. eat	17. own	30. rooms	43. key
5. odd	18. hit	31. knee	44. now
6. ill	19. live (verb)	32. send	45. off
7. jaw	20. move	33. one (won)	46. ice
8. oak	21. ham	34. hurt	47. star
9. else	22. pew	35. tare (tear)	48. ease
10. show	23. die (dye)	36. dumb	49. well
11. cap	24. then	37. with	50. bin (been)
12. tree	25. yore (your)	38. and	
13. young	26. ail (ale)	39. cars	

List 3B

1. year	14. book	27. ate (eight)	40. ten
2. cute	15. use (yews)	28. tan	41. done (dun)
3. though	16. end	29. dull	42. owes
4. hand	17. smooth	30. out	43. he
5. raw	18. jar	31. if	44. knit
6. lie (lye)	19. oil	32. king	45. nest
7. may	20. is	33. no (know)	46. glove
8. pie	21. start	34. farm	47. say
9. have	22. on	35. shove	48. chair
10. this	23. ears	36. camp	49. bill
11. do	24. we	37. tie	50. three
12. wool	25. add (ad)	38. when	
13. aim	26. west	39. are	

List 4B

1. chin	14. so (sew)	26. wood	38. eyes (ayes)
2. all (awl)	15. why	(would)	39. arm
3. who	16. darn	27. bee (be)	40. toy
4. few	17. tea (tee)	28. they	41. cook
5. stiff	18. men	29. dust	42. shoe
6. my	19. of	30. ought (aught)	43. hang
7. nuts	20. pale (pail)	31. jump	44. near
8. save	21. our (hour)	32. leave	45. go
9. his	22. through	33. in (inn)	46. can
10. tin	(thru)	34. ear	47. net
11. aid	23. dolls	35. than	48. clothes
12. yet	24. yes	36. bread (bred)	49. where
13. art	25. at	37. will	50. am

List 1C

1. felt	14. not (knot)	27. thing	40. you (ewe)
2. bells	15. skin	28. ran	41. she
3. owl	16. us	29. law	42. dad
4. jam	17. earn (urn)	30. high	43. true
5. what	18. deaf	31. chew	44. could
6. them	19. wet	32. me	45. give
7. isle (aisle)	20. as	33. ace	46. low
8. bathe	21. or (oar)	34. see (sea)	47. poor
9. none (nun)	22. there (their)	35. mew	48. twins
10. it	23. east	36. him	49. wire
11. up	24. knees	37. day	50. toe
12. stove	25. carve	38. ache	
13. an	26. yard	39. hunt	

List 2C

1. smart	14. yore (your)	27. eat	40. pew
2. well	15. knee	28. ice	41. own
3. jaw	16. ham	29. oak	42. hit
4. off	17. tare (tear)	30. send	43. dumb
5. cap	18. new (knew)	31. tree	44. air (heir)
6. does	19. cars	32. and	45. too (two, to)
7. that	20. young	33. flat	46. show
8. with	21. key	34. hurt	47. now
9. live (verb)	22. else	35. move	48. ill
10. one (won)	23. star	36. rooms	49. ease
11. die (dye)	24. odd	37. then	50. by (buy)
12. gave	25. way (weigh)	38. ail (ale)	
13. chest	26. bin (been)	39. thin	

List 3C

1. though	14. if	27. hand	40. on
2. bill	15. start	28. glove	41. king
3. may	16. add (ad)	29. pie	42. when
4. nest	17. shove	30. owes	43. camp
5. do	18. are	31. wool	44. book
6. use (yews)	19. he	32. end	45. ten
7. tie	20. raw	33. jar	46. knit
8. done (dun)	21. smooth	34. farm	47. this
9. oil	22. year	35. is	48. lie (lye)
10. no (know)	23. aim	36. out	49. chair
11. ears	24. have	37. we	50. cute
12. dull	25. say	38. west	
13. ate (eight)	26. three	39. tan	

List 4C

1. wood (would)
2. bee (be)
3. they
4. dust
5. ought (aught)
6. jump
7. leave
8. in (inn)
9. ear
10. than
11. bread (bred)
12. will
13. darn
14. of
15. toy
16. cook
17. shoe
18. hang
19. near
20. go
21. aid
22. net
23. clothes
24. where
25. am
26. chin
27. all (awl)
28. who
29. few
30. stiff
31. my
32. nuts
33. save
34. his
35. tin
36. so (sew)
37. yet
38. art
39. can
40. why
41. eyes (ayes)
42. tea (tee)
43. men
44. arm
45. pale (pail)
46. our (hour)
47. through (thru)
48. dolls
49. yes
50. at

List 1D

1. owl
2. wire
3. isle (aisle)
4. give
5. up
6. she
7. wet
8. ace
9. skin
10. day
11. east
12. law
13. thing
14. carve
15. mew
16. earn (urn)
17. chew
18. or (oar)
19. hunt
20. an
21. true
22. none (nun)
23. poor
24. what
25. felt
26. toe
27. jam
28. low
29. bathe
30. dad
31. stove
32. ache
33. us
34. see (sea)
35. as
36. high
37. knees
38. yard
39. ran
40. there (their)
41. you (ewe)
42. deaf
43. him
44. not (knot)
45. me
46. it
47. twins
48. bells
49. could
50. them

List 2D

1. jaw
2. ease
3. that
4. die (dye)
5. new (knew)
6. with
7. knee
8. then
9. cars
10. does
11. star
12. oak
13. eat
14. way (weigh)
15. tree
16. and
17. move
18. tare (tear)
19. dumb
20. live (verb)
21. now
22. cap
23. smart
24. by (buy)
25. thin
26. chest
27. off
28. show
29. too (two, to)
30. hit
31. well
32. ail (ale)
33. ham
34. young
35. send
36. hurt
37. odd
38. bin (been)
39. ice
40. else
41. key
42. own
43. rooms
44. yore (your)
45. pew
46. one (won)
47. air (heir)
48. flat
49. ill
50. gave

List 3D

1. may	14. say	27. nest	40. year
2. chair	15. wool	28. knit	41. end
3. tie	16. smooth	29. done (dun)	42. are
4. ears	17. is	30. jar	43. cut
5. king	18. shove	31. dull	44. if
6. ten	19. tan	32. west	45. on
7. start	20. ate (eight)	33. he	46. no (know)
8. we	21. camp	34. farm	47. book
9. add (ad)	22. oil	35. raw	48. use (yews)
10. when	23. this	36. owes	49. lie (lye)
11. aim	24. do	37. have	50. bill
12. pie	25. though	38. three	
13. hand	26. cute	39. glove	

List 4D

1. they	14. my	26. at	39. who
2. yes	15. so (sew)	27. dust	40. net
3. leave	16. am	28. our (hour)	41. hang
4. pale (pail)	17. tin	29. in (inn)	42. aid
5. bread (bred)	18. shoe	30. tea (tee)	43. nuts
6. eyes (ayes)	19. can	31. will	44. arm
7. toy	20. darn	32. art	45. why
8. yet	21. men	33. cook	46. than
9. near	22. ear	34. his	47. of
10. save	23. through	35. go	48. jump
11. clothes	(thru)	36. stiff	49. dolls
12. few	24. ought (aught)	37. where	50. bee (be)
13. all (awl)	25. wood (would)	38. chin	

List 1E

1. them	14. jam	27. up	40. skin
2. give	15. none (nun)	28. twins	41. us
3. it	16. ache	29. poor	42. hunt
4. ace	17. or (oar)	30. him	43. knees
5. deaf	18. high	31. thing	44. mew
6. law	19. carve	32. ran	45. you (ewe)
7. yard	20. there (their)	33. chew	46. east
8. earn (urn)	21. day	34. as	47. me
9. see (sea)	22. not (knot)	35. true	48. wet
10. an	23. she	36. stove	49. could
11. dad	24. bells	37. felt	50. isle (aisle)
12. what	25. wire	38. low	
13. toe	26. owl	39. bathe	

List 2E

1. that	14. thin	27. die (dye)	40. cap
2. ill	15. gave	28. one (won)	41. ail (ale)
3. knee	16. now	29. then	42. tare (tear)
4. pew	17. send	30. own	43. hurt
5. star	18. move	31. bin (been)	44. way (weigh)
6. and	19. ice	32. key	45. else
7. tree	20. eat	33. oak	46. does
8. odd	21. rooms	34. young	47. yore (your)
9. dumb	22. cars	35. live (verb)	48. too (two, to)
10. ham	23. air (heir)	36. hit	49. flat
11. smart	24. new (knew)	37. by (buy)	50. ease
12. with	25. jaw	38. chest	
13. off	26. well	39. show	

List 3E

1. add (ad)	14. wool	27. bill	40. camp
2. we	15. do	28. chair	41. shove
3. ears	16. this	29. say	42. knit
4. start	17. have	30. glove	43. no (know)
5. is	18. pie	31. nest	44. king
6. on	19. may	32. farm	45. if
7. jar	20. lie (lye)	33. he	46. out
8. oil	21. raw	34. owes	47. dull
9. smooth	22. hand	35. done (dun)	48. tan
10. end	23. though	36. ten	49. ate (eight)
11. use (yews)	24. cute	37. are	50. west
12. book	25. year	38. when	
13. aim	26. three	39. tie	

List 4E

1. ought (aught)	13. few	26. be (bee)	39. where
2. wood (would)	14. all (awl)	27. dolls	40. stiff
3. through (thru)	15. clothes	28. jump	41. go
	16. save	29. of	42. his
4. ear	17. near	30. than	43. cook
5. men	18. yet	31. why	44. art
6. darn	19. toy	32. arm	45. will
7. can	20. eyes (ayes)	33. hang	46. tea (tee)
8. shoe	21. bread (bred)	34. nuts	47. in (inn)
9. tin	22. pale (pail)	35. aid	48. our (hour)
10. so (sew)	23. leave	36. net	49. dust
11. my	24. yes	37. who	50. at
12. am	25. they	38. chin	

List 1F

1. isle (aisle)	14. there (their)	27. could	40. day
2. ace	15. not (knot)	28. yard	41. skin
3. east	16. ran	29. dad	42. true
4. hunt	17. high	30. us	43. or (oar)
5. earn (urn)	18. stove	31. you (ewe)	44. bathe
6. what	19. low	32. none (nun)	45. toe
7. jam	20. poor	33. felt	46. knees
8. ache	21. an	34. carve	47. see (sea)
9. him	22. mew	35. up	48. me
10. bells	23. law	36. wire	49. deaf
11. owl	24. wet	37. she	50. them
12. twins	25. give	38. chew	
13. as	26. it	39. thing	

List 2F

1. knee	14. jaw	27. pew	40. cars
2. flat	15. bin (been)	28. does	41. key
3. tree	16. rooms	29. odd	42. move
4. else	17. live (verb)	30. tare (tear)	43. hit
5. smart	18. send	31. with	44. show
6. ail (ale)	19. thin	32. chest	45. cap
7. gave	20. off	33. now	46. ham
8. by (buy)	21. hurt	34. young	47. way (weigh)
9. ice	22. dumb	35. eat	48. and
10. oak	23. yore (your)	36. own	49. too (two, to)
11. air (heir)	24. star	37. new (knew)	50. ill
12. then	25. that	38. well	
13. die (dye)	26. ease	39. one (won)	

List 3F

1. west	14. chair	27. ate (eight)	40. nest
2. start	15. hand	28. jar	41. raw
3. farm	16. knit	29. if	42. done (dun)
4. out	17. pie	30. use (yews)	43. have
5. book	18. ten	31. shove	44. tie
6. when	19. wool	32. do	45. aim
7. this	20. camp	33. are	46. no (know)
8. oil	21. end	34. may	47. smooth
9. lie (lye)	22. king	35. he	48. dull
10. owes	23. on	36. though	49. is
11. glove	24. tan	37. say	50. add (ad)
12. cute	25. we	38. bill	
13. three	26. ears	39. year	

List 4F

1. our (hour)
2. art
3. darn
4. ought (aught)
5. stiff
6. am
7. go
8. few
9. arm
10. yet
11. jump
12. pale (pail)
13. yes
14. bee (be)
15. eyes (ayes)
16. than
17. save
18. toy
19. my
20. chin
21. show
22. his
23. ear
24. tea (tee)
25. at
26. wood (would)
27. in (inn)
28. men
29. cook
30. tin
31. where
32. all (awl)
33. hang
34. near
35. why
36. bread (bred)
37. dolls
38. they
39. leave
40. of
41. aid
42. nuts
43. clothes
44. who
45. so (sew)
46. net
47. can
48. will
49. through (thru)
50. dust

CHILDREN'S SPONDEE LIST[3]

1. sidewalk
2. birthday
3. cupcake
4. airplane
5. headlight
6. blackboard
7. shotgun
8. eyebrow
9. railroad
10. baseball
11. stairway
12. armchair
13. playground
14. doorstep
15. mousetrap
16. cowboy
17. wigwam
18. coughdrop
19. churchbell
20. sunset
21. daylight
22. footstool
23. pancake
24. hotdog
25. outside
26. scarecrow
27. playmate
28. rainbow
29. toothbrush
30. dishpan
31. bathtub
32. jackknife
33. ice cream
34. schoolroom
35. backyard
36. doorbell
37. drugstore
38. streetcar
39. hopscotch
40. jump rope
41. shoelace
42. hairbrush
43. necktie
44. ash tray
45. bedroom
46. toy shop
47. playpen
48. dollhouse
49. highchair
50. downtown
51. meatball
52. sunshine
53. barnyard
54. bus stop
55. football
56. bluejay
57. birdnest

[3] The first eight spondee words are taken from Jean Utley, *What's Its Name* (Urbana, Ill., University of Illinois Press, 1951), p. 126, and the second series of eight spondees is from *ibid.*, p. 127.

KINDERGARTEN PB WORD LISTS[4]

List 1

1. please	14. rag	27. bath	40. neck
2. great	15. put	28. slip	41. beef
3. sled	16. fed	29. ride	42. few
4. pants	17. fold	30. end	43. use
5. rat	18. hunt	31. pink	44. did
6. bad	19. no	32. thank	45. hit
7. pinch	20. box	33. take	46. pond
8. such	21. are	34. cart	47. hot
9. bus	22. teach	35. scab	48. own
10. need	23. slice	36. lay	49. bead
11. ways	24. is	37. class	50. shop
12. five	25. tree	38. me	
13. mouth	26. smile	39. dish	

List 2

1. laugh	14. turn	27. feed	40. as
2. falls	15. grab	28. next	41. grew
3. paste	16. rose	29. wreck	42. knee
4. plow	17. lip	30. waste	43. fresh
5. page	18. bee	31. crab	44. tray
6. weed	19. bet	32. peg	45. cat
7. gray	20. his	33. freeze	46. on
8. park	21. sing	34. race	47. camp
9. wait	22. all	35. bud	48. find
10. fat	23. bless	36. darn	49. yes
11. ax	24. suit	37. fair	50. loud
12. cage	25. splash	38. sack	
13. knife	26. path	39. got	

[4] These three kindergarten PB word lists were devised by Miss Harriet L. Haskins of Johns Hopkins Hospital, as a part of her M.A. thesis at Northwestern University, and are reproduced here with her permission. A fourth list of these PBK words (the original List 2) was discarded for clinical use because it was found to be too easy (personal communication from Miss Haskins).

List 3

1. tire
2. seed
3. purse
4. quick
5. room
6. bug
7. that
8. sell
9. low
10. rich
11. those
12. ache
13. black

14. else
15. nest
16. jay
17. raw
18. true
19. had
20. cost
21. vase
22. press
23. fit
24. bounce
25. wide
26. most

27. thick
28. if
29. them
30. sheep
31. air
32. set
33. dad
34. ship
35. case
36. you
37. may
38. choose
39. white

40. frog
41. bush
42. clown
43. cab
44. hurt
45. pass
46. grade
47. blind
48. drop
49. leave
50. nuts

NAME INDEX

SUBJECT INDEX